Nontuberculous Mycobacterial Pulmonary Disease

Editors

SHANNON KASPERBAUER
RACHEL THOMSON

CLINICS IN
CHEST MEDICINE

www.chestmed.theclinics.com

December 2023 • Volume 44 • Number 4

ELSEVIER

1600 John F. Kennedy Boulevard • Suite 1800 • Philadelphia, Pennsylvania, 19103-2899

http://www.theclinics.com

CLINICS IN CHEST MEDICINE Volume 44, Number 4
December 2023 ISSN 0272-5231, ISBN-13: 978-0-323-93911-9

Editor: Joanna Gascoine
Developmental Editor: Nitesh Barthwal

Clinics in Chest Medicine (ISSN 0272-5231) is published quarterly by Elsevier Inc., 360 Park Avenue South, New York, NY 10010-1710. Months of issue are March, June, September, and December. Periodicals postage paid at New York, NY and additional mailing offices. Subscription prices are $420.00 per year (domestic individuals), $895.00 per year (domestic institutions), $100.00 per year (domestic students/residents), $449.00 per year (Canadian individuals), $1112.00 per year (Canadian institutions), $514.00 per year (international individuals), $1112.00 per year (international institutions), $100.00 per year (Canadian Students), and $230.00 per year (International Students). International air speed delivery is included in all Clinics subscription prices. All prices are subject to change without notice. **POSTMASTER:** Send address changes to Clinics in Chest Medicine, Elsevier Health Sciences Division, Subscription Customer Service, 3251 Riverport Lane, Maryland Heights, MO 63043. **Customer Service: Telephone: 1-800-654-2452** (U.S. and Canada); **1-314-447-8871** (outside U.S. and Canada). **Fax: 1-314-447-8029. E-mail: journalscustomerservice-usa@elsevier.com (for print support); journalsonlinesupport-usa@elsevier.com (for online support).**

Reprints. For copies of 100 or more of articles in this publication, please contact the Commercial Reprints Department, Elsevier Inc., 360 Park Avenue South, New York, NY 10010-1710. Tel.: 212-633-3874; Fax: 212-633-3820; E-mail: reprints@elsevier.com.

Clinics in Chest Medicine is covered in *MEDLINE/PubMed (Index Medicus), Current Contents/Clinical Medicine, EMBASE/ Excerpta Medica, Science Citation Index,* and *ISI/BIOMED.*

Contributors

EDITORS

SHANNON KASPERBAUER, MD
Associate Professor, Department of Medicine, National Jewish Health, Denver, Colorado, USA

RACHEL THOMSON, MBBS, Grad Dip (Clin Epi), PhD, FRACP
Professor, Gallipoli Medical Research Institute, The University of Queensland, Queensland, Australia

AUTHORS

TIMOTHY R. AKSAMIT, MD
Consultant, Pulmonary Disease and Critical Care Medicine, Mayo Clinic, Rochester, Minnesota, USA

IFEANYICHUKWU U. ANIDI, MD, PhD
Pulmonologist, Pulmonary Division, National Heart, Lung and Blood Institute, National Institutes of Health, Bethesda, Maryland, USA

AMANDA M. BAIR, PharmD
Surgery Clinical Pharmacist, Department of Pharmacy Services, Oregon Health & Science University, Portland, OR, USA

TIMOTHY BAIRD, BSc, MBBS, DTM&H, FRACP
Respiratory and Sleep Physician, Sunshine Coast Health Institute, University of the Sunshine Coast, Department of Respiratory Medicine, Sunshine Coast University Hospital, Birtinya, Sunshine Coast, Queensland, Australia

SCOTT BELL, MBBS, FRACP, MD
Professor, Department of Thoracic Medicine, The Prince Charles Hospital, Children's Health Research Centre, Faculty of Medicine, The University of Queensland, Translational Research Institute, Brisbane, Queensland, Australia; Department of Thoracic Medicine, The Prince Charles Hospital, Chermside, Queensland, Australia

SARAH K. BRODE, MD, MPH
Assistant Professor, Department of Medicine, University of Toronto, Division of Respirology, University Health Network, Division of Respiratory Medicine, West Park Healthcare Centre, Toronto, Ontario, Canada

BARBARA A. BROWN-ELLIOTT, MS, MT(ASCP) SM
Professor of Microbiology, The University of Texas Health Science Center at Tyler, Mycobacteria/Nocardia Laboratory, Tyler, Texas, USA

ANDREW BURKE, MBBS, FRACP
University of Queensland Centre for Clinical Research, Faculty of Medicine, The University of Queensland, Department of Thoracic Medicine, The Prince Charles Hospital, Brisbane, Queensland, Australia

CHARLES L. DALEY, MD
Chief of the Division of Mycobacterial and Respiratory Infection, Professor of Medicine, National Jewish Health, University of Colorado School of Medicine, Icahn School of Medicine at Mt. Sinai, Denver, Colorado, USA

DAVID E. GRIFFITH, MD
Professor, Department of Medicine, Division of Mycobacterial Disease and Pulmonary Infections, National Jewish Health, Denver, Colorado, USA

STEVEN M. HOLLAND, MD
Director, Division of Intramural Research,
Laboratory of Clinical Immunology and
Microbiology, National Institute of Allergy
and Infectious Diseases, National
Institutes of Health, Bethesda, Maryland,
USA

MICHAEL R. HOLT, BSC, MBBS, FRACP
Gallipoli Medical Research Foundation, The
University of Queensland, Department of
Thoracic Medicine, Royal Brisbane and
Women's Hospital, Brisbane, Queensland,
Australia

JENNIFER R. HONDA, PhD, ATSF
Associate Professor, Director, Center for
Mycobacterial Treatment and Discovery,
Department of Cellular and Molecular Biology,
School of Medicine, The University of Texas
Health Science Center at Tyler, Tyler, Texas,
USA

REETI KHARE, PhD, D(ABMM)
Associate Professor, Mycobacteriology
Laboratory, National Jewish Health, Denver,
Colorado, USA

THEODORE K. MARRAS, MD, MSc
Department of Medicine, University of
Toronto, Division of Respirology, University
Health Network, Toronto, Ontario,
Canada

JULIA E. MARSHALL, BS
Epidemiology and Population Studies Unit,
Division of Intramural Research, National
Institute of Allergy and Infectious Diseases,
National Institutes of Health, Bethesda,
Maryland, USA

PAMELA J. MCSHANE, MD
Associate Professor, Department of Medicine,
The University of Texas Health Science Center
at Tyler, Tyler, Texas, USA

JOHN D. MITCHELL, MD
Courtenay C. and Lucy Patten Davis Endowed
Chair in Thoracic Surgery, Professor and Chief,
General Thoracic Surgery, Department of
Surgery, Division of Cardiothoracic Surgery,
University of Colorado, Aurora, Colorado,
USA

KOZO MORIMOTO, MD
Chief Doctor, Division of Clinical Research,
Fukujuji Hospital, Japan Anti-Tuberculosis
Association, Kiyose, Tokyo, Japan

HO NAMKOONG, MD, PhD, MPH
Assistant Professor, Department of Infectious
Diseases, Keio University School of Medicine,
Tokyo, Japan

MINH-VU H. NGUYEN, MD, MSc
Lowerre Fellow and Clinical Instructor of
Medicine, Division of Mycobacterial and
Respiratory Infections, National Jewish Health,
Denver, Colorado, USA

KENNETH N. OLIVIER, MD, MPH
Professor of Medicine, Division of Pulmonary
Diseases and Critical Care Medicine,
University of North Carolina School of
Medicine, Chapel Hill, North Carolina, USA

D. REBECCA PREVOTS, PhD, MPH
Epidemiologist and Associate Scientist,
Epidemiology and Population Studies Unit,
Division of Intramural Research, National
Institute of Allergy and Infectious Diseases,
National Institutes of Health, Bethesda,
Maryland, USA

ALICE SAWKA, MBBS, MPH, FRACP
Department of Thoracic Medicine,
Royal Adelaide Hospital, University of
Adelaide, Adelaide, South Australia,
Australia

AMBER C. STREIFEL, PharmD
Infectious Disease Clinical Pharmacist,
Department of Pharmacy Services, Oregon
Health & Science University, Portland, Oregon,
USA

LAUREN J. TAYLOR, MD
General Surgeon, Department of Surgery,
Division of Cardiothoracic Surgery,
University of Colorado, Aurora, Colorado,
USA

CARA D. VARLEY, MD, MPH
Assistant Professor, Department of Medicine,
Division of Infectious Diseases, Oregon Health
& Science University, Program in
Epidemiology, Oregon Health & Science
University-Portland State University School of
Public Health

DIRK WAGNER, MD
Division of Infectious Diseases, Department of
Internal Medicine II, Medical Center - University
of Freiburg, Freiburg, Germany

KEVIN L. WINTHROP, MD, MPH
Professor, Department of Medicine, Division of
Infectious Diseases, Oregon Health & Science
University, Program in Epidemiology, Oregon
Health & Science University-Portland State
University School of Public Health

MARIE YAN, MD
Department of Medicine, University of Toronto,
Toronto, Ontario, Canada; Clinician
Investigator Program, University of British
Columbia, Vancouver, British Columbia,
Canada

Contents

Patients with nontuberculous mycobacterial (NTM) lung infection require life-long attention to their bronchiectasis, whether or not their NTM infection has been cured. The identification of the cause of bronchiectasis and/or coexisting diseases is important because it may affect therapeutic strategies. Airway clearance is the mainstay of bronchiectasis management. It can include multiple breathing techniques, devices, and mucoactive agents. The exact airway clearance regimen should be customized to each individual patient. Chronic pathogenic airway bacteria, such as *Pseudomonas aeruginosa*, may warrant consideration of eradication therapy and/or chronic use of maintenance inhaled antibiotics.

Nontuberculous mycobacteria (NTM) typically cause opportunistic pulmonary infections and reliable laboratory results can assist with diagnosis of disease. Microscopy can detect acid-fast bacilli from specimens though it has poor sensitivity. Solid and liquid culture are used to grow NTM, which are identified by molecular or protein-based assays. Because culture has a long turnaround time, some assays are designed to identify NTM directly from sputum specimens. When indicated, phenotypic susceptibility testing should be performed by broth microdilution as per the guidelines from the Clinical Laboratory Standards Institute. Genotypic susceptibility methods may be used to decrease the turnaround time for some antimicrobials.

The diagnosis of nontuberculous mycobacterial (NTM) pulmonary disease is based on three criteria: patient's symptoms, radiographic findings, and microbiologic results. The microbiologic criterion is the most complicated because it requires more than one positive sputum acid-fast bacilli culture. Clinicians are challenged to apply the diagnostic criteria in the context of variable patient symptoms, NTM pathogenicity, and host susceptibility. The decision to treat NTM pulmonary disease entails assessment of the risks and benefits of therapy and the patient's wishes and ability to receive treatment.

Treatment of M avium pulmonary disease requires a three-drug, macrolide-based regimen that is administered for 12 months beyond culture conversion. The regimen can be administered 3 days a week in non-cavitary, nodular bronchiectatic disease but should be given daily when cavitary disease is present. For treatment refractory disease, amikacin liposome inhalation suspension is added to the regimen. Parenteral amikacin or streptomycin should be administered in the setting of extensive radiographic involvement or macrolide resistance. Recurrence of disease is common and often due to reinfection. Novel and repurposed agents are being evaluated in clinical trials.

Mycobacterium abscessus pulmonary disease is highly antibiotic-resistant, and the current armamentarium of antibiotics yields poor treatment outcomes with significant drug toxicity. Macrolide susceptibility is a key prognostic factor. Optimal drug combinations, duration of therapy, and management of refractory disease are unknown. Surgical resection, performed at centers with experience in surgical management of nontuberculous mycobacterial pulmonary disease, may produce favorable outcomes in select patients. Multiple emerging therapeutic candidates hold promise for more efficacious and tolerable treatment options.

Nontuberculous mycobacterial pulmonary disease caused by the less common nontuberculous mycobacteria have distinct features depending on the species. Diagnostic evaluation follows the established criteria for all nontuberculous mycobacteria, but with certain qualifications given species-specific and regional differences in pathogenicity. Clinicians should first institute nonpharmacologic management and evaluate clinical, radiologic, and microbiologic factors in the decision regarding antimycobacterial therapy. Treatment is challenging, and evidence-based recommendations are limited for most species. Drug susceptibility testing is used to help with regimen selection; however, this approach is imperfect given the uncertain correlation between in vitro activity and clinical response for most drugs.

In the treatment of nontuberculous mycobacteria (NTM) lung disease, clinicians must consider potential toxicities that may occur as a result of prolonged exposure to a multidrug antibiotic regimen. Frequent clinical and microbiological monitoring is required to assess response and guide treatment duration. This article summarizes toxicity profiles of the antibiotics that are most frequently prescribed for the treatment of NTM lung disease. The role of therapeutic drug monitoring during use of amikacin and linezolid is discussed. The available evidence to guide frequency and extent of medication monitoring during NTM treatment is provided.

The immunocompromised host is at an increased risk for pulmonary and extrapulmonary NTM infections. Where data are available in these specific populations, increased mortality is observed with NTM disease. Prior to starting therapy for NTM disease, providers should ensure diagnostic criteria are met as treatment is long and often associated with significant side effects and toxicities. Treatment should involve 2 to 4 agents and be guided by cultures and antimicrobial susceptibilities.

Drug interactions are important to consider, especially in those with HIV or transplant recipients. Whenever possible, immunosuppression should be reduced or changed.

Standard treatment of nontuberculous mycobacterial pulmonary disease (NTM-PD) infection involves a multi-drug antimicrobial regimen for at least 12 months. The length, complexity, and side effect profile of antibiotic therapy for NTM-PD pose significant difficulties for maintaining patient adherence. Furthermore, physician adherence to NTM guidelines suffers for similar reasons to the extent that a study evaluating treatment approaches across multiple specialties found that only 13% of antibiotic regimens met ATS/IDSA guidelines. For this reason, a great need exists for therapy that augments the current armamentarium of antimicrobial chemotherapeutics or provides an alternative approach for decreasing host mycobacterial burden. As our knowledge of the mechanisms driving protective responses to NTM-PD infections by mammalian hosts expand, these processes provide novel therapeutic targets. These agents, which are commonly referred to as host-directed therapies (HDTs) have the potential of providing the much-needed boost to the nontuberculous mycobacterial therapeutic pipeline. In this review, we will focus on translational research and clinical trial data that detail the creation of therapeutic modalities developed to improve host mechanical protection and immunologic responses to PNTM infection.

Non-tuberculous mycobacteria (NTM) infection is a major cause of morbidity in people with cystic fibrosis (pwCF) with rates of infection increasing worldwide. Accurate diagnosis and decisions surrounding best management remain challenging. Treatment guidelines have been developed to assist physicians in managing NTM in pwCF, but involve prolonged and complex mycobacterial regimens, often associated with significant toxicity. Fortunately, current management and outcomes of NTM in CF are likely to evolve due to improved understanding of disease acquisition, better diagnostics, emerging antimycobacterial therapies, and the widespread uptake of cystic fibrosis transmembrane conductance regulator (CFTR) modulator therapies.

Rates of nontuberculous mycobacterial pulmonary disease are increasing worldwide, particularly in the United States and other developed countries. While multi-drug antimicrobial therapy is the mainstay of treatment, surgical resection has emerged as an important adjunct. In this article, we will review the indications for surgery, preoperative considerations, surgical techniques, and postoperative outcomes.

CLINICS IN CHEST MEDICINE

FORTHCOMING ISSUES

March 2024
Sarcoidosis
Robert P. Baughman, Elyse E. Lower, and
Marc A. Judson, *Editors*

June 2024
Thoracic Imaging
Jane P. Ko, *Editor*

September 2024
Pediatric Respiratory Disease
Erick Forno and Gregory Sawicki, *Editors*

RECENT ISSUES

September 2023
Aiming to Improve Equity in Pulmonary Health
Drew Harris, Emily Brigham and Juan Celedon, *Editors*

June 2023
COVID-19 Lung Disease: Lessons Learned
Guang-Shing Cheng and Charles Dela Cruz, *Editors*

March 2023
Lung Transplantation
Luis Angel and Stephanie M. Levine, *Editors*

SERIES OF RELATED INTEREST

Critical Care Clinics
Available at: https://www.criticalcare.theclinics.com/

THE CLINICS ARE AVAILABLE ONLINE!
Access your subscription at:
www.theclinics.com

Preface
Things They Are a Changing in the Field of Nontuberculous Mycobacteria

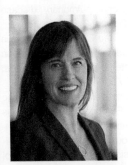

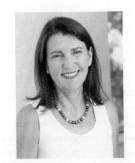

Shannon Kasperbauer, MD

Rachel Thomson, MBBS, Grad Dip (Clin Epi), PhD, FRACP

Editors

This issue of *Clinics in Chest Medicine* is dedicated to Nontuberculous Mycobacterial Pulmonary Disease (NTM-PD). There has been an exponential increase in NTM-PD in many regions of the world over the past 20 years. The last review on Nontuberculous Mycobacteria in *Clinics in Chest Medicine* was published in 2015. Since that issue, we have witnessed a historical milestone in the field of NTM-PD. The first drug was approved by the FDA for the treatment of refractory *Mycobacterium avium* complex (MAC) pulmonary disease. This same agent is now being studied in treatment-naïve MAC. In parallel, research around NTM-PD has also increased, and we now have an improved understanding of environmental sources and contributors to disease epidemiology, host susceptibility, prognosis, and mortality rates. Significant advances in diagnostics and therapeutics have been made with now multiple clinical trials of novel therapeutics contributing to improved outcomes for patients.

We have also seen multiple new guideline statements, including the multisociety guidelines for the treatment of MAC,[1,2] as well as the treatment of the other less common NTM that cause disease in humans.[3] In addition, the US Cystic Fibrosis Foundation and the European Respiratory Society published a consensus recommendation to treat NTM in cystic fibrosis patients.[4] Finally, as most patients with NTM-PD have concomitant bronchiectasis, we would draw your attention to the recent bronchiectasis guideline statement published by the British Thoracic Society.[5]

And yet, with all the advances in the last eight years, there is a tremendous unmet need in our patients. At-risk patients with known bronchiectasis are infrequently monitored with mycobacterial sputum cultures. The average time from symptom onset to diagnosis is over two years. The heterogeneity in presentation begs the question related to who needs to be treated? We continue to rely on antiquated markers of disease severity, such as smear status and cavitation. Once patients finally have the diagnosis, only a minority receive guideline-based therapy. Treatment is measured in years and fraught with toxicity. Outcomes on treatment pale in comparison to its formative cousin *Mycobacterium tuberculosis*. Finally, we lack a validated tool to measure patient-reported outcomes, as regulatory agencies emphasize this as an important endpoint in therapeutic studies.

In the articles that follow, our contributors summarize the current state of knowledge of important aspects of NTM-PD and outline the gaps in our understanding that need further exploration. We would like to thank the authors for their excellent contributions and Karen Solomon and the Elsevier staff

Clin Chest Med 44 (2023) xiii–xiv
https://doi.org/10.1016/j.ccm.2023.09.001
0272-5231/23/© 2023 Published by Elsevier Inc.

for their patience and commitment to bringing this issue to publication. We hope that you enjoy this issue and that it provides useful information for clinicians, patients, and researchers to further enhance awareness and understanding of this important disease.

Shannon Kasperbauer, MD
Department of Medicine
National Jewish Health
1400 Jackson Street
Denver, CO 80206, USA

Rachel Thomson, MBBS, Grad Dip (Clin Epi),
PhD, FRACP
Gallipoli Medical Research Institute
University of Queensland
121 Newdegate Street
Greenslopes, Queensland 4120, Australia

E-mail addresses:
KasperbauerS@NJHealth.org (S. Kasperbauer)
r.thomson@uq.edu.au (R. Thomson)

REFERENCES

1. Daley CL, Iaccarino JM, Lange C, et al. Treatment of nontuberculous mycobacterial pulmonary disease: an official ATS/ERS/ESCMID/IDSA clinical practice guideline. Clin Infect Dis 2020;71(4):e1–36.
2. Haworth CS, Banks J, Capstick T, et al. British Thoracic Society guidelines for the management of non-tuberculous mycobacterial pulmonary disease (NTM-PD). Thorax 2017;72(suppl 2):ii1–64.
3. Lange C, Böttger EC, Cambau E, et al. Consensus management recommendations for less common non-tuberculous mycobacterial pulmonary diseases. Lancet Infect Dis 2022;22(7):e178–90.
4. Floto RA, Olivier KN, Saiman L, et al. US Cystic Fibrosis Foundation and European Cystic Fibrosis Society consensus recommendations for the management of non-tuberculous mycobacteria in individuals with cystic fibrosis. Thorax 2016;71(suppl 1):i1–22.
5. Hill AT, Sullivan AL, Chalmers JD, et al. British Thoracic Society Guideline for bronchiectasis in adults. Thorax 2019;74(suppl 1):1–69.

Environmental Sources and Transmission of Nontuberculous Mycobacteria

Jennifer R. Honda, PhD

KEYWORDS

- Nontuberculous mycobacteria • Environment • Genomics • Transmission • Climate change

KEY POINTS

- The fields of microbiology and comparative bacterial genomics have facilitated the identification of human built environments as hot spots for NTM colonization.
- The combination of microbiology and comparative bacterial genomics should be applied even more regularly to reveal new niches including animal reservoirs involved in NTM transmission.
- Hastened climate changes will likely increase the risk for environmentally transmissible respiratory NTM infections as formidable public health threats globally.

INTRODUCTION

Expanding the Field of Environmental Nontuberculous Mycobacteria Biology

Recognition of environmental nontuberculous mycobacteria (NTM) as human pathogens began in the 1960s and grew in notoriety in the HIV era.[1,2] NTM are now widely recognized as inhabitants of soil and dust but are also categorized as important drinking water-associated opportunistic pathogens that thrive in human-built water systems with the capacity to cause problematic disease in susceptible individuals.[3]

It has been suggested that NTM simply "surround people."[4–7] In 1979, Gruft and colleagues[8] demonstrated that aerosols from estuaries and ocean water in the southeast (SE) portions of the United States harbor NTM, demonstrating their innate survival in natural water sources.[9] By the mid-1980s, acidic soil from United States floodplains were reported as NTM niches.[10] High densities of NTM have been recovered from chicken farms in the SE United States, but low densities of NTM from chicken litter[11] hint to the potential of animals as possible reservoirs for NTM infection.[9] In 1995, *Mycobacterium avium* complex (MAC) was isolated from cigarettes, suggesting environmental smoke and pollutants that harm the lung may also carry infectious NTM.[12] It is clear, NTM are inhabitants of natural and human-engineered environments that survive, in part, due to selection by human actions[13] mixed with their intrinsic capacity for adherence and disinfectant tolerance that promote high numbers in homes and enrichment in plumbing systems.[6] Numerous reports reinforce potable water and drinking water distribution systems as important sources of NTM exposures.[14,15] In another study of people with MAC pulmonary disease and bronchiectasis controls in Japan, exposure to residential soil was a likely source of pulmonary MAC infection.[16] Thomson and colleagues[17,18] found pathogenic NTM including *Mycobacterium abscessus* in large urban water distribution systems in Australia. Falkinham and colleagues[6,19] reported low NTM counts from homes with wells and water heaters

Department of Cellular and Molecular Biology, University of Texas Health Science Center at Tyler, 11937 US Hwy 271, BMR Building, Tyler, TX 75708, USA

E-mail address: Jennifer.Honda@UTTyler.edu

Clin Chest Med 44 (2023) 661–674
https://doi.org/10.1016/j.ccm.2023.07.001
0272-5231/23/

set to greater than 130°F and advocate that NTM are flexible adaptors that adeptly adjust to their changing environments.[7]

These earlier studies established fundamental information regarding the generalizable environmental niches of NTM using phenotypic and biochemical typing, DNA probe kits, and PCR–RFLP (polymerase chain reaction - restriction fragment length polymorphism) for NTM species identification.[20,21] As the field moves to investigate more specialized, novel NTM niches that go beyond freshwater and soil, such as outbreak investigations and large-scale environmental hazards to NTM transmission events, higher resolution techniques that apply both microbiological culture of environmental samples and bacterial genomics are now favored by the scientific community. Whole genome sequencing (WGS) has been used to study NTM transmission for nearly a decade. As a genotyping tool, comparative genomics now allows for a detailed examination of isolate relatedness and determination of whether isolates were derived from a common source or ancestor. Thus, there continues to be a pressing need to learn more about these organisms and applying NTM genomics at a broad scale will significantly accelerate the current understanding of environmental NTM biology, pathogenesis, and transmission.

Despite growing concerns of NTM as a significant public health problem and greater availability and accessibility to genomic tools, NTM niches and the role of the environment in the acquisition of infection and outbreaks remain understudied. Tracking these infections may help to understand how disease spreads within populations. These factors showcase the need for increased surveillance through mandatory pulmonary disease reporting on a global scale.[22]

The current review highlights and summarizes recent literature and new knowledge regarding the environmental sources of NTM, the newly described factors that likely influence the presence of NTM in the environment and demonstrate the application of NTM genomics to learn a great deal more about the breadth and diversity of NTM in their innate niches. It has been inherently difficult to pinpoint infection and outbreak drivers, and while the ubiquity of NTM is generalized, not all NTM are equally pathogenic. As more studies come to light, there will be a pressing need to know more about which NTM species colonize environments and how their genomes are studied to reveal a new understanding for the capacity of NTM to survive in the environment and infect the human lung and how to mitigate exposures with increased surveillance.

Nontuberculous Mycobacteria and the Environmental Features that Drive Diversity

Nontuberculous mycobacteria distribution varies by geographic region

The worldwide geographic diversity of NTM infections has been well described.[23] In the United States, several geographic areas including California and Florida are NTM hot spots with Hawai'i a top area of NTM pulmonary disease and interest.[24–29] A team of microbiologists, geochemists, bioinformaticians, molecular biologists, epidemiologists, volcano research scientists, clinicians, and an extended community science network, performed the first large-scale NTM environmental sampling campaign across highly populated and natural areas within the State of Hawai'i to understand the unique island features that drive NTM prevalence and diversity.[30–34] Applying microbiological culture of environmental samples and comparative genomics, it was revealed that NTM are not as pan-ubiquitous as predicted, as microbiological recovery rates for environmental NTM were modest even in this geographic hot spot at 27% (764/2,831 environmental samples) (Honda, 2023, unpublished). More importantly, this island archipelago, while isolated in the middle of the Pacific Ocean, harbored a preponderance of clinically relevant NTM compared with species of NTM that do not cause human infections. In addition, clinically relevant NTM species frequently inhabited selected niches within broad environments, suggesting that the diversity of NTM species is critically important to understanding potential environmental risks for infection. In Hawai'i, the most frequently recovered NTM species from households were the opportunistic pathogens *Mycobacterium chimaera*, *Mycobacterium chelonae*, *Mycobacterium porcinum*, and *M. abscessus* compared with less frequently recovered and less pathogenic *Mycobacterium interjectum*, *Mycobacterium alvei*, and *Mycobacterium paraffinicum*.[34] These studies and others that apply microbiological culture of environmental samples for viable NTM isolates rely on gold-standard approaches but are limited by the inability of culture media and conditions to capture the total representation of all NTM isolates present in any sample. Yet, these data suggest that delineating which NTM species are in environment matters because each sampled niche did not necessarily harbor NTM or pathogenic NTM species by culture methods. By inference, NTM of human significance are not as pervasive in expansive environments initially described. Rather, NTM are more likely to be ubiquitous in selected niches within broad environments, an important distinction. Phylogenetic and sequence variant network analyses were used to evaluate whether genetic diversity among environmental NTM species from Hawai'i differed from the continental United States revealing high or low genetic diversity varied among the species.[34]

New discoveries connecting nontuberculous mycobacteria, showers, and freshwater

Piping within built environments such as office buildings, schools, hotels, shopping malls, airports, and other similar structures may be colonization sites for NTM. Stagnant and unused water in these structures because of the recent COVID-19 pandemic may have created an enrichment of NTM in these systems. Hozalski and colleagues[35] applied a combination of culture-based assays, quantitative PCR, and quantitative microbial risk assessments to show flushing of stagnant shower water may reduce NTM concentration to below detection limits within 6 minutes. In homes, showers are a frequently sampled site to probe for environmental NTM.[4,34,36–40] Moving beyond NTM diversity reporting in showers, Shen and colleagues recently applied mass balance models to quantify the proportion of NTM transferred from building water to indoor air during showering. Then, estimations of live cells were performed using live cell sorting and flow cytometry, discovering NTM showed damaged membranes but retained their ability to grow in culture media, imitating respiratory secretions of people with cystic fibrosis (pwCF).[41]

Owing to multiple access challenges, documenting the presence of colonizing NTM upwards from the home to possible exogenous inoculation sites such as natural water or soil remains difficult to study and track. Conversely, it is presumed that water run-off from soil leads to inoculation of NTM into surface water or ground aquifers that enter water treatment plants, distribution systems, and innervate into homes and other human-built sites.[13] To address these gaps in knowledge, Nelson and colleagues[31] recently leveraged microbiology and geological partnerships, a combination of the microbiological culture of NTM in riparian environments, freshwater stream sediments and flow analyses, stream discharge calculations, and groundwater modeling to report evidence of NTM transport from Hawai'i streams into losing stream stretches and aquifers that enter public water supplies and home plumbing.

Metals and minerals are features that modulate nontuberculous mycobacteria presence in the environment

Over 10 years ago, epidemiological studies applying logistic regression and univariate models using county-level environmental and sociodemographic data were performed to identify low and high-risk US areas for NTM pulmonary infections. Through this work, environmental features such as greater precipitation, high evapotranspiration levels, low elevation, percent of land covered by surface water, soil with greater levels of copper and sodium, and lower manganese levels were characteristics linked to increased risk for pulmonary NTM infections in the United States.[24] More recently, there is growing support showing high atmospheric moisture in certain geographic areas including Hawai'i, California, Florida, and Louisiana increase the risk for environmental NTM exposures.[42] Using the annualized registry data from the cystic fibrosis (CF) foundation, geospatial analyses revealed annual precipitation and soil mineral levels were associated with NTM sputum positivity in Florida.[43] In the context of soil, Glickman and colleagues[32] reported in vitro growth of environmentally derived M. abscessus isolates from Hawai'i was promoted in the presence of soil hematite, an iron oxide mineral. A multivariate, population-based study demonstrated that risk factors for pulmonary NTM isolation in North Carolina were more related to exposure to hydric and acidic soils rather than population density or road network density.[44]

In the past, high numbers of Mycobacterium kansasii lung infection cases were often observed in geographic areas with intense mining activity as in Australia.[45] Lipner and colleagues featured a variety of epidemiological models including geospatial, ecological models, population-based case–control studies, and population-based cohort studies using patient incidence data to evaluate the environmental minerals and trace metals role in NTM infections. This includes a Colorado-focused study reporting that for every 1 log unit increase in calcium and molybdenum concentrations in source water, NTM disease risk increased by 19% and 17%, respectively, compared with people who did not have NTM infections.[46] For those with CF in Colorado, the odds of M. abscessus infection was 79% for every 1 unit log increase of molybdenum in surface water compared with people who did not have NTM infections.[47] In Oregon, every unit increase in the log concentration of vanadium and molybdenum in surface water increased the risk for MAC and M. abscessus infection by 49% and 41%, respectively.[48] Although this new knowledge is important to the field, in vitro mineral and NTM studies to validate these findings alongside ecological studies to recover viable CF NTM pathogens from areas of high calcium and molybdenum concentrations remain missing areas of scientific research.

Revisiting animals as important nontuberculous mycobacteria reservoirs

Although not as widely studied as the built environment, animals may be important reservoirs for NTM. *Mycobacterium marinum* is associated with cold and warm freshwater and saltwater sources and can cause disease in fish, oysters, snakes, and eels.[49] The first human cases of *M. marinum* infection were reported in 1951 from Sweden as skin lesions on swimmers who frequented contaminated pools.[50] *Mycobacterium szulgai* is responsible for infections in fish and animals that live in or in close association with freshwater including crocodiles and clawed frogs, while *M,. avium* infections occur in dwarf cichlids, *Mycobacterium lentiflavum* in swordtails, and *M. abscessus* in zebrafish and milkfish.[51] The first report of *M. chelonae* was its isolation from sea turtles with pulmonary disease in 1903.[52] *Mycobacterium fortuitum* was originally isolated from neon tetra in 1953.[53] *M. avium* subspecies *hominissuis* was recovered from ornamental fish[54] and public aquarium long-tailed carpet sharks in the Netherlands.[55] Recently, Komine and colleagues[56] applied WGS to perform a phylogenetic analysis demonstrating the transmission of *M. marinum* among fish, invertebrates, seagrass, periphytons, biofilms, sand, and water.

Land animals may also be zoonotic reservoirs associated with the emergence and spread of NTM. In areas of the Iberian Peninsula, *M. avium* subsp *avium* and *hominissuis* were documented in wildlife including badgers and wild pigs.[57–59] In a recent study from Spain, a collaboration between researchers and veterinarians showed both wild and livestock pigs harbored potentially pathogenic NTM, suggesting ungulates as a primary animal reservoir for NTM.[60] Additionally, population genomics studies have revealed the dominant strains and transmission of *M avium* subsp *paratuberculosis* within dairy herds, even reporting the frequency of mixed-strain infections.[61–63]

Classical molecular and biochemical tests were applied to identify *Mycobacterium gastri* from abdominal organs and lymph nodes of a 9 year old captive and immune-suppressed red panda from a Japan zoo, but was unable to identify point sources of exposure, prevalence, and gene analyses.[64] *M. avium* subsp *hominissuis* was identified using 16S rRNA and IS1245 and IS901 sequencing of bronchoalveolar lavage samples collected from zoo tapirs with the protracted disease in Germany, which was also detected in tapir swimming pool water, pool walls, and sleeping beds.[65] To clarify the taxonomy and host ranges of the various subspecies of *M. avium*[66] and *Mycobacterium*

intracellulare[67,68] known to infect humans, animals, and birds, comparative genomic studies have been performed. For example, a recent study applied WGS to investigate NTM isolates from birds diagnosed with avian mycobacteriosis at the San Diego Zoo over a 12 year period, and uncovered transmission patterns of *M. avium* subsp *avium*.[69]

Overall, applying comparative genomics to understand the role of animals in the zoonotic transmission of environmental NTM is a burgeoning field that would benefit from increased numbers of studies focused on NTM genetic diversity in animals and studies to determine the molecular and drug resistance correlates associated with disease using NTM isolates recovered from the environment, animals, and humans. Such studies would improve our understanding of the interconnectedness of these important NTM infections.

Applying Genomics to Demonstrate Matched Environmental and Clinical Nontuberculous Mycobacteria Isolates

To understand where in the environment people acquire their infections, most prior studies have applied molecular tools including DNA probe kits, PCR–RFLP, and culture multilocus enzyme electrophoresis to differentiate and match environmental to clinical isolates. These studies were tabulated and summarized in 2015 in a literature review by Halstrom and colleagues.[70] In **Table 1**, studies since the Halstrom review are summarized that transition to using combinations of molecular and genomic genotyping methods to determine genetically matched environmental and clinical NTM isolates. These include studies from the United States and Korea applying dual variable-number tandem repeat genotyping and WGS or WGS alone to show genetic similarities between household and clinical isolates of NTM (eg, *M. avium*, *M. fortuitum*, *M. chimaera*, *M. abscessus*, and *M. intracellulare*).[71–78]

Utility of Genomic Sequencing to Understand the Dominant Circulating Clones of M. abscessus, Global Disease Transmission Patterns and Outbreak Investigations

WGS and comparative genomics have advanced our understanding the genetic diversity of global clinical *M. abscessus* isolates, and to a lesser extent, MAC isolates. Dominant circulating clones (DCCs) of *M abscessus* have been observed in geographically diverse locations[79] first described among widely separated outbreaks of *M. abscessus* subsp *massiliense*,[80–82] among CF pulmonary

Table 1
Summary of PubMed studies since 2016 that have matched environmental to clinical isolates using genomics

Country	Clinical Samples	Environment Investigated	NTM + Environmental Samples: No. of Environmental Samples Collected	Matched Occurred Between Environment and Clinical Sample	Species Matched	Species Characterization Method	References
United States	Patient (n = 120) respiratory isolates	Water biofilm from 5 US states (n = 80)	19:80	13:57 (environment: environment + clinical)	M. avium	Culture Variable-number tandem repeat genotyping; whole genome sequencing	Iakhiaeva et al[71]
United States	Patients (n = 38), skin biopsy (n = 9/13 with test results), isolates (n = 13)	Tattoo studio tap water (n = 10), bottles of gray wash ink (n = 5), faucet swabs (n = 2)	11:13	1:1 (tattoo ink:skin biopsy) 8:4:3 (tattoo ink:skin biopsy:tap water)	M. fortuitum, M. abscessus	Culture Whole genome sequencing	Griffin[70]
United States	Patient (n = 26) control (n = 11) sputum or BAL	Variety of household plumbing, humidifiers	95:334	11:21 (respiratory: environment)	M. avium	Culture Variable-number tandem repeat genotyping; whole genome sequencing	Lande et al[71]
United States	Hospital outbreak patients (n = 11); clinical controls (n = 11)	Hospital water outlets (n = 4)	N/A	4:7:1 (environmental isolates: outbreak hospital clinical isolates: control clinical isolates)	M. abscessus	Culture Whole genome sequencing	Davidson et al[72]

(continued on next page)

Table 1
(continued)

Country	Clinical Samples	Environment Investigated	NTM + Environmental Samples: No. of Environmental Samples Collected	Matched Occurred Between Environment and Clinical Sample	Species Matched	Species Characterization Method	References
United States	Isolates from patients with left ventricular assist devices (n = 4)	Water specimens (sink, shower) (n = 14); Ice machines (n = 2)	2:14 2:2	8:0 (M. abscessus isolates from water and ice machines:clinical isolates) by culture 16:16 (Samples from water and ice machines:clinical) by culture independent	M. abscessus	Culture Whole genome sequencing and subsequent Culture independent	Klompas et al[73]
United States	Patients with CF (n = 80 isolates)	Health care setting (biofilm, dust) (n = 161)	11:161	0:11 (environment: patient isolates)	M. abscessus , M. avium (no match)	Culture Whole genomic sequencing	Gross et al[74]
United States	Patients with CF (n = 11 isolates)	Health care setting (biofilm, dust) (n = 132)	8:132	1:8 (environment: patient isolates)	M. chimaera, M. avium (no match)	Culture Whole genomic sequencing	Gross et al[75]
Korea	NTM patients cohabitating for > 15 yrs (n = 3 pairs); sputum (n = 4); bronchial washings (n = 2)		(Home 1) 7:12 (Home 2): 0:15 (Home 3): 1:15	1:1 (environment: patient isolates) 1:1 (environment: patient isolates) 1:1 (environment: patient isolates)	(Pair 1) M. avium (Pair 2) M. intracellulare (Pair 3) M. intracellulare, and M. abscessus	Culture Whole genomic sequencing	Yoon et al[76]

isolates across Europe and Australia,[83] and in the United States CF Centers.[84,85]

Owing to the increased awareness of M. abscessus DCCs and access to WGS, a plethora of retrospective studies have been published using WGS to evaluate the potential for person-to-person or health care-associated transmission of NTM. Recent M. abscessus studies were performed as single or multi-site investigations in Europe,[86–89] Australia,[90] Canada,[91] and Asia[92–94] with findings of genetically similar isolate clusters in a subset of patients. For most clusters, there was limited evidence for health care overlaps or social connections between patients that pointed to widespread person-to-person transmission, although it could not be ruled out in some cases. In the most extensive study of clinical M. abscessus isolates to date, the authors analyzed ~2300 isolates from 906 patients sequenced as part of the routine Public Health England diagnostic service.[95] This unbiased sample set included CF and non-CF isolates, and genomic analyses revealed high-density clusters distributed over a wide geographic area. Epidemiologic studies showed that CF and non-CF patients were equally likely to have clustered isolates, and there were few identifiable links between patients in clusters. One intriguing finding was that patients were 1.14 times more likely to have clustered isolates for each 10 years in age, regardless of underlying condition. The authors suggested that this could be due to repeated exposures to an unknown environmental vector, which is an important and key hypothesis yet to be explored on any large scale.

More recent studies showed that DCCs represent a substantial proportion of non-CF isolates derived from both pulmonary and extrapulmonary infections in the United States, Europe, Australia, and Asia.[95–99] The widespread presence of DCCs has led to intense speculation about the extent of person-to-person transmission of M. abscessus as well as the evolutionary origins and trajectory of DCCs.[100] A study analyzed mutational signatures in M. abscessus genomes and proposed that non-CF carriers, particularly smokers, helped disseminate DCCs globally in the mid-to-late 20th century, which led to subsequent clonal expansions in the CF population.[98]

Hospitals are increasingly recognized as bone fide sites of NTM colonization and possible outbreaks.[101] Hospital water and surgical sources have been associated with severe NTM infections including M. chelonae infections associated with LASIK eye and plastic surgeries.[102] At least 17 published reports show NTM isolation from hospital ice or ice-making machines.[103] WGS was recently applied to confirm the genetic similarity between M. abscessus isolates recovered from ice machines of a US hospital and cardiac surgery patient specimens associated with commercial water purification systems.[75] A 2 phase hospital-associated outbreak of M. abscessus occurred among lung transplant and cardiac surgery patients and was linked to contaminated water sources from the addition of a new hospital wing,[74,104] resolving with the successful implementation of water engineering interventions and tap water avoidance protocols.[104,105] A separate outbreak of M. abscessus was reported among pwCF in a hospital in Hawai'i, and improved adherence to infection control practices reduced future cases.[106]

Within the hospital environment, equipment pieces are point sources for pathogenic NTM exposure. M. fortuitum outbreaks have been associated with hospital bronchoscopy units.[102,107] But the highest profile scenarios in recent time are the well-documented global outbreaks of M. chimaera infections associated with open-chest heart surgeries and medical devices, that is, heater–cooler units (HCUs), with more than 140 cases of severe infections identified worldwide.[108–112] A recent review summarized WGS applications related to M. chimaera and HCU infections; thus, these studies are not discussed at length here.[113] Dental procedure rooms are also not immune to NTM colonization, as contaminated tap water used for pediatric pulpectomies during dental procedures was identified as a point source for M abscessus outbreaks.[114] Promising research in statistical process control methods are currently being evaluated to improve NTM surveillance and early outbreak detection in health care environments.[115]

Recently, a standardized approach for NTM outbreak investigations at US CF Centers was developed by Gross and colleagues,[116] focusing on all clinically relevant NTM species through a multi-site study called healthcare-associated links in transmission of NTM. Using combined environmental sampling, the microbiological culture of NTM isolates, watershed analyses, and integrated pan-genome analyses, the health care-associated transmission of M. abscessus was found to be rare in a Colorado Adult CF Center.[76] M. avium transmission events may be possible among pwCF and a cluster of M. intracellulare subsp chimaera pulmonary infection was linked to a health care water source.[77] These studies reinforce the notion that genomic comparisons alone are insufficient to conclude transmission and underscore MAC species as important yet understudied NTM that may be acquired in CF health care environments.

Overall, there have been fewer genomic studies focused exclusively on the global transmission of MAC compared with M. abscessus. Two large studies evaluating clinical MAC isolates were recently performed in the United States[117] and England.[118] The US study focused on clinical isolates from CF Centers in 23 states and reported that *M. avium* and *M. intracellulare* populations were genetically diverse. Only a few isolated clusters among pwCF were identified. The English study included CF and non-CF isolates from a London hospital and identified both *M. avium* subsp *hominissuis* and *avium* in the clinical isolate population. This study also observed a small proportion of isolated clusters among patients. In both studies, clinical *M. avium* and *M. intracellulare* populations did not have DCCs like *M. abscessus*, but most *M. chimaera* isolates belonged to few high-density clades suggesting narrow genetic diversity in this subspecies. A common theme among clinical MAC WGS studies was the observation of mixed strain or mixed species infections in up to 30% of cases that was also observed when sequencing colony sweeps derived from sputum samples.[119] This contrasts with *M. abscessus* infections that are primarily clonal.[83,85,120] The ability to determine infection status (ie, single vs. mixed infections, relapse vs. reinfection) is a clear benefit of WGS and critically important for understanding potential inoculum sources of different NTM species and designing prevention and treatment strategies moving forward.

To begin to identify factors that facilitate the survival of *M. avium* in diverse niches, Keen and colleagues[121] compared and annotated the genomes of 65 human clinical isolates, 31 animal, and 13 soil *M. avium* isolates to generate a core genome alignment to construct a maximum phylogenetic tree. From these analyses, specific *M. avium* genotypes associated with human infections, animals, and free-standing environments and isolates could be distinguished by their core and accessory genomes, patterns of horizontal gene transfer, and virulence factors. To identify genomic processes that facilitate *M. abscessus* survival in diverse niches, this same group sequenced 175 isolates longitudinally collected from 30 people with *M. abscessus* infection and found highly related isolate pairs across hospital centers with a low likelihood for transmission.[122] A mercury resistance plasmid, likely needed for environmental survival, was detected in early isolates but lost from later isolates suggesting a fitness compromise for survival in the lung.

Environmental Threat Events that Influence Nontuberculous Mycobacteria Colonization

As colonizing bacteria of water, soil, and dust, NTM distribution, abundance, diversity, and transmission may be significantly impacted in a variety of ways, elevating the consideration of NTM as climate-sensitive respiratory pathogens. Already, increased moisture in the air has been linked to higher NTM disease prevalence rates.[24] Tsunamis, typhoons, and other natural disasters such as flooding and earthquakes cause large-scale movement of water, soil, and dust and can increase exposures and exacerbate disease risk.[123] As such, increased NTM incidence and prevalence rates have been reported in Florida during times of hurricanes.[124] Dried soil caused by severe droughts may more easily aerosolize NTM into long-distance traveling plumes. *Mycobacterium* 16S gene sequences have been detected in dust caused by natural desert dust events.[125] Warmer climates melt snow and glaciers which may become a new source of NTM dissemination into freshwater conduits. In Asia, a high abundance of *Mycobacterium* sequences has been detected from snow collected from high altitude sites of Mt. Tateyama in Japan contaminated with pollutants from neighboring industrial areas of Beijing.[125] Thawing glaciers due to climate changes have been linked to increased frequency of volcanic eruptions[126] and viable *M. abscessus*, *M. avium*, and *M. chimaera* have been recovered from freshly erupted ash from the Kilauea volcano, Hawai'i after its largest eruption in 250 years.[127]

DISCUSSION

The role of the environment in human NTM acquisition remains a hot topic among those in the NTM community and those who endure these infections. There will likely be no single, globally applicable checklist of equally important defining environmental determinants associated with NTM pulmonary disease emergence. However, regional and worldwide climatic and environmental factors will determine NTM diversity and personalize risk for infection to each location. As such, pulmonary disease surveillance in locations globally is increasingly needed. A significant barrier is the inability to accurately pinpoint exposure sources due to the lengthy lag time between environmental exposure and clinical presentation. International health security in the context of NTM requires dramatic improvement, but the game-changing recent advances in NTM genomics and transmission as discussed are creating positive leaps forward. Finding ways to intervene, reduce, and/or control environmentally acquired NTM infections will be the next field for which solutions are needed.

SUMMARY

NTM resilience in diverse environments ideally positions these opportunistic pathogens as formidable public health challenges and warrants innovative and equitable management solutions to reduce infections.[128] Future studies should focus on moving beyond retrospective studies or single snapshots in time studies to favor prospective, longitudinal studies and increased disease surveillance to exponentially improve our ability to forecast environmental features that promote or reduce environmental NTM prevalence.

CLINICS CARE POINTS

- Successful management of NTM pulmonary disease requires a multifaceted approach including a keen awareness of possible environmental niches, knowledge of reported features that promote NTM in the environment, and cognizance of the geographic hot spots for infection.

- The combination of microbiology and comparative bacterial genomics has begun to uncover the contribution of zoonotic transmission to the interconnectedness of NTM diseases.

- Studies of *M. abscessus* outbreaks using genomic sequencing have revealed the global circulation of dominant clones.

- Microbiological, molecular, and genomic tools have been used in combination to identify possible environmental sources of exposure by genetically matching environmental isolates to respiratory isolates.

- Evidence based results concerning the usefulness of interventions to reduce and/or control environmentally acquired NTM infections will certainly empower clinical care and improve patient outcomes.

DISCLOSURE

J.R. Honda is supported by the Cystic Fibrosis Foundation, National Institutes of Health, National Science Foundation, Shoot for the Cure, and Padosi Foundation.

ACKNOWLEDGMENTS

Many thanks to Rebecca Davidson, PhD for reviewing the article.

REFERENCES

1. Christianson LC, Dewlett HJ. Pulmonary disease in adults associated with unclassified mycobacteria. Am J Med 1960;29:980–91.
2. Johnson MM, Odell JA. Nontuberculous mycobacterial pulmonary infections. J Thorac Dis 2014;6(3):210–20.
3. Proctor C, Garner E, Hamilton KA, et al. Tenets of a holistic approach to drinking water-associated pathogen research, management, and communication. Water Res 2022;211:117997.
4. Feazel LM, Baumgartner LK, Peterson KL, et al. Opportunistic pathogens enriched in showerhead biofilms. Proc Natl Acad Sci U S A 2009;106(38):16393–9.
5. Falkinham JO 3rd, Iseman MD, de Haas P, et al. *Mycobacterium avium* in a shower linked to pulmonary disease. J Water Health 2008;6(2):209–13.
6. Falkinham JO 3rd. Nontuberculous mycobacteria from household plumbing of patients with nontuberculous mycobacteria disease. Emerg Infect Dis 2011;17(3):419–24.
7. Falkinham JO, 3rd, Ecology of nontuberculous mycobacteria, *Microorganisms*, 9 (11), 2021, 1-10.
8. Gruft H, Loder A, Osterhout M, et al. Postulated sources of Mycobacterium intracellulare and Mycobacterium scrofulaceum infection: isolation of mycobacteria from estuaries and ocean waters. Am Rev Respir Dis 1979;120(6):1385–8.
9. Falkinham JO 3rd, Parker BC, Gruft H. Epidemiology of infection by nontuberculous mycobacteria. I. Geographic distribution in the eastern United States. Am Rev Respir Dis 1980;121(6):931–7.
10. Brooks RW, Parker BC, Gruft H, et al. Epidemiology of infection by nontuberculous mycobacteria. V. Numbers in eastern United States soils and correlation with soil characteristics. Am Rev Respir Dis 1984;130(4):630–3.
11. Falkinham JO 3rd, George KL, Parker BC. Epidemiology of infection by nontuberculous mycobacteria. VIII. Absence of mycobacteria in chicken litter. Am Rev Respir Dis 1989;139(6):1347–9.
12. Eaton T, Falkinham JO 3rd, von Reyn CF. Recovery of mycobacterium avium from cigarettes. J Clin Microbiol 1995;33(10):2757–8.
13. Falkinham JO 3rd. Nontuberculous mycobacteria in the environment. Tuberculosis 2022;137:102267.
14. von Reyn CF, Maslow JN, Barber TW, et al. Persistent colonisation of potable water as a source of Mycobacterium avium infection in AIDS. Lancet 1994;343(8906):1137–41.
15. Falkinham JO, Norton CD, LeChevallier MW. Factors influencing numbers of mycobacterium avium, mycobacterium intracellulare, and other mycobacteria in drinking water distribution systems. Appl Environ Microbiol 2001;67:1225–31.

16. Fujita K, Ito Y, Hirai T, et al. Genetic relatedness of Mycobacterium avium-intracellulare complex isolates from patients with pulmonary MAC disease and their residential soils. Clin Microbiol Infect 2013;19(6):537–41.

17. Thomson RM, Carter R, Tolson C, et al. Factors associated with the isolation of Nontuberculous mycobacteria (NTM) from a large municipal water system in Brisbane, Australia. BMC Microbiol 2013;13:89.

18. Thomson R, Tolson C, Sidjabat H, et al. Mycobacterium abscessus isolated from municipal water - a potential source of human infection. BMC Infect Dis 2013;13:241.

19. Martin EC, Parker BC, Falkinham JO 3rd. Epidemiology of infection by nontuberculous mycobacteria. VII. Absence of mycobacteria in southeastern groundwaters. Am Rev Respir Dis 1987;136(2):344–8.

20. Taillard C, Greub G, Weber R, et al. Clinical implications of Mycobacterium kansasii species heterogeneity: swiss national survey. J Clin Microbiol 2003;41(3):1240–4.

21. Nash KA, Brown-Elliott BA, Wallace RJ Jr. A novel gene, erm(41), confers inducible macrolide resistance to clinical isolates of Mycobacterium abscessus but is absent from Mycobacterium chelonae. Antimicrobial Agents Chemother 2009;53(4):1367–76.

22. Winthrop KL, Henkle E, Walker A, et al. On the reportability of nontuberculous mycobacterial disease to public health authorities. Ann Am Thorac Soc 2017;14(3):314–7.

23. Hoefsloot W, van Ingen J, Andrejak C, et al. The geographic diversity of nontuberculous mycobacteria isolated from pulmonary samples: an NTM-NET collaborative study. Eur Respir J 2013;42(6):1604–13.

24. Adjemian J, Olivier KN, Seitz AE, et al. Spatial clusters of nontuberculous mycobacterial lung disease in the United States. Am J Respir Crit Care Med 2012;186(6):553–8.

25. Adjemian J, Olivier KN, Seitz AE, et al. Prevalence of nontuberculous mycobacterial lung disease in U.S. Medicare beneficiaries. Am J Respir Crit Care Med 2012;185(8):881–6.

26. Adjemian J, Frankland TB, Daida YG, et al. Epidemiology of nontuberculous mycobacterial lung disease and tuberculosis, Hawaii, USA. Emerg Infect Dis 2017;23(3):439–47.

27. Adjemian J, Olivier KN, Prevots DR. Nontuberculous mycobacteria among cystic fibrosis patients in the United States: screening practices and environmental risk. Am J Respir Crit Care Med 2014;190(5):581–6.

28. Adjemian J, Olivier KN, Prevots DR. Epidemiology of pulmonary nontuberculous mycobacterial sputum positivity in patients with cystic fibrosis in the United States, 2010-2014. Ann Am Thorac Soc 2018;15(9):1114–5.

29. Mirsaeidi M, Machado RF, Garcia JG, et al. Nontuberculous mycobacterial disease mortality in the United States, 1999-2010: a population-based comparative study. PLoS One 2014;9(3):1–9.

30. Parsons AW, Dawrs SN, Nelson ST, et al. Soil Properties and moisture synergistically influence nontuberculous mycobacterial prevalence in natural environments of hawai'i. Appl Environ Microbiol 2022;88(9):e0001822.

31. Nelson ST, Robinson S, Rey K, et al. Exposure pathways of nontuberculous mycobacteria through soil, streams, and groundwater, hawai'i, USA. Geohealth 2021;5(4). e2020GH000350.

32. Glickman CM, Virdi R, Hasan NA, et al. Assessment of soil features on the growth of environmental nontuberculous mycobacterial isolates from Hawai'i. Appl Environ Microbiol 2020;86(21). 001211-20.

33. Virdi R, Lowe ME, Norton GJ, et al. Lower Recovery of nontuberculous mycobacteria from outdoor hawai'i environmental water biofilms compared to indoor samples. Microorganisms 2021;9(2):224.

34. Honda JR, Hasan NA, Davidson RM, et al. Environmental nontuberculous mycobacteria in the Hawaiian Islands. PLoS Neglected Trop Dis 2016;10(10):e0005068.

35. Hozalski RM, LaPara TM, Zhao X, et al. Flushing of stagnant premise water systems after the COVID-19 shutdown can reduce infection risk by legionella and mycobacterium spp. Environ Sci Technol 2020;54(24):15914–24.

36. Virdi R, Lowe ME, Norton GJ, et al. Lower recovery of nontuberculous mycobacteria from outdoor hawai'i environmental water biofilms compared to indoor samples, Microorganisms, 9 (2), 2021, 1-16.

37. Gebert MJ, Delgado-Baquerizo M, Oliverio AM, et al. Ecological analyses of mycobacteria in showerhead biofilms and their relevance to human health. mBio 2018;9(5).

38. Thomson R, Tolson C, Carter R, et al. Isolation of nontuberculous mycobacteria (NTM) from household water and shower aerosols in patients with pulmonary disease caused by NTM. J Clin Microbiol 2013;51(9):3006–11.

39. van Ingen J, Blaak H, de Beer J, et al. Rapidly growing nontuberculous mycobacteria cultured from home tap and shower water. Appl Environ Microbiol 2010;76(17):6017–9.

40. Tzou CL, Dirac MA, Becker AL, et al. Association between mycobacterium avium complex pulmonary disease and mycobacteria in home water and soil. Ann Am Thorac Soc 2020;17(1):57–62.

41. Shen Y, Haig S-J, Prussin AJ, II, et al. Shower water contributes viable nontuberculous mycobacteria to indoor air, PNAS Nexus, 1 (5), 2022, 1-14.

42. Adjemian J, Daniel-Wayman S, Ricotta E, et al. Epidemiology of nontuberculous mycobacteriosis. Semin Respir Crit Care Med 2018;39(3):325–35.

43. Foote SL, Lipner EM, Prevots DR, et al. Environmental predictors of pulmonary nontuberculous mycobacteria (NTM) sputum positivity among persons with cystic fibrosis in the state of Florida. PLoS One 2021;16(12):e0259964.

44. DeFlorio-Barker S, Egorov A, Smith GS, et al. Environmental risk factors associated with pulmonary isolation of nontuberculous mycobacteria, a population-based study in the southeastern United States. Sci Total Environ 2021;763:144552.

45. Thomson RM, Furuya-Kanamori L, Coffey C, et al. Influence of climate variables on the rising incidence of nontuberculous mycobacterial (NTM) infections in Queensland, Australia 2001-2016. Sci Total Environ 2020;740:139796.

46. Lipner EM, French J, Bern CR, et al. Nontuberculous mycobacterial disease and molybdenum in Colorado watersheds, *Int J Environ Res Publ Health*, 17 (11), 2020, 1-15.

47. Lipner EM, Crooks JL, French J, et al. Nontuberculous mycobacterial infection and environmental molybdenum in persons with cystic fibrosis: a case-control study in Colorado. J Expo Sci Environ Epidemiol 2022;32(2):289–94.

48. Lipner EM, French JP, Falkinham JO 3rd, et al. Nontuberculous mycobacteria infection risk and trace metals in surface water: a population-based ecologic epidemiologic study in Oregon. Ann Am Thorac Soc 2022;19(4):543–50.

49. Canetti D, Riccardi N, Antonello RM, et al. Mycobacterium marinum: a brief update for clinical purposes. Eur J Intern Med 2022;105:15–9.

50. Hashish E, Merwad A, Elgaml S, et al. Mycobacterium marinum infection in fish and man: epidemiology, pathophysiology and management; a review. Vet Q 2018;38(1):35–46.

51. Delghandi MR, El-Matbouli M. and Menanteau-Ledouble S., Mycobacteriosis and Infections with non-tuberculous mycobacteria in aquatic organisms: a review, *Microorganisms*, 8 (9), 2020, 1-18.

52. Grange JM. Mycobacterium chelonei. Tubercle. 1981;62(4):273–6.

53. Ross AJ, Brancato FP. Mycobacterium fortuitum cruz from the tropical fish hyphessobrycon innesi. J Bacteriol 1959;78(3):392–5.

54. Lescenko P, Matlova L, Dvorska L, et al. Mycobacterial infection in aquarium fish. Vet Med - Czech 2003;48(3):71–8.

55. Janse M, Kik MJ. Mycobacterium avium granulomas in a captive epaulette shark, hemiscyllium ocellatum (bonnaterre). J Fish Dis 2012;35(12):935–40.

56. Komine T, Srivorakul S, Yoshida M, et al. Core single nucleotide polymorphism analysis reveals transmission of mycobacterium marinum between animal and environmental sources in two aquaria. J Fish Dis 2023;46(5):507–16.

57. Balseiro A, Rodriguez O, Gonzalez-Quiros P, et al. Infection of Eurasian badgers (Meles meles) with Mycobacterium bovis and Mycobacterium avium complex in Spain. Vet J 2011;190(2):e21–5.

58. Domingos M, Amado A, Botelho A. IS1245 RFLP analysis of strains of Mycobacterium avium subspecies hominissuis isolated from pigs with tuberculosis lymphadenitis in Portugal. Vet Rec 2009; 164(4):116–20.

59. Munoz-Mendoza M, Marreros N, Boadella M, et al. Wild boar tuberculosis in iberian atlantic Spain: a different picture from Mediterranean habitats. BMC Vet Res 2013;9:176.

60. Varela-Castro L, Barral M, Arnal MC, et al. Beyond tuberculosis: diversity and implications of non-tuberculous mycobacteria at the wildlife-livestock interface. Transbound Emerg Dis 2022;69(5): e2978–93.

61. Conde C, Theze J, Cochard T, et al. Genetic features of Mycobacterium avium subsp. paratuberculosis strains circulating in the west of France deciphered by whole-genome sequencing. Microbiol Spectr 2022;10(6):e0339222.

62. Nigsch A, Robbe-Austerman S, Stuber TP, et al. Who infects whom?-Reconstructing infection chains of Mycobacterium avium ssp. paratuberculosis in an endemically infected dairy herd by use of genomic data. PLoS One 2021;16(5):e0246983.

63. Perets V, Allen A, Crispell J, et al. Evidence for local and international spread of Mycobacterium avium subspecies paratuberculosis through whole genome sequencing of isolates from the island of Ireland. Vet Microbiol 2022;268:109416.

64. Fuke N, Hirai T, Makimura N, et al. Non-tuberculous mycobacteriosis with T-cell lymphoma in a red panda (ailurus fulgens). J Comp Pathol 2016; 155(2–3):263–6.

65. Marcordes S, Lueders I, Grund L, et al. Clinical outcome and diagnostic methods of atypical mycobacteriosis due to Mycobacterium avium ssp. hominissuis in a group of captive lowland tapirs (Tapirus terrestris). Transbound Emerg Dis 2021; 68(3):1305–13.

66. Mizzi R, Plain KM, Whittington R, et al. Global phylogeny of Mycobacterium avium and identification of mutation hotspots during niche adaptation. Front Microbiol 2022;13:892333.

67. Song Y, Ge X, Chen Y, et al. Mycobacterium bovis induces mitophagy to suppress host xenophagy for its intracellular survival. Autophagy 2022;18(6): 1401–15.

68. Tortoli E, Meehan CJ, Grottola A, et al. Genome-based taxonomic revision detects a number of synonymous taxa in the genus Mycobacterium. Infect Genet Evol 2019;75:103983.

69. Witte C, Fowler JH, Pfeiffer W, et al. Social network analysis and whole-genome sequencing to evaluate disease transmission in a large, dynamic population: a study of avian mycobacteriosis in zoo birds. PLoS One 2021;16(6):e0252152.

70. Halstrom S, Price P, Thomson R. Review: environmental mycobacteria as a cause of human infection. Int J Mycobacteriol 2015;4(2):81–91.

71. Iakhiaeva E, Howard ST, Brown Elliott BA, et al. Variable-number tandem-repeat analysis of respiratory and household water biofilm isolates of "mycobacterium avium subsp. hominissuis" with establishment of a PCR database. J Clin Microbiol 2016;54(4):891–901.

72. Griffin I, Schmitz A, Oliver C, et al. Outbreak of tattoo-associated nontuberculous mycobacterial skin infections. Clin Infect Dis 2019;69(6):949–55.

73. Lande L, Alexander DC, Wallace RJ Jr, et al. Mycobacterium avium in community and household water, suburban philadelphia, Pennsylvania, USA, 2010-2012. Emerg Infect Dis 2019;25(3):473–81.

74. Davidson RM, Nick SE, Kammlade SM, et al. Genomic analysis of a hospital-associated outbreak of mycobacterium abscessus: implications on transmission. J Clin Microbiol 2022;60(1): e0154721.

75. Klompas M, Akusobi C, Boyer J, et al. Mycobacterium abscessus cluster in cardiac surgery patients potentially attributable to a commercial water purification system. Ann Intern Med 2023;176(3): 333–9.

76. Gross JE, Caceres S, Poch K, et al. Investigating nontuberculous mycobacteria transmission at the Colorado adult cystic fibrosis program. Am J Respir Crit Care Med 2022;205(9):1064–74.

77. Gross JE, Teneback CC, Sweet JG, et al. Molecular epidemiologic investigation of mycobacterium intracellulare subspecies chimaera lung infections at an adult cystic fibrosis program. Ann Am Thorac Soc 2023;20(5):677–86.

78. Yoon JK, Kim TS, Kim JI, et al. Whole genome sequencing of nontuberculous mycobacterium (NTM) isolates from sputum specimens of cohabiting patients with NTM pulmonary disease and NTM isolates from their environment. BMC Genom 2020;21(1):322.

79. Davidson RM. A closer look at the genomic variation of geographically diverse mycobacterium abscessus clones that cause human infection and disease. Front Microbiol 2018;9:2988.

80. Everall I, Nogueira CL, Bryant JM, et al. Genomic epidemiology of a national outbreak of postsurgical Mycobacterium abscessus wound infections in Brazil. Microb Genom 2017;3(5):e000111.

81. Davidson RM, Hasan NA, de Moura VC, et al. Phylogenomics of Brazilian epidemic isolates of Mycobacterium abscessus subsp. bolletii reveals relationships of global outbreak strains. Infect Genet Evol 2013;20:292–7.

82. Tettelin H, Davidson RM, Agrawal S, et al. High-level relatedness among Mycobacterium abscessus subsp. massiliense strains from widely separated outbreaks. Emerg Infect Dis 2014; 20(3):364–71.

83. Bryant JM, Grogono DM, Rodriguez-Rincon D, et al. Emergence and spread of a human-transmissible multidrug-resistant nontuberculous mycobacterium. Science 2016;354(6313): 751–7.

84. Davidson RM, Hasan NA, Reynolds PR, et al. Genome sequencing of Mycobacterium abscessus isolates from patients in the United States and comparisons to globally diverse clinical strains. J Clin Microbiol 2014;52(10):3573–82.

85. Davidson RM, Hasan NA, Epperson LE, et al. Population genomics of mycobacterium abscessus from United States cystic fibrosis care centers. Ann Am Thorac Soc 2021;18(12):1960–9.

86. Tortoli E, Kohl TA, Trovato A, et al. Mycobacterium abscessus in patients with cystic fibrosis: low impact of inter-human transmission in Italy, *Eur Respir J*, 50 (1), 2017, 1-4.

87. Doyle RM, Rubio M, Dixon G, et al. Cross-transmission is not the source of new mycobacterium abscessus infections in a multicenter cohort of cystic fibrosis patients. Clin Infect Dis 2020;70(9): 1855–64.

88. Redondo N, Mok S, Montgomery L, et al. Genomic analysis of mycobacterium abscessus complex isolates collected in Ireland between 2006 and 2017, *J Clin Microbiol*, 58 (7), 2020, 1-8.

89. Wetzstein N, Diricks M, Kohl TA, et al. Molecular epidemiology of mycobacterium abscessus isolates recovered from German cystic fibrosis patients. Microbiol Spectr 2022;10(4):e0171422.

90. Yan J, Kevat A, Martinez E, et al. Investigating transmission of Mycobacterium abscessus amongst children in an Australian cystic fibrosis centre. J Cyst Fibros 2020;19(2):219–24.

91. Waglechner N, Tullis E, Stephenson AL, et al. Genomic epidemiology of Mycobacterium abscessus in a Canadian cystic fibrosis centre. Sci Rep 2022;12(1):16116.

92. Fujiwara K, Yoshida M, Murase Y, et al. Potential cross-transmission of mycobacterium abscessus among non-cystic fibrosis patients at a tertiary hospital in Japan. Microbiol Spectr 2022;10(3): e0009722.

93. Kaewprasert O, Nonghanphithak D, Chetchotisakd P, et al. Whole-genome sequencing and drug-susceptibility analysis of serial mycobacterium abscessus isolates from Thai patients, *Biology*, 11 (9), 2022, 1-13.

94. Chew KL, Octavia S, Jureen R, et al. Molecular epidemiology and phylogenomic analysis of

Mycobacterium abscessus clinical isolates in an Asian population, *Microb Genom*, 7 (11), 2021, 1-9.

95. Lipworth S, Hough N, Weston N, et al. Epidemiology of Mycobacterium abscessus in England: an observational study. Lancet Microbe 2021; 2(10):e498–507.

96. Davidson RM, Benoit JB, Kammlade SM, et al. Genomic characterization of sporadic isolates of the dominant clone of Mycobacterium abscessus subspecies massiliense. Sci Rep 2021;11(1):15336.

97. Jin P, Dai J, Guo Y, et al. Genomic analysis of mycobacterium abscessus complex isolates from patients with pulmonary infection in China. Microbiol Spectr 2022;10(4):e0011822.

98. Ruis C, Bryant JM, Bell SC, et al. Dissemination of mycobacterium abscessus via global transmission networks. Nature microbiology 2021;6(10):1279–88.

99. Bronson RA, Gupta C, Manson AL, et al. Global phylogenomic analyses of Mycobacterium abscessus provide context for non cystic fibrosis infections and the evolution of antibiotic resistance. Nat Commun 2021;12(1):5145.

100. Bryant JM, Brown KP, Burbaud S, et al. Stepwise pathogenic evolution of Mycobacterium abscessus. Science 2021;372(6541).

101. Sood G, Parrish N. Outbreaks of nontuberculous mycobacteria. Curr Opin Infect Dis 2017;30(4): 404–9.

102. Edens C, Liebich L, Halpin AL, et al. Mycobacterium chelonae eye infections associated with humidifier use in an outpatient LASIK Clinic–Ohio, 2015. MMWR Morb Mortal Wkly Rep 2015;64(41): 1177.

103. Evans TW, Kalambokidis MJ, Jungblut AD, et al. Lipid biomarkers from microbial mats on the McMurdo Ice Shelf, Antarctica: signatures for life in the cryosphere. Front Microbiol 2022;13:903621.

104. Baker AW, Lewis SS, Alexander BD, et al. Two-phase hospital-associated outbreak of mycobacterium abscessus: investigation and mitigation. Clin Infect Dis 2017;64(7):902–11.

105. Baker AW, Stout JE, Anderson DJ, et al. Tap water avoidance decreases rates of hospital-onset pulmonary nontuberculous mycobacteria. Clin Infect Dis 2021;73(3):524–7.

106. Johnston DI, Chisty Z, Gross JE, et al. Investigation of Mycobacterium abscessus outbreak among cystic fibrosis patients, Hawaii 2012. J Hosp Infect 2016;94(2):198–200.

107. Campos-Gutierrez S, Ramos-Real MJ, Abreu R, et al. Pseudo-outbreak of Mycobacterium fortuitum in a hospital bronchoscopy unit. Am J Infect Control 2020;48(7):765–9.

108. Hasan NA, Epperson LE, Lawsin A, et al. Genomic analysis of cardiac surgery-associated mycobacterium chimaera infections, United States. Emerg Infect Dis 2019;25(3):559–63.

109. Perkins KM, Lawsin A, Hasan NA, et al. Notes from the field: mycobacterium chimaera contamination of heater-cooler devices used in cardiac surgery - United States. MMWR Morb Mortal Wkly Rep 2016;65(40):1117–8.

110. Campins Marti M, Borras Bermejo B, Armadans Gil L. Infections with Mycobacterium chimaera and open chest surgery. An unresolved problem. Med Clin 2019;152(8):317–23.

111. Sax H, Bloemberg G, Hasse B, et al. Prolonged outbreak of mycobacterium chimaera infection after open-chest heart surgery. Clin Infect Dis 2015; 61(1):67–75.

112. Chand M, Lamagni T, Kranzer K, et al. Insidious risk of severe mycobacterium chimaera infection in cardiac surgery patients. Clin Infect Dis 2017; 64(3):335–42.

113. Schreiber PW, Kohl TA, Kuster SP, et al. The global outbreak of Mycobacterium chimaera infections in cardiac surgery-a systematic review of whole-genome sequencing studies and joint analysis. Clin Microbiol Infect 2021;27(11):1613–20.

114. Besinis A, De Peralta T, Tredwin CJ, et al. Review of nanomaterials in dentistry: interactions with the oral microenvironment, clinical applications, hazards, and benefits. ACS Nano 2015;9(3): 2255–89.

115. Baker AW, Maged A, Haridy S, et al. Use of statistical process control methods for early detection of healthcare facility-associated nontuberculous mycobacterial outbreaks: a single center pilot study, Clin Infect Dis, 76(8), 2022, 1459-1467.

116. Gross JE, Caceres S, Poch K, et al. Healthcare-associated links in transmission of nontuberculous mycobacteria among people with cystic fibrosis (HALT NTM) study: rationale and study design. PLoS One 2021;16(12):e0261628.

117. Hasan NA, Davidson RM, Epperson LE, et al. Population genomics and inference of mycobacterium avium complex clusters in cystic fibrosis care centers, United States. Emerg Infect Dis 2021;27(11): 2836–46.

118. van Tonder AJ, Ellis HC, Churchward CP, et al. Mycobacterium avium complex (MAC) genomics and transmission in a London hospital, *Eur Respir J*, 61(4), 2022, 1–15.

119. Operario DJ, Pholwat S, Koeppel AF, et al. Mycobacterium avium complex diversity within lung disease, as revealed by whole-genome sequencing. Am J Respir Crit Care Med 2019;200(3):393–6.

120. Nick JA, Dedrick RM, Gray AL, et al. Host and pathogen response to bacteriophage engineered against Mycobacterium abscessus lung infection. Cell 2022;185(11):1860–1874 e1812.

121. Keen EC, Choi J, Wallace MA, et al. Comparative genomics of mycobacterium avium complex reveals signatures of environment-specific

adaptation and community acquisition. mSystems 2021;6(5):e0119421.

122. Choi J, Keen EC, Wallace MA, et al. Genomic analyses of longitudinal mycobacterium abscessus isolates in a multi-center cohort reveal parallel signatures of in-host adaptation. J Infect Dis 2023;187:1–11.

123. Honda JR, Bernhard JN, Chan ED. Natural disasters and nontuberculous mycobacteria: a recipe for increased disease? Chest 2015;147(2):304–8.

124. Kambali S, Quinonez E, Sharifi A, et al. Pulmonary nontuberculous mycobacterial disease in Florida and association with large-scale natural disasters. BMC Publ Health 2021;21(1):2058.

125. Maki T, Noda J, Morimoto K, et al. Long-range transport of airborne bacteria over East Asia: asian dust events carry potentially nontuberculous Mycobacterium populations. Environ Int 2022;168: 107471.

126. Gloor; GTSEJWIPSITLASAHCLCCBCM. Climatic control on Icelandic volcanic activity during the mid-Holocene. Geology 2018;46(1):47–50.

127. Dawrs SN, Virdi R, Norton GJ, et al. Nontuberculous mycobacteria and volcanic ash from the Kilauea volcano, Hawai'i 2019;A1037–A1037.

128. Blanc S, Robinson D, Fahrenfeld N. Potential for nontuberculous mycobacteria proliferation in natural and engineered water systems due to climate change: a literature review. City and Environmental Interactions 2021;11:1–12.

Global Epidemiology of Nontuberculous Mycobacterial Pulmonary Disease: A Review

D. Rebecca Prevots, PhD, MPH[a],*, Julia E. Marshall, BS[a], Dirk Wagner, MD[b,1], Kozo Morimoto, MD[c,1]

KEYWORDS

- Epidemiology • Nontuberculous mycobacteria • *Mycobacterium avium* • *Mycobacterium abscessus*
- Pulmonary disease • Global • Exposome

KEY POINTS

- Population-based data from North America, Europe, and East Asia demonstrate continued increases in NTM isolation and disease across regions and in most countries.
- In countries and regions where population-based data are not available, NTM species identification among persons screened for TB provides a measure of the unrecognized burden of NTM.
- NTM-PD incidence and prevalence remain generally higher in East Asia, North America, and Australia than in Europe.
- Species-specific differences exist in prevalence, trends, and distribution within countries and regions, and should be considered when analyzing trends data:
- Cumulative exposure to soil and water aerosols increases the risk of infection , as do water quality and composition
- Water quality and composition influences the risk for NTM infection, as has been shown in a study analyzing the concentrations of vanadium and molybdenum in source water for municipal water systems that are associated with an increased risk of MAC and *Mycobacterium abscessus* complex in the United States.

INTRODUCTION

In this article, we review approaches to studying the epidemiology of nontuberculous mycobacterial (NTM) pulmonary disease (NTM-PD) and update advances in the field since the last review published in 2015.[1]

The Importance of Epidemiology: Surveillance and Research

Defining the NTM-PD disease burden is critical for justifying the need for resource allocation, both for clinical resources such as health care, as well as for the development of new therapeutics. A fuller

[a] Epidemiology and Population Studies Unit, Division of Intramural Research, National Institute of Allergy and Infectious Diseases, National Institutes of Health, 5601 Fishers Lane, Bethesda, MD 20852, USA; [b] Division of Infectious Diseases, Department of Internal Medicine II, Medical Center- University of Freiburg, Faculty of Medicine, Hugstetter Street. 55, Freiburg b106, Germany; [c] Division of Clinical Research, Fukujuji Hospital, Japan Anti-Tuberculosis Association (JATA), 3-1-24, Matsuyama, Kiyose, Tokyo, Japan
[1] These authors shared equally in the development of this work.
* Corresponding author.
E-mail address: rprevots@nih.gov

Clin Chest Med 44 (2023) 675–721
https://doi.org/10.1016/j.ccm.2023.08.012
0272-5231/23/Published by Elsevier Inc.

understanding of the risk factors that contribute to changes in disease frequency is important for guiding and evaluating interventions, at either the individual-level through modification of behaviors or through structural interventions beyond the individual. Epidemiologic surveillance is key for estimating the burden of disease (prevalence) as well as the frequency of new cases (incidence) in a given population,[2] which in turn can lead to developing hypotheses regarding individual or general environmental risk factors for infection and disease.[3,4]

We here present a new approach for understanding the external and internal exposures that may lead to an increased risk of NTM disease[5] (**Fig. 1**). This paradigm is adapted from the fields of environmental epidemiology[5] and cancer epidemiology,[6] whereby cumulative exposures to a variety of types of exposures will increase the risk of infection and disease. With respect to NTM-PD, specific environmental factors include those in an individual's environment, such as those exposures from high-risk activities such as gardening, with aerosolization of soil. General environmental exposures include those beyond the control of a single individual, which affect an entire population. Both factors interact with the human host, and host susceptibility, including biologic response, will influence the risk of developing NTM-PD[5] (see **Fig. 1**).

Methodologic Challenges

A key methodologic challenge is the lack of a global surveillance system with standard case definitions that would allow comparison within and across countries and regions. The NTM-PD case definition, which includes microbiologic, radiographic, and clinical criteria, was developed by ATS/IDSA in 2007 for diagnostic and treatment purposes,[7] and was endorsed in the more recent American Thoracic Society (ATS)/ European Respiratory Society (ERS)/ European Society of Clinical Microbiology and Infectious Diseases (ESCMID) /Infectious Disease Society of American (IDSA)guidelines.[8] In this review, we will use the simplified term "ATS-criteria" acknowledging the equal contribution of the other societies. However, different case definitions may be used for epidemiologic purposes of monitoring infection rates and risk factor identification because the decision about whether and when to treat is different from the surveillance goal of identifying patterns of infection and disease.

Ascertaining the radiographic and clinical criteria for NTM-PD is generally time consuming and costly and, therefore, not feasible at the scale needed to study national and regional patterns, particularly in areas with a higher disease burden. Therefore, microbiology data from centralized public health laboratory systems, as well as administrative claims data with International Classification of Disease (ICD) codes have been increasingly used to better understand the epidemiology of NTM-PD. Each approach has strengths and limitations. Microbiologic data provide an indicator of exposure from the environment but will overestimate the true disease prevalence because not all

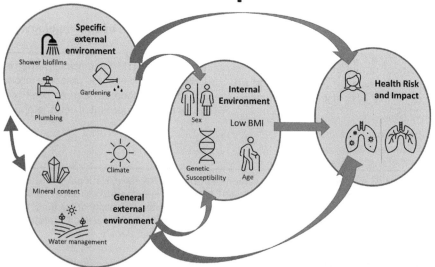

Fig. 1. NTM exosome framework. (*Adapted from* The exposome: a new paradigm to study the impact of environment on health, Vrijheid M., 69, 876-8, 2014 with permission from BMJ Publishing Group Ltd.)

isolates from respiratory secretions are clinically significant. In this review, we use the term "isolation" or "isolates" to refer to culture positivity of respiratory specimens for NTM without necessarily attributing these isolates to a disease status in a specific patient. We therefore also avoid the term "colonization," which suggests "no disease," a status, which has not been well studied. Although the term "NTM infection" has often been used to refer to cases that satisfy the ATS microbiologic criteria,[9–14] we generally avoid the use of this term because the definition of this term has not been standardized.

The microbiologic component of the ATS criteria, as well as ICD codes (9 or 10), have been evaluated and found to have a high-predictive value for NTM-PD (meeting the full ATS diagnostic criteria). In a large, population-based cohort from a centralized provincial laboratory in Ontario, Canada, 46% of those with an isolate of NTM met the microbiologic component of the ATS disease diagnostic criteria.[14] Within the subset of patients being followed in a clinic setting, 73% of the patients who fulfilled the ATS microbiologic criteria met the full ATS disease criteria, indicating a high-predictive value.[14] Similarly, in a large national study using NTM isolates from the national referral laboratory in Denmark, among a small subset with isolates meeting ATS microbiologic criteria (termed "possible NTM disease"), 90% met the full ATS disease criteria.[13] In a study in North Carolina, United States, based on mycobacterial isolation and full chart review, 55.7% of those with an isolate met the ATS microbiologic criteria, and 60.9% of these met the full criteria including microbiologic, clinical, and radiographic criteria.[15] Thus, although analysis of isolates is important for understanding patterns and trends, case definitions based on 1 or 2 isolates will usually overestimate the burden of ATS defined NTM-PD.

ICD codes provide a more useful indicator of true disease, although they will tend to underestimate true disease prevalence because administrative codes tend to lack sensitivity for rare disease. The sensitivity of the ICD codes relative to the ATS microbiologic criteria has been found to range from 27%[16] in a general population to 50% among persons with rheumatoid arthritis[17] and up to 69% among persons with bronchiectasis[18]; the positive predictive value across various studies has ranged from 77% to 100%.[17–19] Although these codes may underestimate true disease rates, the direction of this bias is unlikely to change substantially across time and populations, such that these codes are useful tools for epidemiologic purposes.

Two noteworthy examples of implementation of NTM-PD surveillance are from Queensland, Australia, and the state of Oregon, United States. In Queensland, laboratory-based notification of NTM isolates has been mandated since the inception of the Tuberculosis control program in the 1950s, and all cases of NTM isolation are notifiable under the Public Health Act.[3] Data from this surveillance system has since facilitated the characterization of NTM-PD epidemiology, particularly with respect to geographic distribution, environmental risk factors, and increasing burden.[3] In the state of Oregon, United States, a pilot surveillance program was implemented from 2005 to 2006 and provided important insights regarding NTM epidemiology.[4,19] Currently, in the United States, only 4 states have mandated notification of NTM-PD, as part of Centers for Disease Control and Prevention (CDC) through an Emerging Infections Network pilot program.[20,21]

Despite the known limitations of death certificate data, in the United States, recent data have shown an increase in non–human immunodeficiency virus (HIV)-associated NTM-related deaths from 1999 to 2014, during a period in which both HIV-associated NTM-related mortality decreased, and TB-associated mortality also decreased significantly.[22] In Japan, in the absence of nationally representative data, mortality data were useful for providing insight into patterns by age, sex, and region, and for estimating prevalence.[23] Several studies have identified the increased risk of mortality associated with NTM-PD.[24,25] In one study, persons with NTM-PD had a 4-fold increased risk of death after adjusting for all other factors (HR = 3.64).[26]

Risk Factors: Environment

General and specific environmental risk factors identified to date are summarized in **Table 1**. Specific exposures refer to those estimated from studies which associate individual behaviors or household factors with human NTM pulmonary isolation or disease. General exposures refer to those not unique to a single individual but rather which affect the broader population.

Case-control studies in the United States, South Korea, and Japan have identified individual factors related to water and soil exposure. A recent study in Oregon, United States, found that the NTM isolation in the household shower aerosols was significantly associated with NTM-PD[27] but that other home water and soil exposure were not. This finding is supported by a study in Queensland, Australia, which found genetic matches between patient isolates and species identified from shower aerosols and household water supplies.[28] In the initial Oregon study, the only household-level

Table 1
Environmental risk factors for nontuberculous mycobacterial infection and disease

Risk Factor	Relative Risk, Odds Ratio, Relative Prevalence, or Other Measure	Case Definition
Environmental: specific individual exposures		
NTM isolation from shower aerosols, OR, United States	4.0 [OR][27]	MAC-PD, case-control study
Use of spray bottle to spray house plants, OR, United States	2.7 [OR][29]	MAC-PD, case-control study
Use of public baths ≥1/wk, South Korea	4.0 [OR][30]	MAC-PD, case-control study
Indoor swimming pool use (in the past 4 mo), United States	5.9 [OR][31]	Incident pulmonary isolation among persons with CF (pwCF)
Soil exposure, Japan (bronchiectasis with MAC vs bronchiectasis with no MAC)	5.9 [OR][33]	MAC-PD, case-control study
Environment-general exposures, measured at population level: climate, soil, and water related		
Relative abundance of NTM in showerhead biofilm and population prevalence	Significant correlation, $P < .0001$[35]	NTM-PD and NTM pulmonary isolation (Medicare with ICD codes; CF ≥ 1 pulmonary isolate)
Higher average annual precipitation, FL, United States	1.34[130]	Incident pulmonary isolation (≥1 isolate) among persons with CF
Increased soil sodium, FL, United States	1.92[130]	Incident pulmonary isolation (≥1 isolate) among persons with CF
Increased soil manganese, FL, United States	0.59[130]	Incident pulmonary isolation (≥1 isolate) among persons with CF
Increased molybdenum concentrations in source water	1.41[12] 1.79[11]	M abscessus incident pulmonary isolation (≥2 isolates), non-CF M abscessus pulmonary isolation in persons with CF (≥1 isolate)
Increased vanadium concentrations in source water	1.49[12] 1.22[36]	Incident MAC isolation (≥2 isolates), non-CF Incident MAC pulmonary isolation, non-CF (≥2 isolates)
Percent hydric soil in census blocks, NC, United States	26.8[38]	NTM pulmonary isolation (≥1 isolate), non-CF
Proportion of area as surface water, United States	4.6[39]	NTM-PD (ICD codes)
Mean daily potential evapotranspiration, United States	4.0[39]	NTM-PD (ICD codes)
Copper soil levels, per 1 ppm increase, United States	1.2[39]	NTM-PD (ICD codes)
Sodium soil levels, per 0.1 ppm increase, United States	1.9[39]	NTM-PD (ICD codes)
Manganese soil levels, per 100 ppm increase, United States	0.7[39]	NTM-PD (ICD codes)
Increased average topsoil depth, Australia	0.87 (M intracellulare)[42]	NTM isolation (≥1 isolate), non-CF
Soil bulk density, Australia	1.8 (M kansasii)[42]	NTM isolation (≥1 isolate), non-CF

factors significantly associated with NTM-PD risk was spraying plants with a spray bottle [OR = 2.7].[29] In South Korea, the use of public baths at least weekly was associated with a 4-fold increased risk of NTM-PD.[30] In the United States, a national study of NTM-PD among persons with cystic fibrosis (CF) found that indoor swimming pool use at least monthly was significantly associated with incident NTM isolation[31] (see **Table 1**), and that other behavioral factors, including showering frequency, were not. A study among children with CF in Florida found that those who lived in households that were within 500 m of a body of water had a significant 9.4-fold increased odds of having NTM pulmonary isolation.[32] In Japan, exposure to soil more than twice weekly was significantly associated with the NTM-PD.[33] The high risk associated with frequent soil exposure is consistent with a population-based study of agriculture workers in Florida, which found that cumulative occupational exposure was significantly associated with infection, as defined by *M avium* skin test sensitivity.[34] The risk associated with any given behavior will depend on the intensity of the exposure and the NTM abundance in environmental exposure source—generally soil or water. The risk associated with household NTM isolation from shower aerosols in the NTM-PD study in Oregon is supported by a national study of shower biofilms, which found a significant correlation between the relative abundance of NTM in showerhead biofilms and state-level NTM-PD prevalence in both the CF population and the US Medicare beneficiary population aged 65 years or older.[35]

Ecologic epidemiologic studies have found water, soil, and climate factors associated with an increased risk of NTM-PD; these studies have been conducted primarily in the United States and Australia (see **Table 1**). In several studies conducted in the United States from 2020 to 2022, a consistently significant and strong association has been found between concentrations of molybdenum and *Mycobacterium abscessus* infection and vanadium and *Mycobacterium avium* complex (MAC) infections in natural water sources (ground or surface) supplying municipal water systems: for every log increase in molybdenum concentrations, the risk of *M abscessus* isolation increased by 41%[12] to 79%[11] and for every log increase in the concentration of vanadium, the risk of MAC isolation ($\geq$2 isolates) increased 22%[36] to 49%[12] (see **Table 1**). Interestingly, a case-control study in South Korea found NTM-PD patients had significantly higher median blood serum concentrations of molybdenum than controls.[37]

Several other studies have identified risks related to soil, land use, and other climate factors. In North Carolina, United States, the percent hydric soil in census blocks was significantly associated with NTM isolation: census blocks with 20% or greater hydric soils had a significant 26.8% increased adjusted mean patient count relative to those with 20% or lesser hydric soils.[38] In Florida, in the CF population, increased soil sodium in the zip code of residence was associated with an increased risk of incident NTM isolation, whereas increased soil manganese was protective.[39] In the same study, persons living in counties with above average annual levels of precipitation were also at increased risk of incident infection.[39] In 2 national studies in the United States, vapor pressure (a measure of the water in the atmosphere at a given temperature) was predictive of disease prevalence among patients with CF[31] as well as Medicare beneficiaries aged 65 years or older.[31,40] In addition, in the national Medicare study, evapotranspiration (the potential of the atmosphere to absorb water), and the proportion of the area as surface water were predictive of high-risk areas.[39] In the Medicare study, higher manganese soil levels in the county were associated with lower incidence of NTM-PD, whereas higher copper and sodium levels in soil were associated with an increased risk.[39] In Queensland, Australia, an effect of temperature and rainfall was observed but this varied by region: cyclic incidence patterns were associated with temperature and rainfall.[41] In a prior study in Australia, increased average topsoil depth was protective against *Mycobacterium intracellulare*, whereas increased soil bulk density was positively associated with *Mycobacterium kansasii* disease.[42] In Japan, NTM-PD mortality, a surrogate measure for disease prevalence and distribution, was higher in the warmer and more humid coastal areas and in an area with a large amount of surface water (lake).[23] A recent study found dust bioaerosols as a source of NTM, with higher relative abundance in East Asian inland cities in Japan and China than in desert areas.[43]

EPIDEMIOLOGY OF NONTUBERCULOUS MYCOBACTERIAL ISOLATION AND DISEASE BY GLOBAL REGION

In our review of epidemiological data of NTM-PD, we strive to include the highest quality data published since 2014. Ideal studies comprise population-based investigations including both clinical and microbiologic data and encompassing an adequate temporal period to best capture the burden of infection in the population. However, because these types of data are often not available, other data sources are used as described previously.

SYSTEMATIC REVIEW AND META-ANALYSIS—GLOBAL

A systematic review and meta-analysis was recently conducted for global, culture-based, microbiologic data, indicating an overall increase worldwide in the frequency of isolation, including that which satisfies the ATS microbiologic criteria.[9] This review included only those studies with culture-based data for at least 3 years, and with at least 200 samples, representing findings from 47 publications in more than 18 countries. Overall, 82% of studies reported increasing isolation, and 66.7% reported increasing disease, using either the adapted ATS microbiologic criteria or the full radiographic and clinical criteria. The overall rate of increase was 4% (3.2–4.8) per year for isolation and 4.1% (3.2–5) per year for disease, which was

most often defined using the ATS microbiologic criteria. Most of these studies focused on MAC, the predominant species, and to a lesser degree the *M abscessus* group[9] (**Fig. 2**).

A recent Delphi survey including a physician survey as well as chart review allowed comparison of prevalence rates across 4 European countries (France, Germany, Spain, and United Kingdom) and Japan, and found a remarkably similar prevalence of NTM-PD of 6.1/100,000 to 6.6/100,000 across European countries but with a 4-fold increased prevalence in Japan, suggesting true differences in prevalence.[44]

North America

In North America, national and subnational studies indicate increasing prevalence and incidence, and continue to demonstrate geographic heterogeneity in NTM isolation and disease. This section is based on 5 national studies from the United States, 1 provincial level study from Ontario, Canada, and 9

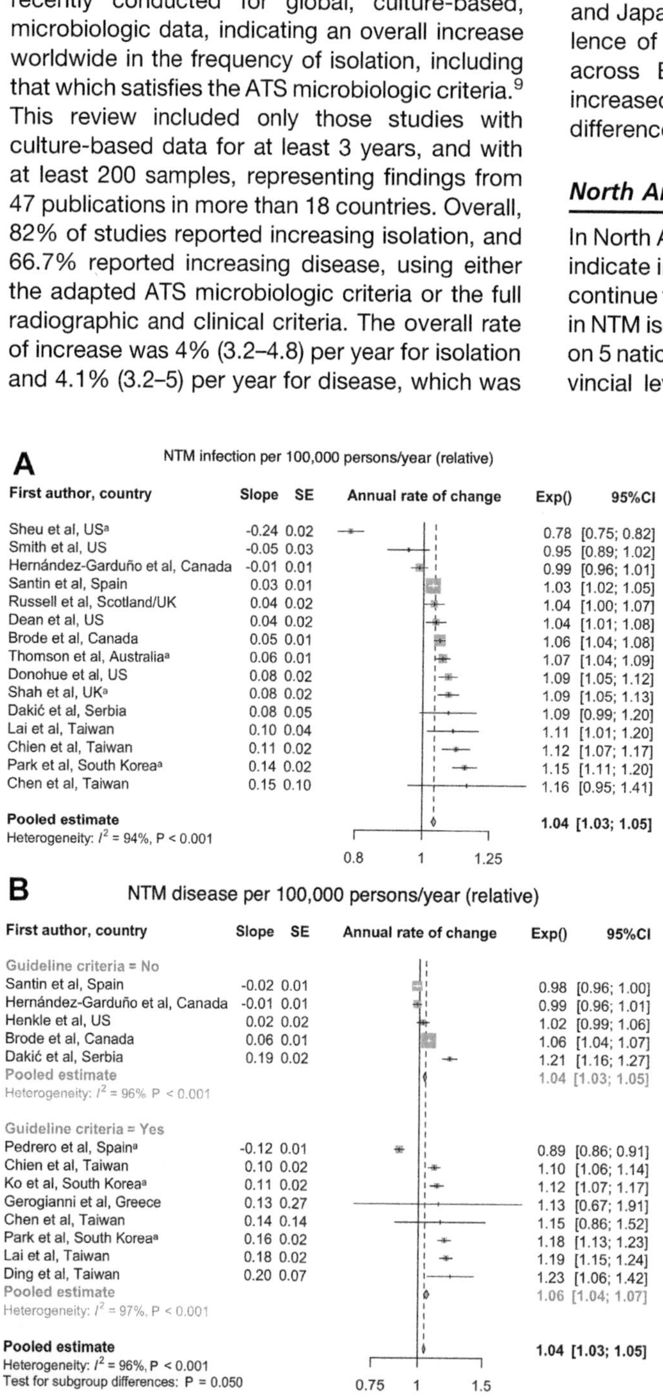

Fig. 2. (A) Forest plot of annual change of NTM infection per 100,000 persons/y. (B) Forest plot of annual change of NTM disease per 100,000 persons/y (Dahl and colleagues, 2022); with permission (see Fig. 6 in original). (*From* Dahl VN, Mølhave M, Fløe A, et al. Global trends of pulmonary infections with nontuberculous mycobacteria: a systematic review. *Int J Infect Dis.* Oct 13 2022;125:120-131. doi:10.1016/j.ijid.2022.10.013; with permission. (see Fig. 3 in original).)

state or territorial level studies in the United States. The national studies include 3 based on ICD codes to define disease and 2 based on microbiologic data. The heterogeneity of methodologic approaches makes comparisons difficult but, overall, these studies indicate a picture of increasing prevalence dominated by MAC infections.

In the United States, a national study to estimate prevalence and incidence of NTM-PD defined this as 2 claims with NTM-PD ICD codes separated by 30 days. This study estimated a prevalence of 6.8/100,000 in 2008, increasing to 11.7/100,000 in 2015, with an estimated annual incidence from 3.1/100,000 to 4.7/100,000 during the same time period[45] (**Fig. 3**). A separate study, which estimated prevalence using a single ICD code for NTM to define a case, estimated a prevalence of 27.9/100,000 in 2010, with a projected estimate of 181,037 cases in 2014, assuming a continued 8% annual prevalence increase.[46] The discrepancy in estimates between the 2 studies for a similar year (2014/2015) is due to the more specific case definition in the former study. The geographic heterogeneity across states was consistent with prior reports and historic patterns, with the highest prevalence in the warm, humid areas in the Southeast and Southwest.[46] A study in a high-risk population, among veterans with chronic obstructive pulmonary disease (COPD), also used 2 ICD codes for NTM-PD to define disease and found an increasing incidence and prevalence NTM-PD from 2001 to 2015, with incidence increasing from 34.2/100,000 to 70.3/100,000 and prevalence from 93.1/100,000 to 277.6/100,000 patients.[47]

Two national, microbiologic studies based on electronic health records demonstrated geographic variation in NTM species as well as increasing trends in acid fast bacilli (AFB testing and NTM isolation prevalence in high-risk groups.[48,49] Among 5 million unique patients of whom 7812 had at least one isolate, MAC was the most common species,

ranging from 61% to 91% of isolates, and was most frequent in the South and Northeast regions; *M abscessus/Mycobacterium chelonae* ranged from 2% to 18% of isolates and were most frequent in the West. A separate national study using microbiology data from a different large EHR system to study frequency of AFB testing and pulmonary NTM isolation during 2009 to 2015 found an overall AFB testing rate of 45/10,000 population with an increasing annual percent change (APC) of 3.2%.[49] The isolation rate for pathogenic NTM also increased with an APC of 4.5% and was highest among persons with CF and those with bronchiectasis.[49]

One subnational study used population-based surveillance data from 2014 in 4 states (Mississippi, Missouri, Ohio, and Wisconsin) to describe NTM isolation. Overall prevalence was 13.3/100,000 population (after excluding *Mycobacterium gordonae*), with a predominance of MAC, at a prevalence of 8.5/100,000.[50] An earlier study, which estimated trends from 2008 to 2013 in the same 4 states plus Maryland found an increasing trend, with an APC of 9.9%.[51]

Hawaii and Florida have been identified as "hotspots" for NTM in the United States. In Hawaii, microbiologic data from a large, linked health-care system were used to associate microbiologic data with demographic and clinical factors for the period 2005 and 2013. Isolation was based on at least one pulmonary isolate, and the ATS microbiologic criteria were used to define NTM-PD.[52] Isolation prevalence increased significantly during the study period, from 20/100,000 in 2005 to 44/100,000 in 2013, with an APC of 6% and a period prevalence of 122/100,000; MAC was the most commonly isolated species, comprising 64% of isolates. NTM-PD (ATS microbiologic criteria) increased from 9/100,000 in 2005 to 19/100,000 in 2013 (**Table 2**). NTM isolation prevalence varied by ethnic group, with NTM isolation rates approximately 2-fold

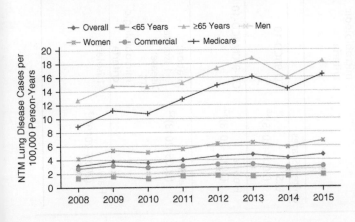

Fig. 3. Annual incidence of NTM-PD in national US health insurance plan (Optum EHR database) 2008 to 2015. (Reprinted with permission of the American Thoracic Society. Copyright © 2023 American Thoracic Society. All rights reserved. Cite: Winthrop KL, Marras TK, Adjemian J, Zhang H, Wang P, Zhang Q./2020/Incidence and Prevalence of Nontuberculous Mycobacterial Lung Disease in a Large U.S. Managed Care Health Plan, 2008-2015/*Ann Am Thorac Soc*./17/178-185. Annals of the American Thoracic Society is an official journal of the American Thoracic Society.(see Fig. 2 in original).)

Table 2
Studies of rates of pulmonary nontuberculous mycobacterial isolation and disease by region

Location (dates)[a]	Case Definition	Data Source/Cohort	Annual Prevalence (per 100,000 population)		Period Prevalence		Incidence (per 100,000 population)
			Isolation (dates)	Disease (dates)	Period Duration (years)	Prevalence (per 100,000 population)	
North America							
Canada							
Ontario, Canada (1998-2010)[131]	Isolation: ≥1 isolate Disease: ATS microbiologic criteria	Public Health Ontario Laboratory Database	11.4-22.2 (1998-2010) (APC: 6.3%); Annual Change (MAC: 0.291, M xenopi: 0.059, M abscessus: 0.019)	4.65-9.08 (1998-2010) (APC: 8.0%)[b,c]	-	-	-
United States							
U.S. (2008-2015)[45]	ICD-9/ICD-10	Optum Clinformatics Data Mart Care Claims database	-	6.78-11.70 (APC: 7.5%) (2008-2015)	8	-	3.13-4.73 (2008-2015) (APC: 5.2%) (D)
Florida (2012-2018)[55]	ICD-9-CM/ICD-10	OneFlorida Clinical Research Consortium database	-	14.3-22.6 (2012-2018)	7	-	6.5-5.4 (2012-2018) (D)
Hawaii (2005-2013)[52]	Isolation: ≥1 isolate Disease: ATS microbiologic criteria	Kaiser Permanente Hawaii databases	20-44 (2005-2013) (APC: 6%)[b]	9-19 (2005-2013)[b,c]	9	Range by ethnic group: 50-300 (I)[b]	-
Hawaii (2005-2019)[53]	≥1 isolate	Kaiser Permanente Hawaii EHR databases	-	-	15	-	Overall annualized: 44.8 (I)[b], Range by ethnic group: 17-63 (I)[b], Cumulative: 247 (I)[b]

Maryland, Mississippi, Missouri, Ohio, Wisconsin (2008–2013)[51]	≥1 isolate	Surveillance data from Maryland, Mississippi, Missouri, Ohio, Wisconsin	Overall: 8.7–13.9 (2008–2013)[9,h] (APC: 9.9%)[9,h], Maryland: 9.5–9.29 (2008–2013)[9,h] Mississippi: 10.2–13.69 (2008–2013)[9,h], Missouri: 5.5–13.39 (2008–2013)[9,h], Ohio: 5.8–11.39 (2008–2013)[9,h], Wisconsin: 15.4–24.69 (2008–2013)[9,h]	-	-
North Carolina (2006–2010)[58]	≥1 isolate	All labs that test for NTM in 3 counties (hospital, commercial, public health)	Overall: 9.4[b]	-	-
North Carolina (2006–2010)[38]	≥1 isolate	All labs that test for NTM in 3 counties (hospital, commercial, public health)	-	5	Cumulative: 8.8 (I)
Oregon (2007–2012)[10]	ATS microbiologic criteria	All laboratories that test for NTM in Oregon	5.9 (2011–2012)[c]	6	5.0 (APC: 2.2%) (D)[c]; 3.8 (D)[c,h]
US-Affiliated Pacific Island Jurisdictions (2007–2011)[54]	≥1 isolate	Diagnostic Laboratory Services data	2–48 (2007–2011) (adjusted rate ratio: 1.65)	4	Overall: 106 (I); American Samoa (22) (I), Federated States of Micronesia (164) (I)

(continued on next page)

Table 2
(continued)

Location (dates)[a]	Case Definition	Data Source/Cohort	Annual Prevalence (per 100,000 population)		Period Prevalence		Incidence (per 100,000 population)
			Isolation (dates)	Disease (dates)	Period Duration (years)	Prevalence (per 100,000 population)	
Central and South America							
French Guiana (2008–2018)[61]	Isolation: ≥1 isolate Disease: Full ATS criteria	Three general hospitals EHR data	-	-	11	-	6.17 (I); 1.07 (D)
Mexico City, Mexico (2001–2017)[62]	Full ATS criteria	Tertiary care referral medical center EHR data	-	-	17	-	SGM: 0.6/1000 admissions (2001–2011)-1.9 (2012–2017) (D)[9]; RGM: 0.3/1000 (2001–2011)–1.1/1000 (2012–2017) (D)[9]
Uruguay (2006–2018)[67]	≥1 isolate	National tuberculosis reference laboratory EHR data	0.33–1.57 (2006–2018) (4.79-fold increase)[9]	-	-	-	-
Europe							
Czech Republic (2012–2018)[81]	Full ATS criteria	Public Health Institute Ostrava database for Moravian and Silesian Regions	-	-	7	-	1.1 (D)[9]
Denmark (1991–2015)[68]	Isolation: ≥1 isolate Disease: Modified ATS microbiologic criteria	International Reference Laboratory data	-	-	25	-	2.14 (I); Definite and Possible NTM-PD: 1.10 (D)[c,9]

Location (year)	Criteria	Database					
England, Wales and Northern Ireland (January 2007–July 2012)[77]	≥1 isolate	Public Health England database	-	6	-	-	3.4–5.0 (2007–2012) (I)[b]
France (2010–2017)[69]	ICD-10 or suggestive medication	National Health System database	-	8	5.92 (D)	-	1.025–1.096 (2010–2017) (D)
Germany (2009–2014)[72]	ICD-10	Health Risk Institute health services research database	-	-	-	2.3–3.3 (2009–2014)[h]	-
Germany (2010–2011)[26]	ICD-10	German statutory health insurances claims database	-	2	-	-	1.12–1.48 (2010–2011) (D); Cumulative: 2.6 (D)
Germany (2011–2016)[71]	ICD-10 (German modification)	InGef research database of statutory health insurances claims	-	5	-	ICD-10 coded: 3.79[h]; Predicted: 19.05[h]	ICD-10 coded: 1.56 (D)[h]; Predicted: 15.33 (D)[h]
Greece (January 2007–May 2013)[84]	Isolation: ≥1 isolate Disease: Full (12 pts) ATS criteria and ATS microbiologic criteria (56 pts)	Sismanoglio-A. Fleming General Hospital of Attiki EHR data	-	7	-	-	Cumulative:18.9 (I); Cumulative: 8.8 (D)[d]
Portugal (2002–2012)[73]	Treatment of NTM-PD	National Tuberculosis Surveillance System database	-	11	-	-	0.54 (D)[g]
Scotland (2000–2010)[86]	ATS microbiologic criteria	Scottish Mycobacteria Reference Laboratory data	-	11	-	-	2.43 (D)[b,c,g]

(continued on next page)

Table 2
(continued)

Location (dates)[a]	Case Definition	Data Source/Cohort	Annual Prevalence (per 100,000 population)		Period Prevalence		Incidence (per 100,000 population)
			Isolation (dates)	Disease (dates)	Period Duration (years)	Prevalence (per 100,000 population)	
Serbia (2010–2015)[74]	Isolation: 1 isolate Disease: ATS microbiologic criteria	The National Reference Laboratory of Serbia database	-	0.31 (2011–2012)–0.47 (2014–2015)[b,c]	6	-	1.3 (I); 0.29 (D)[b,c]
Spain (1994–2014)[75]	Isolation: ≥1 isolate Disease: ≥2 positive cultures or antimicrobial chemotherapy	Referral Hospital (Bellvitge University Hospital) Laboratory data	-	-	21	113.2 (I)[b]; 42.8 (D)[b,e]	-
Spain (1994–2015)[76]	Isolation: ≥1 isolate Disease: Full ATS criteria (only RGM)	Referral Hospital (Bellvitge University Hospital) Laboratory data	-	-	22	-	0.34–1.73 (2003–2015) (APC: 8.3%) (I)[g]
Spain (1997–2016)[78]	Full ATS criteria	Microbiology Laboratory of Cruces University Hospital data	-	-	20	-	10.6–1.8 (2016) (APC: 3.3% (MAC), −6.5% [M kansasii]) (D)
The United Kingdom (2006–2016)[79]	"Strict cohort," highly likely to have NTM-PD; "Expanded cohort" possible NTM-PD[f]	Clinical Practice Research Datalink	-	Strict cohort: 7.68–4.70 (2006–2016)[g]	10	Strict cohort: 6.38 (D)[g]	Strict cohort: 3.85–1.28 (2006–2016) (D)[g]; Expanded cohort: 22.9–40.9 (2006–2016) (D)[g]

The Netherlands (2012–2019)[70]	Drug combination in drug dispensing database, ICD-10	IQVIA's Real-World Data Longitudinal Prescription database, Outpatient Pharmacy Database of the PHARMO Database Network, IQVIA's health insurance claims database, Hospitalization Database of the PHARMO Database Network	-	2.3–5.9 (databases); 6.2–9.9 (pulmonologist survey)	-	-	-
East Asia							
Japan (2001–2009)[132]	Full ATS criteria	Microbiological database of 11 hospitals in Nagasaki prefecture	-	-	9	-	4.6–10.1 (2001–2009) (D)
Japan (2004–2006)[23]	ICD-8-10, estimated from Death Statistics	Vital Statistics of Japan database	-	33–65 (2005)[h]	-	-	-
Japan (2009–2014)[107]	ICD-10	The Japanese National Database of Health Insurance Claims	-	29 (2011)	6	-	8.6 (2011) (D)
Japan (2012–2013)[105]	ATS microbiologic criteria	3 major laboratories (SRL, Inc., LSI Medience Corporation, BML, Inc)	-	12 (2012–2013)[b,c]	2	24 (D)[b,c]	-
South Korea (2001–2015)[104]	Full ATS criteria	NTM Registry of Tertiary Referral Hospital (Samsung Medical Center)	-	-	15	-	7.0–55.6 (2001–2015) (D)

(continued on next page)

Table 2
(continued)

Location (dates)[a]	Case Definition	Data Source/Cohort	Annual Prevalence (per 100,000 population)		Period Prevalence		Incidence (per 100,000 population)
			Isolation (dates)	Disease (dates)	Period Duration (years)	Prevalence (per 100,000 population)	
South Korea (2003–2016)[98]	ICD-10	NHIS database	-	1.2–33.3[h]	14	-	1.0–17.9 (2003–2019) (D)[g]
South Korea (2006–2016)[100]	Full ATS criteria	Tertiary Referral Hospital (Severance Hospital) EHR data	-	-	11	-	4.6–19.6 (2006–2016) (I); 1.2–4.8 (2006–2016) (APC: 14%) (D)
South Korea (2007–2018)[99]	ICD-10	Health Insurance Review and Assessment Service database	-	5.3–41.7	12	-	Diagnostic-based: 3.5–18.0 (2008–2018) (APC: 16.7%) (D); Clinically refined: 2.9–12.3 (2008–2018) (APC: 13.2%) (D)
South Korea (2009–2015)[133]	ICD-10	Health Insurance Review and Assessment service database	-	-	7	-	6.6–26.6 (2009–2015) (D)
South Korea (2009–2015)[103]	Full ATS criteria	Tertiary care Hospitals (Pusan National University, Pusan National University Yangsan) EHR data	-	-	7	-	6.8–12.9 (2009–2015) (D)[9]
Taiwan (2000–2012)[115]	Full ATS criteria	Tertiary Medical Center (National Taiwan University) data	-	-	-	-	3.4–13 (D)

Location (period)	Database	Case definition				
Taiwan (2003–2018)[113]	National Health Insurance Research database	ICD-9-CM, treatment	-	0.68–7.17[9] (Treatment Case)	-	0.54–3.35 (2003–2018) (D) (Treatment case)[9]
Taiwan (2005–2013)[112]	National Health Insurance Research database	ICD-9-CM, ≥2 cultures, treatment	-	-	-	5.3–14.8 (2005–2013) (D)[9,h]
Taiwan (2007–2010)[114]	National TB Registry of Taiwan CDC	≥1 isolate	-	-	8.6 (I)	-
Taiwan (2010–2014)[116]	6-Hospital EHR database	Full ATS criteria	-	-	46 (D)	-
West and Central Asia						
Iran (1990–2014)[134]	-	-	25	-	9.6–10.6 (D)[9]	-
Oceania						
Australia (2001–2016)[41]	Queensland Notifiable Conditions database	≥1 isolate	16	-	11.1–25.88 (I)[9]	-
Australia (2012–2015)[3]	Queensland Notifiable Conditions database	≥1 isolate	4	-	25.9 (I)[9]	-

Abbreviations: APC, annual percent change; EHR, electronic health records; ICD-10, International diagnostic classification of diseases–tenth revision; ICD-9, International diagnostic classification of diseases–ninth revision; RGM, rapid-growing mycobacteria; SGM, slow-growing mycobacteria.

a Rates expressed as annual rates per 100,000 population, averaged over study period unless otherwise specified.
b Studies which excluded *M gordonae*.
c NTM-PD is defined using ATS microbiologic criteria.
d NTM-PD is defined using ATS microbiologic criteria and full ATS criteria.
e NTM-PD is defined using ATS microbiologic criteria or antimicrobial chemotherapy.
f NTM-PD is defined ≥2 positive cultures or antimicrobial chemotherapy.
f "Strict cohort" is defined using evidence of treatment and/or monitoring of NTM-PD and "expanded cohort" is defined using NTM disease clinical terminology codes.
g Included patients with NTM isolated from extrapulmonary sites/specimens from extrapulmonary sites.
h Adjusted.

higher among persons who identified as Chinese, Korean, Japanese, and Vietnamese relative to those who identified as White, and the prevalence was 2-fold lower among Native Hawaiian and other Pacific Islander relative to Whites[52] (**Table 3**). Another study used kaiser permanente Hawaii (KPH) data to estimate NTM infection incidence by ethnic group during the period 2005 to 2019 (see **Table 2**).[53] Cases were defined as 1 or greater pulmonary isolate. Average annual isolation incidence was 44.8 cases/100,000 beneficiaries, with a cumulative incidence of 247 cases/100,000 during the study period. Beneficiaries who self-identified with only Asian ethnic groups had the highest NTM pulmonary isolation incidence (46 cases/100,000 person-years) and had a 30% increased risk after controlling for all other clinical and demographic factors.[53] A separate study from the US Affiliated Pacific Islands, based on samples submitted to the Diagnostic Laboratory Services in Hawaii, typically for the evaluation of suspected TB, found a significantly increasing rate of NTM isolation, increasing from 0.5% of isolates screened in 2007% to 11.3% in 2011, corresponding to an NTM isolation prevalence increase of 2/100,000 to 48/100,000. MTB isolation remained stable during the same period.[54]

In Florida, a study using the statewide clinical network and defining cases based on a single ICD code found an increasing disease prevalence, from 14.3/100,000 in 2012 to 22.6/100,000 in 2018.[55] A second study in Florida at a single large academic medical center with NTM defined by pulmonary isolation found that *M abscessus* was the predominant species, representing 39.1% of pulmonary isolates[56] (see **Table 3**). The finding of a predominance of *M abscessus* in Florida is consistent with a recent study showing that the South had the highest proportion of *M abscessus* isolates, and Florida had the highest 5-year period prevalence of *M abscessus* (17%).[57]

A population-based study in 3 counties of North Carolina (Durham, Wake, and Orange) estimated the prevalence of NTM isolation from 2006 through 2010 using primarily laboratory reports, for an average annual isolation prevalence of 9.4/100,000 (excluding *M gordonae*; 11.5 including *M gordonae*).[58] MAC comprised 50.9% of isolates, followed by *M gordonae* (20.4%) and *M abscessus* complex (13.6) (see **Table 3**).[58] Cumulative incidence of NTM isolation was 8.8/100,000 across Durham County, Orange County, and Wake County (see **Table 2**).[38] A statewide study in Oregon from 2007 to 2012 used the ATS microbiologic criteria to define NTM-PD and found an average annual incidence of 5/100,000, ranging from 4.8/100,000

in 2007 to 5.6/100,000 in 2012.[10] The predominant species were MAC (85.7%), followed by rapidly growing mycobacteria (8.1%: *M abscessus/M chelonae* complex; *M chelonae*; *Mycobacterium fortuitum* complex)[10] (see **Tables 2** and **3**).

Ontario, Canada

An earlier report[59] showed a significant increase in NTM isolation and disease (ATS microbiologic criteria) from 1998 to 2010, based on analysis of isolates from the Public Health Ontario Laboratory, which represents approximately 95% of NTM isolates in Ontario. A more recent analysis in a subset of patients being treated for NTM-PD in a tertiary care center and who met the full ATS NTM disease diagnostic criteria found a significant increase in *M avium*-PD between the periods 2009 to 2012 and 2015 to 2018 and no significant change in non-*M avium* species in the same period, demonstrating that the increase in NTM-PD is being driven by *M avium*.[60]

Central and South America

We identified 6 studies published between 2014 and 2022 from French Guiana,[61] Mexico,[62] Brazil,[63–65] and Panama.[66] All studies, apart from one, were single-center studies. The results of these studies may be influenced by referral bias. In addition, many studies lack a denominator in a defined population, which the limits the comparability of results.

In French Guiana, a retrospective, observational study of 3 hospitals during the period 2008 to 2018, identified 178 patients with NTM-positive sputum cultures and 31 patients with NTM-PD. Incidence of NTM isolation and disease was 6.17/100,000 and 1.07/1,000,000. This study defined disease using the full ATS diagnostic criteria. *M avium* (52%) was the most common species among patients with NTM-PD, followed by *M intracellulare* (29%), and *M abscessus* (16%). Among patients with NTM isolates, *M fortuitum* (23%) was most commonly identified, followed by *M intracellulare* (17%), and *M avium* (12%).[61]

A single center, retrospective study in Mexico City identified 158 patients that met the ATS criteria. The average annual isolation incidence increased for slow growing species from 0.6/1000 admissions (2001–2011) to 1.9/1000 admissions (2012–2017) and for rapidly growing species from 0.3/1000 admissions (2001–2011) to 1.1/1000 admissions (2012–2017) (see **Table 2**). From these patients, the most common species were MAC (47%), *M abscessus* (27.3%), and *M fortuitum* (27.3%) (see **Table 3**).[62]

Many studies on NTM in Brazil occur at the state-level and evaluate patient records at large,

Table 3
Nontuberculous mycobacterial isolations from respiratory specimen (I) and nontuberculous mycobacterial pulmonary disease (D) by species and region

Location (dates)	N	Most Common Species (%)				
North America						
Canada						
Ontario, Canada (1998–2010)[131]	I: 2631	MAC (50.5)	M xenopi (21.6)	M gordonae (12.8)	M fortuitum (5)	M abscessus (2.2) M chelonae (1.5)
Toronto, Ontario, Canada (2003–2019)[60]	D: 252	M avium (87.3)	M xenopi (12.7)	-	-	-
United States						
Florida (2011–2017)[56]	I: 396	M abscessus subsp abscessus (24.8), M abscessus subsp bolletii (<1) M abscessus subsp massiliense (4.5) M chelonae (1.8)	M gordonae (18.7)	M avium (1.6) M chimaera (4.7) M intracellulare (1.8); M kansasii (4.7)	M szulgai (3.9)	Mfortuitum(3.3)
Hawaii (2005–2013)[52]	455 (I: 201, D: 254[f])	MAC (63.7)	M fortuitum (24)	M abscessus (19.1)	-	-
Hawaii (2005–2019)[53]	I: 739	MAC (69)	M fortuitum group (24)	M abscessus (21)	M kansasii (2)	-
Illinois, U.S. (2000–2012)[135]	I: 448	M avium (54) M chimera (28) M intracellulare (18)	-	-	-	-
Iowa (1996–2017)[136]	D: 185	MAC (68.6)	M kansasii (8.1)	M abscessus (7.6) M chelonae (5.4)	M fortuitum (2.2); M xenopi (2.2)	-
North Carolina (2006–2010)[58]	I: 750	MAC (50.9)	M gordonae (20.4)	M abscessus complex (13.6)	M fortuitum (5)	M mucogenicum (3.9)
Oregon (2007–2012)[10]	I: 806	M avium/intracellulare complex (82.8)	M abscessus/chelonae complex (4.1) M chelonae (<1)	M fortuitum complex (2.9)	M lentiflavum (1)	M kansasii (<1)
	D: 1146[f]	M avium/intracellulare complex (85.7)	M abscessus/chelonae complex (5.9) M chelonae (1.2)	M kansasii (1.2)	M lentiflavum (1)	M fortuitum complex (<1)

(continued on next page)

Table 3
(continued)

	N					
United States (2009–2013)[48]	I: 487	MAC (77)	M abscessus/M chelonae (9)	M kansasii (6)	M fortuitum (5)	-
US-Affiliated Pacific Island Jurisdictions (2007–2011)[54]	I: 35[e]	MAC (31.4)	M fortuitum (20)	M gordonae (14.3)	M abscessus/chelonae (5.7); M parascrofulaceum/M fortuitum (5.7)	M florentinum (2.9); M kansasii (2.9); M mucogenicum (2.9); M paraffinicum (2.9); M simiae (2.9); M terrae (2.9)
Central and South America						
Ceará, Brazil (2005–2016)[65]	I: 42	M abscessus (4.8); M avium (4.8); M fortuitum (4.8)	M kansasii (2.4); M szulgai (2.4)	-	-	-
French Guiana (2008–2018)[61]	I: 147	M fortuitum (23)	M avium (12) M intracellulare (17) M abscessus (16)	M gordonae (5); M scrofulaceum (5) M genavense (3)	M abscessus (3); M smegmatis (3)	M interjectum (2); M kansasii (2)
	D: 31	M avium (52) M intracellulare (29)				-
Mexico City, Mexico (2001–2017)[62]	D: 66	MAC (47)	M abscessus (27.3); M fortuitum (27.3)	M kansasii (7.6); M scrofulaceum (7.6)	-	-
Panama (2012–2014)[66]	I: 7	M avium (57.1)	M haemophilum (28.6)	M tusciae (14.3)	-	-
Rio Grande do Sul, Brazil (2003–2013)[63]	D: 100	M avium (26) M intracellulare (9)	M kansasii (17)	M abscessus (12)	M fortuitum (4)	M gordonae (3)
São Paulo, Brazil (2011–2014)[64]	I: 2843	M avium (18.3) M intracellulare (14.9)	M kansasii (15.9)	M gordonae (13.2)	M fortuitum (10.9)	M abscessus (7.7) M chelonae (3.4)
	D: 448[f]	M kansasii (29.2)	M avium (20.8) M intracellulare (19.6)	M abscessus (17.2) M chelonae (<1)	M gordonae (4.5)	M fortuitum (3.6)
Uruguay (2006–2018)[67]	I: 255[d]	M avium (23.9) M intracellulare (33.7)	M kansasii (8.2)	M gordonae (5.9)	M peregrinum (4.7)	M abscessus (1.2) M chelonae (3.1); M fortuitum (3.1)

Europe

Location	No.						
Belgium (2015–2018)[137]	I: 264	*M avium* (12.1)	*M chimaera/M intracellulare* (20.8)	*M abscessus* (12.9) *M chelonae* (6.1)	*M gordonae* (3.4)	*M fortuitum* (1.9); *M xenopi* (1.9)	*M paragordonae* (1.5)
Belgium (2010–2017)[138]	I: 384	*M avium* (25)	*M chimaera* (4.4) *M intracellulare* (16.7)	*M gordonae* (14.6)	*M xenopi* (7.6)	*M fortuitum* (3.9)	*M abscessus* (3.1) *M chelonae* (2.9)
	D: 165	*M marseillense* (<1) *M avium* (31.5) *M chimaera* (4.2) *M intracellulare* (24.8) *M marseillense* (<1)	*M xenopi* (8.5)	*M abscessus* (6.7) *M chelonae* (<1)	*M kansasii* (4.2)	*M malmoense* (3.6)	
Croatia (2006–2015)[139]	I: 1926	*M gordonae* (42.6)	*M xenopi* (15.3)	*M fortuitum* (11.4)	*M terrae* (6.6)	*M abscessus* (2.1) *M chelonae* (5) *M fortuitum* (1.5); *M gordonae* (1.5)	
	D: 137	*M xenopi* (39.4)	*M avium* (22.6) *M chimaera* (1.5) *M intracellulare* (14.6)	*M kansasii* (5.8)	*M abscessus* (4.4)		
Czech Republic (2012–2018)[81]	I: 2176[d]	*M xenopi* (36.4)	*M avium-intracellulare complex* (17.7)	*M gordonae* (15.7)	*M fortuitum* (9.7)	*M kansasii* (6.2)	
	D: 303[d]	*M avium-intracellulare complex* (47.2)	*M kansasii* (23.8)	*M xenopi* (18.2)	*M abscessus* (1.3) *M chelonae* (2.3)	*M fortuitum* (2); *M malmoense* (2)	
England, Wales and Northern Ireland (January 2007–July 2012)[77]	I: 16294	MAC (35.6)	*M gordonae* (16.7)	*M abscessus* (5) *M chelonae* (9.7)	*M fortuitum* (8.2)	*M kansasii* (5.9); *M xenopi* (5.9)	
France (2002–2013)[140]	D: 92	*M avium* (29.3) *M intracellulare* (29.3)	*M kansasii* (17.4)	*M xenopi* (16.3)	*M abscessus* (2.2)	*M fortuitum* (1.1); *M gordonae* (1.1); *M interjectum* (1.1); *M scrofulaceum* (1.1); *M simiae* (1.1)	

(continued on next page)

Table 3
(continued)

Location	N					
France (2009–2014)[141]	D: 477	M avium (31.2) M intracellulare (28.1)	M xenopi (19.7)	M kansasii (5.7)	M abscessus complex (3.8) M chelonae (<1)	M fortuitum (2.7)
Germany (2006–2016)[142]	I: 216	MAC (33.3)	M gordonae (23.6)	M xenopi (15.2)	M abscessus complex (9.3)	-
Greece (January 2007–May 2013)[84]	I: 122	M gordonae (13.9)	M avium (13.1) M intracellulare (9.8)	M fortuitum (12.2)	M lentiflavum (4.9); M peregrinum (4.9)	M abscessus (1.6) M chelonae (2.4); M xenopi (2.4)
	D: 12	M avium (25) M intracellulare (25)	M abscessus (8.3); M fortuitum (8.3); M gordonae (8.3); M xenopi (8.3)	-	-	-
Ireland (January 2007–July 2012)[143]	I: 37	M avium (59.5) M intracellulare (10.8)	M gordonae (10.8)	M abscessus (5.4) M chelonae (5.4); M szulgai (5.4)	M malmoense (2.7)	-
The Netherlands (2008–2013)[144]	D: 63	M avium (36.5) M chimera (4.8) M intracellulare (12.7)	M malmoense (11.1)	M kansasii (9.5)	M abscessus (6.3)	M simiae (4.8)
Poland (2010–2015)[145]	I: 73	M avium (22) M intracellulare (8); M kansasii (22)	M gordonae (19)	M xenopi (11)	M fortuitum (6)	M abscessus (3)
	D: 36	M kansasii (36)	M avium (28) M intracellulare (11)	M xenopi (8)	M abscessus (6)	M gordonae (3)
Poland (2013–2017)[146]	I: 2799[d]	M kansasii (27.2)	M avium (22) M intracellulare (6.2)	M xenopi (16)	M gordonae (14.5)	M fortuitum (5.9)
Portugal (2005–2014)[147]	I: 365	MAC (48.2)	M gordonae (13.7)	M peregrinum (11)	M abscessus (1.6) M chelonae (7.9)	M kansasii (5.8)
Scotland (2000–2010)[86]	I: 933	MAC (44.8)	M malmoense (21.7)	M abscessus (13.7) M chelonae (2.6)	M xenopi (4.5)	M kansasii (3.9)
Serbia (2009–2016)[148]	I: 296[d] D: 83	M gordonae (22.3) MAC (30.1)	M fortuitum (21.3) M xenopi (24.1)	M xenopi (13.5) M kansasii (18.1)	M peregrinum (12.2) -	MAC (9.8) -

Region (period)	N					
Serbia (2010–2015)[74]	I: 565	M xenopi (17.3)	M gordonae (12.9)	M fortuitum (11.3)	M abscessus (4.6) / M chelonae (4.1)	M kansasii (4.2)
	D: 126[f]	M xenopi (28.6)	M abscessus (15.1) / M chelonae (2.4)	M kansasii (11.1)	M fortuitum (10.3)	M avium (7.9) / M intracellulare (6.3)
Spain (1994–2014)[75]	I: 680	M kansasii (28.5)	MAC (20.4)	M xenopi (14.1)	M abscessus (2.5)	-
	D: 257[b,c]	M kansasii (59.9)	MAC (26.1)	M xenopi (6.2)	M abscessus (4.3)	-
Spain (1994–2015)[76] (only RGM)	I:116	M fortuitum (45.7)	M abscessus (5.2) / M chelonae (33.6) / M fortuitum (26.7)	M mucogenicum (8.6)	M mageritense (1.7); M peregrinum (1.7)	-
	D: 15	M abscessus (40) / M chelonae (26.7)	M fortuitum (26.7)	M mucogenicum (6.7)	-	-
Spain (1997–2016)[78]	D: 327	M kansasii (83.8)	MAC (13.1)	-	-	
Spain (2007–2013)[149]	I: 156	MAC (64.1)	M gordonae (12.2)	M abscessus (1.9) / M chelonae (8.3)	M fortuitum (5.8)	M lentiflavum (4.5); M scrofulaceum (4.5)
	D: 34[f]	MAC (79.4)	M genavense (8.8)	M abscessus (2.9) / M chelonae (5.9)	M malmoense (2.9); M xenopi (2.9)	-
Spain (2013–2017)[150]	I: 314	M avium (48.4) / M intracellulare (16.6)	M fortuitum (12.1)	M gordonae (8)	M lentiflavum (4.1)	M abscessus (<1) / M chelonae (3.2)
Switzerland (2015–2020)[151]	I: 236[d]	M gordonae (24.6)	M avium (23.3) / M chimera (3.4) / M intracellulare (6.8)	M xenopi (11.9)	M abscessus subsp. abscessus (6.4) / M chelonae (4.2)	M fortuitum (4.2)
The United Kingdom (2007–2014)[152]	I: 853	M avium (21.2) / M intracellulare (31.3)	M gordonae (15.2)	M abscessus (8.4) / M chelonae (8.4)	M xenopi (7.9)	M malmoense (4.7)
Africa						
Botswana (Aug 2012–Nov 2014) (HIV-infected)[89]	I: 228	M avium (2.2) / M intracellulare (47.8)	M gordonae (7)	M malmoense (3.9)	M simiae (3.5)	M asiaticum (2.6); M fortuitum (2.6); M scrofulaceum (2.6)

(continued on next page)

Table 3
(continued)

Study	I:					
Ethiopia (2017)[93]	I: 35	M simiae (42.9)	M abscessus complex (14.3)	M fortuitum (11.4)	M avium complex (5.7) M intracellulare (8.6); M gordonae (8.6)	M kansasii (2.9); M scrofulaceum (2.9); M szulgai (2.9)
Gabon (Jan 2018–Dec 2020)[97]	I: 137	M avium (5.1) M intracellulare (54)	M fortuitum (21.9)	M abscessus (6.6) M chelonae (2.2)	M kansasii (4.4)	M mucogenicum (1.5)
Ghana (2012–2014)[90]	I: 43	M avium subsp. paratuberculosis (30.2); M colombiense (7); M intracellulare (41.9)	M abscessus (11.3)	M mucogenicum (7)	M simiae (2.3)	-
Ghana (Jan 2013–Mar 2014)[91]	I: 38	MAC (23.7)	M chelonae complex (7.9); M simiae (7.9)	M fortuitum complex (5.3)	M arupense (2.6); M flavescens (2.6); M kansasii (2.6); M terrae (2.6)	-
Kenya (2020)[94]	I: 146	MAC (31)	M fortuitum complex (20)	M abscessus complex (14)	-	-
Mali (2006–2013)[92]	I:41	M avium (24.4)	M specie (7.3)	M simiae (4.9)	-	-
Nigeria, Cameroon, Ghana (Jan-Dec 2017)[153]	I: 14	M fortuitum (35.7)	M engbaekii (14.3); M avium (7.1) M colombiense (7.1) M intracellulare (14.3)	M gordonae (7.1); M paraense (7.1); M peregrinum (7.1)	-	-
Tanzania (Nov 2012–Jan 2013)[95]	I: 36	M gordonae (16.7); M interjectum (16.7)	M avium (5.5) M colombiense (2.8) M intracellulare (11.1)	M scrofulaceum (8.3)	M fortuitum (5.5); M kumamotonense (5.5)	-
Tanzania (Nov 2019–Aug 2020)[154]	I: 24	M avium (8.3) M intracellulare (16.7)	M abscessus subsp. abscessus (12.5) M abscessus subsp. bolletii (4.2)	M fortuitum group (8.3)	M kansasii (4.2); M simiae (4.2); M szulgai (4.2)	-

Tunisia (2002–2016)[88]	I: 30	M kansasii (23.3)	M fortuitum (16.7); M novocastrense (16.7)	M chelonae (10)	M gadium (6. 6); M gordonae (6. 6)	M flavescens (3.3); M peregrinum (3.3); M porcinum (3.3)
East Asia					
China (2008–2012)[155]	I: 616	M kansasii (45)	M avium (3.6) M intracellulare (20.8)	M chelonae-abscessus complex (14.9)	M fortuitum (4.5)	-
China (2009–2019)[156]	I: 1102	M avium (13.2) M intracellulare (54.8)	M chelonae-abscessus complex (16.5)	M kansasii (8.2)	M gordonae (3.3)	M fortuitum (<1)
China (2010–2015)[120]	I: 232	M avium (4.7) M intracellulare (40.5)	M abscessus (28.4)	M kansasii (9.9)	M fortuitum (8.6)	M gordonae (4.3)
	D: 72[a]	M avium (2.8) M intracellulare (52.8)	M abscessus (33.3)	M kansasii (9.7)	M szulgai (1.4)	-
China (2013–2016)[157]	D: 607	M avium (16.3) M intracellulare (28.2)	M abscessus subsp. abscessus (23.9) M abscessus subsp. massiliense (16.6)	M kansasii (10)	M fortuitum (2.8)	M gordonae (1)
China (2014–2021)[119]	I: 1755	M avium (7.8) M intracellulare (51.6)	M abscessus (22.2)	M kansasii (8.3)	M fortuitum (2.1); M gordonae (2.1)	M paragordonae (1.3)
China (2015–2020)[118]	I: 789	M abscessus (35.1)	M avium (6.8) M intracellulare (12.8)	M fortuitum (10.1)	M kansasii (10)	M gordonae (9.4)
China (2017–2018)[158]	D: 87	M avium (11.5) M intracellulare (70.1)	M chelonae-abscessus complex (11.5)	M kansasii (7.5)	M gordonae (1.1)	-
China (2018)[159]	I: 24	M avium (4.2) M intracellulare (66.7)	M abscessus (12.5)	M kansasii (8.3)	M fortuitum (4.2); M szulgai (4.2)	-
China (2019–2020)[117]	D: 458	M avium (8.5) M intracellulare (52.6)	M abscessus complex (23.1)	M kansasii (8.1)	M szulgai (2.6)	-

(continued on next page)

Table 3 *(continued)*

Location (years)	n					
Japan (2000–2013)[108]	D: 592[f]	M avium (70.6) M intracellulare (22.3)	–	–	–	–
Japan (2001–2009)[132]	D: 975	M avium (42.6) M intracellulare (44.3)	M abscessus (3.1) M chelonae (<1)	M gordonae (2.1); M kansasii (2.1)	–	–
Japan (2006–2016)[109]	I: 3620	MAC (82.2)	M abscessus complex (4.5) M chelonae (<1)	M kansasii (3.7)	M fortuitum (2.1)	M peregrinum (<1)
	D: 2155[f]	MAC (87.2)	M abscessus complex (5.5) M chelonae (<1)	M kansasii (3.9)	M fortuitum (1.3)	M. lentiflavum (<1); M. szulgai (<1)
Japan (2009–2015)[160]	I: 416	M abscessus (31) M chelonae (11)	M avium (5) M intracellulare (20)	M gordonae (18)	M fortuitum (11)	–
	D: 114	M abscessus (36) M chelonae (10)	M avium (6) M intracellulare (27)	M fortuitum (10)	M gordonae (6)	–
Japan (2012–2013)[105]	I: 26059	M avium (61.8) M intracellulare (31.1)	M kansasii (2.1)	M abscessus (2) M chelonae (<1)	M fortuitum (1.1)	M terrae (<1)
	D: 7167[f]	M avium (65.1) M intracellulare (32.4)	M kansasii (3.4)	M abscessus (2.7)	M fortuitum (<1)	–
South Korea (2001–2015)[104]	D: 2329	MAC (75)	M abscessus (22)	M kansasii (3)	–	–
South Korea (2006–2016)[100]	D: 1017	MAC (63.6)	M abscessus complex (10.8)	M fortuitum (2.1); M kansasii (2.1)	–	–
South Korea (2007–2019)[102]	I: 2807	M avium (19.2) M intracellulare (50)	M fortuitum complex (4.7)	M abscessus (4.6) M chelonae (1)	M gordonae (3.5)	M kansasii (1.1)
South Korea (2009–2015)[103]	I: 5558	M avium (23.1) M intracellulare (38.9)	M abscessus (8.4)	M kansasii (7.7)	–	–

Location (period)	N					
South Korea (2014–2019)[101]	I: 4962	M avium (17.5) M intracellulare (42.3)	M abscessus (7) M chelonae (3.3)	M fortuitum (5.5)	M kansasii (3.6)	M mucogenicum (2.7)
Taiwan (2000–2012)[115]	D: 3317	MAC (41.5)	M abscessus (21.4) M chelonae (9.4)	M fortuitum (13.4)	M kansasii (7.1)	M gordonae (5)
Taiwan (2007–2010)[114]	I: 894	MAC (32.4)	M abscessus complex (9.2) M chelonae complex (17.6)	M fortuitum complex (17)	M kansasii (9.8)	M gordonae (7)
Taiwan (2010–2014)[116]	D: 1674	MAC (34.4)	M abscessus (24.3)	M kansasii (11)	M fortuitum (9.8)	M gordonae (4.7)
South and Southeast Asia						
India (1981–2020)[161]	I: 2071	MAC (18.9)	M abscessus (8.8) M chelonae (10.3)	M fortuitum (9.8)	M gordonae (6.9)	M terrae (6.3)
India (2013–2015)[126]	I: 209	M abscessus (31.1) M chelonae (8.1)	M fortuitum (20.6)	M avium (8.1) M intracellulare (13.4)	M interjectum (4.3); M simiae (4.3)	M gordonae (3.3)
India (2014–2015)[127]	I: 164	M chelonae (26.8)	M fortuitum (12.8)	M gordonae (9.1)	M kansasii (6.1)	M simiae (4.9)
India (2015–2020)[125]	I: 43	M abscessus complex (37.2) M chelonae (2.3)	M fortuitum (23.3)	M chimaera (2.3) M colombiense (2.3) M intracellulare (7) M marseillense (2.3)	M parascrofulaceum (4.7); M simiae (4.7)	-
Pakistan (2016–2019)[122]	I: 169	MAC (61)	M abscessus (24)	M fortuitum (5.5); M kansasii (5.5)	M gordonae (1.8); M szulgai (1.8)	-
Singapore (2011–2012)[162]	I: 511	M abscessus (39.5) M chelonae (1.8)	M fortuitum (16.6)	M kansasii (15.5)	M avium (15.1)	M gordonae (7)
Singapore (2012–2016)[163]	I: 2026[d]	M chelonae-abscessus complex (49.9)	M fortuitum (17)	MAC (15.4)	M kansasii (11.5)	M haemophilum (2)
	D: 352	M chelonae-abscessus complex (56)	MAC (28.1)	M fortuitum group (25.9)	M kansasii (20.2)	M scrofulaceum (2.3)

(continued on next page)

Table 3
(continued)

West and Central Asia							
Iran (2011–2017)[124]	I: 236	M abscessus (19.1)	-	-			-
Iran (2016–2018)[123]	I: 95	M fortuitum (48.4)	M simiae (16.8)	M kansasii (15.7)	M abscessus (7.3)		
Turkey (2015–2019)[121]	I: 45[d]	M fortuitum (24.4)	M abscessus (17.7) / M chelonae (8.9)	M lentiflavum (11.1); M simiae (11.1)	M avium (4.4) / M intracellulare (8.9)	M gordonae (6.7)	M thermoresistibile (4.2)
Saudi Arabia (2006–2012)[164]	I: 142	MAC (35)	M fortuitum (24)	M chelonae-abscessus complex (17)	M gordonae (6)	M kansasii (4)	
	D: 40	MAC (47.5)	M abscessus (25)	M kansasii (10)	M fortuitum (7.5)	M szulgai (5)	
Oceania							
Australia (2001–2016)[41]	I: 12,219[d]	M avium (9.8) / M intracellulare (39.1)	M abscessus (8.5) / M chelonae (3.3)	M fortuitum (8.3)	M kansasii (2.4)	-	
French Polynesia (2008–2013)[128]	I: 87[d]	M fortuitum (11.5) / M porcinum (18.4) / M senegalense (13.8)	M abscessus (29.9) / M bolletii (1.1) / M massiliense (1.1)	M mucogenicum complex (9.2)	M avium (1.1) / M chimaera (3.4) / M intracellulare (1.1)	-	
Papua New Guinea (2010–2012)[129]	I: 9	M avium (33.3) / M intracellulare (22.2); M fortuitum (33.3)	M terrae (22.2)	-	-	-	

Abbreviations: MAC, mycobacterium avium complex; RGM, rapidly growing nontuberculous mycobacterial species.

a Included only patients whose radiographic disease pattern could be classified as cavitary, bronochiectatic, or consolidative.
b 2 positive cultures or antimicrobial chemotherapy.
c M avium and M intracellulare concurrently isolated.
d Included patients with NTM isolated from extrapulmonary sites/specimens from extrapulmonary sites.
e Subanalysis of study population.
f NTM-PD defined using ATS microbiologic criteria.

state referral hospitals that treat TB and NTM-related diseases. A retrospective, single institution study of patients in the state of Rio Grande do Sul identified 100 patients that met the full ATS criteria for NTM-PD (2003–2013). The most common NTM species were *M avium* (26%), *M kansasii* (17%), *M abscessus* (12%), and *M intracellulare* (9%) (see **Table 3**).[63] In the state of São Paulo, 448 patients were identified as NTM-PD using the ATS microbiologic criteria. From these patients, *M kansasii* (29.2%), *M avium* (20.8%), *M intracellulare* (19.6%), and *M abscessus* (17.2%) were the most common species (see **Table 3**).[64] In the state of Ceará, NTM was isolated from pulmonary samples from 42 patients between 2005 and 2016. A high proportion of isolates were not sent to the National Reference Laboratory for identification (81%). Of the species that were identified, the most common were *M avium* (4.8%), *M fortuitum* (4.8%), and *M abscessus* (4.8%) (see **Table 3**).[65]

A study at the national tuberculous laboratory in Montevideo, Uruguay identified 255 NTM isolates from 204 TB suspects during 2006 to 2018; 210 isolates were collected from pulmonary samples. Most NTM isolates were identified as MAC species (57.6%), followed by *M kansasii* (8.2%), *M gordonae* (5.9%), and *M peregrinum* (4.7%) (see **Table 3**).[67]

Europe

Studies from 10 European countries published between 2014 and 2022 have calculated the incidence or prevalence of NTM isolation and/or NTM-PD (see **Table 2**). Data sets, study populations, and identification methods of patients with NTM-PD differed significantly; thus, comparison of the incidence or prevalence is difficult. Some of these studies have also calculated trends over the respective study period: either a stable (Denmark,[68] France,[69] and The Netherlands[70]) or increasing NTM-isolation or NTM-PD incidence or prevalence (Germany,[26,71,72] Portugal,[73] Serbia,[74] Spain,[75,76] and United Kingdom[77]) was seen. Decreasing incidences for NTM isolation as reported in one study from Spain[78] and one from United Kingdom[79] are explained by the dominating decrease in *M kansasii* isolation and PD in the Bilbao region[78] and by the selection of the data source, for example, primary care records, where the decrease of the incidence and prevalence of the strictly defined NTM-PD cases probably represented a shift of management of NTM-PD toward secondary care.[79] Species isolated from respiratory secretions or causing NTM-PD varies widely among countries and even within countries (see **Table 3**); of note are the high percentages of

NTM-PD caused by *Mycobacterium xenopi* in Croatia, Czech Republic, and Serbia; by *M kansasii* in Poland and some Spanish regions; and by *M malmoense* in Scotland and The Netherlands, resembling isolation data published by the nontuberculous mycobacteria Network European Trials group (NTM NET).[80] A changing epidemiology of species causing NTM-PD over time is also noted in some regions,[78] such that analysis of aggregate trends may obscure species-specific changes. In Europe, COPD often is a concomitant disease, with a mean age around 60 years and a generally similar overall male:female sex distribution with some exceptions (**Table 4**).

Czech Republic

NTM isolates from the Public Health Institute Ostrava representing the Moravian and Silesian Regions from eastern Czech Republic were classified according to ATS diagnostic criteria and the incidence of each NTM species presented as an average annual incidence in the studied period from 2012 to 2018: The average incidence of patients with NTM-PD was 1.10/100,000 (1.33/100,000 in men and 0.88/100,000 in women) during the study period, with patients with MAC pulmonary disease (MAC-PD) predominantly women and patients with *M kansasii*-PD and *M xenopi*-PD predominantly men, with distinct epidemiology in local districts.[81]

Denmark

A retrospective nationwide cohort study including microbiological data from the Danish International Reference Laboratory (Staten Serum Institute) in Denmark from 1991 to 2015 reported an annual (isolation) incidence rate of NTM isolation from a pulmonary site of 2.14/100,000 in adults aged 15 years and older and (using ATS microbiologic criteria only) an incidence of 1.10/100,000 for cases with definite and possible NTM disease. No significant trend toward an increase or decrease for definite NTM disease incidence (that included patients with definite NTM-PD as defined by the authors, which were not reported separately) was found.[68] However, a more recent study using ICD codes and representing the Central region of Denmark found an increasing trend in NTM-PD, suggesting a potential increase in clinically relevant disease.[82]

France

The National Health System Database (Système National des Données de Santé -SNDS), which covers more than 99% of the French population was used to detect newly diagnosed patients with NTM-PD not previously treated (using outpatient drug consumptions) or hospitalized for

Table 4
Age and sex distribution of nontuberculous mycobacterial isolations from respiratory specimen (I) and nontuberculous mycobacterial pulmonary disease (D) by region

Location (dates)	N	Mean Age (years)	Female (%)	COPD (%)/Bronchiectasis (%)/History of TB (%)	Other Pulmonary Disease (%)
North America					
Florida, United States (2011–2017)[56]	I: 271	60.5	28.5	20.8/2.2/2.2	Asthma (2.8), CF (11.1), ILD (3.6), lung cancer (7.5)
Florida, United States (2012–2018)[55]	D: 7963 (ICD-9/10)	-	54	27.7/30.7/10.6	CF (4.1)
Hawaii, United States (2005–2013)[52]	I: 201 D: 254[d]	65.2 66	50 57	39.8/27.9/- 43/44/-	Lung cancer (12) Lung cancer (11)
Hawaii, United States (2005–2019)[53]	I: 739	Median: 63	54	-/-/-	-
Illinois, United States (2000–2012)[135]	I: 448	63.0	63	11–22[f]/-/5–9[f]	-
Iowa, United States (1996–2017)[136]	D: 185	Median: 63	55	30.3/26.5/-	CF (7.6), ILD (5.9), Structural Lung Disease (60.5)
North Carolina, United States (2006–2010)[58]	I: 750	-	41.2	-/-/-	-
North Carolina, United States (2006–2010)[38]	I: 507	60	51.8	-/-/-	-
Oregon, United States (2007–2012)[10]	I: 806 D: 1146[d]	Median: 66 Median: 69	49.6 55.7	-/-/- -/-/-	- -
United States (2001–2015)[47]	I: 4676 (ICD-9/ICD-10)	-	0.13	100/2.5/2.6	Asthma (12.2), ILD (12.8), Lung Cancer (3.1)
United States (2008–2015)[45]	D: 6280 (ICD-9/ICD-10)	69	67.6	52.6/37/7	Aspergillosis (3.0), Asthma (23.2), CF (1.7)
US-Affiliated Pacific Island Jurisdictions (2007–2011)[54]	I: 35[h]	Median: 34.8	49.2	27.6/-/44.8	-

Central and South America

Ceará, Brazil (2005–2016)[65]	I: 69[c]	38.6	26.1	11.9/-/73.8	All (13)[a]
French Guiana (2008–2018)[61]	178 (D: 31, I: 147)	49	39.3	17/5/16	Chronic pulmonary disease (33)
Mexico City, Mexico (2001–2017)[62]	D: 67	Median: 52–61[g]	48–50[g]	-/-/-	Any (13)[a]
Rio Grande do Sul, Brazil (2003–2013)[63]	D: 100	54.6	49	17/22/85	CF (1), Silicosis (1)

Europe

Belgium (2010–2017)[138]	D: 165	Median: 64	43	41.8/20/7.3	Aspergillosis (4.2), CF (6.1), Prior NTM-PD (13.9)
Croatia (2006–2015)[139]	D: 137	Median: 66	47.5	45.3/29.2/27.7	Asthma (2.2), Prior NTM-PD (5.1)
France (2002–2013)[140]	D: 92	Median: 61.5	42.4	14.1/17.4/12	All (46.7)[a]
France (2009–2014)[141]	D: 477	Median: 65	29.6–56.2[f]	-/-/31.4	All (68)[a]
France (2010–2017)[69]	D: 5628 (ICD-10 or suggestive medication)	60.9	47.1	18.8/10.6/14.1	CF (3.2), lung cancer (5.7)
Germany (2009–2014)[72]	D: 85–126 per year (ICD-10) (2009–2014)	55–61 (2009–2014)	43.4–52.9 (2009–2014)	62.4–79.2 (2009–2014)/ 6.6–18.3 (2009–2014)/ 13.5–24 (2009–2014)	Asthma (20.8–29.2) (2009–2014), Lung cancer (3.5–10.3) (2009–2014)
Germany (2010–2011)[26]	D: 125 (ICD-10)	49.8	50.4	-	-
Germany (2011–2016)[71]	D: 218 (ICD-10, German modification)	61.4	41.3	46.3/10.1/17	Asthma (25.2). ILD (3.7)
Greece (January 2007–May 2013)[84]	I: 62	-	-	42/35/13	Asthma (6.4) CF (1.6)
	D: 12	-	-	50/25/41	Asthma (8.3)
The Netherlands (2008–2013)[144]	D: 63	60.8	50.8	66.7–71.4[f]/-/10.5–14.3[f]	Asthma (1.6–15.8[f]), Lung cancer (5.3–14.3[f])
Poland (2010–2015)[145]	D: 36	58.5	83.3	19/33/28	Asthma (6), CF (8), ILD (28), lung cancer (16.7)
Portugal (2002–2012)[73]	D: 632 (NTM-PD treatment)[c]	Median: 54	39.7	6.3/-/-	ILD (3.3)

(continued on next page)

Table 4
(continued)

Location (dates)	N	Mean Age (years)	Female (%)	COPD (%)/Bronchiectasis (%)/History of TB (%)	Other Pulmonary Disease (%)
Serbia (2009–2016)[148]	D: 85[c]	59.2	34.1	40/10/13	-
Serbia (2010–2015)[74]	D: 126[d]	65.4	47.6	-	-
Spain (1997–2016)[78]	D: 327	56.8	28.8	30.1/29.3/-	Any (56)[a]
The United Kingdom (2007–2014)[152]	D: 112	65	51.8	44.5/38.4/9.8	Asthma (16.9), ILD (5.4)
East Asia					
China (2010–2015)[120]	D: 72	54.1	47.2	8.3/6.9/15.3	Silicosis (2.8)
China (2013–2016)[157]	D: 607	-	56.2	4.1/58.6/59.6	-
China (2014–2021)[119]	I: 1755	-	53.6	-/-/-	-
China (2015–2020)[118]	I: 789	Median: 36	39.0	-/-/22.4	-
China (2017–2018)[158]	D: 87	Median: 60	41.4	6.9/19.5/64.4	-
China (2019–2020)[117]	D: 458	-	34.9	9.2/26.2/45.6	Asthma (2.2)
Japan (2004–2006)[23]	D: 309 (ICD-8-10, estimated from Death Statistics)	67	64.7	3.2/4.2/19.1	Asthma (3.2), ILD (1.3), lung cancer (1.3)
Japan (1999–2010)[165]	D: 782	68.1	68.5	4.3/-/11.6	ILD (3.5)
Japan (2000–2013)[108]	D: 592[d]	66.0	61.1	6.4/-/9.5	Asthma (6.3), ILD (6.6)
Japan (2001–2009)[132]	D: 975	71.2	69.7	5.8/0.3/13.5	Asthma (1.8), ILD (4.0), lung cancer (5.5), silicosis (1.3)
Japan (2006–2016)[109]	D: 2155[d]	Median: 69	66.5	-/-/-	-
Japan (2009–2014)[107]	D (Incident):11,034 (2011) (ICD-10)	69.3	69.6	6.9/23.5/6.3	Aspergillosis (6.1), ILD (9.9), lung cancer (5.3)
Japan (2009–2015)[160]	D: 114	Median: 74–78.5[f]	59–68[f]	(5–24)[f]/(11–15)[f]/(16–17)[f]	Asthma (8–17)[f], ILD (5–8)[f]
Japan (2013–2015)[111]	D: 184[e]	69.5	75.5	-/5.4/8.2	-
Japan (2012–2013)[105]	D: 7167[d]	73.6[b]	65.5[b]	-/-/-	-

					Aspergillosis (1.9), asthma (18.3), DPB (1.6), ILD (6.0), lung cancer (4.5)
Japan (2014)[166]	D: 419 (ICD-10)	Median: 59	68	3.1/-/-	
South Korea (2001–2015)[104]	D: 2329	Median: 60	59	-/-/-	-
South Korea (2003–2016)[98]	D: 46,194 (ICD-10)	55.8	61.1	-/-/-	-
South Korea (2006–2016)[100]	D: 1017	62.7	58.8	13.5/83.9/48.3	Asthma (7.3), lung cancer (4.0)
South Korea (2007–2018)[99]	D: 45,321 (ICD-10)	-	56.9	-/-/-	-
South Korea (2007–2019)[102]	I: 2984[c]	-	42.3	-/-/-	-
South Korea (2009–2015)[133]	D: 52,551 (ICD-10)[c]	53.0	57.2	25.6/21.9/33.7	Asthma (33.2), ILD (2.6), lung cancer (5.8)
Taiwan (2000–2012)[115]	D: 3317	-	42.3	-/-/-	-
Taiwan (2003–2018)[113]	D(treatment case): 558 (ICD-9-CM)[c]	62.5	42.5	-/-/-	Chronic lung disease (42.8)
Taiwan (2005–2013)[112]	D: 450 (ICD-9-CM)[c]	-	38	-/-/-	-
Taiwan (2007–2010)[114]	I: 894	-	44.4	-/-/-	-
Taiwan (2010–2014)[116]	D: 1674	-	44.3	23.4/15.6/25.4	Asthma (5.2), ILD (6)
South-Southeast Asia					
India (1981–2020)[161]	D: 365	-	44	-/3/65	-
India (2013–2015)[126]	I: 263[c]	Median: 48	39.5	-/-/-	-
India (2015–2020)[125]	I: 105[c]	-	50.5	5.7/-/16.2	-
Pakistan (2016–2019)[122]	I: 169	Median: 45	39	-/-/65	-
Singapore (2011–2012)[162]	I: 485	Median: 70	37.9	14.2/28.7/34.4	Asthma (6.6); ILD (3.7)

(continued on next page)

Table 4
(continued)

Location (dates)	N	Mean Age (years)	Female (%)	COPD (%)/Bronchiectasis (%)/History of TB (%)	Other Pulmonary Disease (%)
Singapore (2012–2016)[163]	D: 352	Median: 67	48.3	13.1/36.4/27.6	Asthma (4.0)
Central and West Asia					
Iran (2016–2018)[123]	I: 95	47.4	42.1	-/-/-	-
Saudi Arabia (2006–2012)[164]	D: 40	54	42	7.5/15/12	Asthma (15), CF (2.5), ILD (10)
Oceania					
Australia (2001–2016)[41]	I: 12,219[c]	Median: 66	50.1	-/-/-	-
Australia (2012–2015)[3]	I: 1222[c]	Median: 66	51	-/-/-	-
Papua New Guinea (2010–2012)[129]	I: 9	35.7	88.9	-/-/-	-

Abbreviations: CF, cystic fibrosis; COPD, chronic obstructive pulmonary disease; DPB, diffuse panbrochiolitis; ICD-10, International diagnostic classification of diseases–tenth revision; ICD-9, International diagnostic classification of diseases–ninth revision; ILD, interstitial lung disease; RGM, rapid-growing nontuberculous mycobacteria; SGM, slow-growing nontuberculous mycobacteria; TB, tuberculosis.

a All pulmonary comorbidities, including COPD, bronchiectasis, History of TB.
b MAC patients only.
c Included patients with NTM isolated from extrapulmonary sites/specimens from extrapulmonary sites.
d NTM-PD defined using ATS microbiologic criteria.
e NTM-PD defined using full ATS criteria or 2008 Japanese Society for Tuberculosis/Japanese Respiratory Society Guidelines for the diagnosis of NTM pulmonary infection.
f Range by NTM species.
g Range by RGM and SGM.
h Subanalysis of study population.

NTM-PD in the last 3 years, using ICD-10 codes. A stable incidence of NTM-PD between 1.025/100,000 in 2010 and 1.096/100,000 in 2017 was reported. The NTM-PD prevalence was estimated at 5.92/100,000 inhabitants during 8 years.[69] The dataset did not include untreated patients with NTM-PD (incidence and prevalence probably underestimated); however, the stable incidence is likely valid for France from 2010 through 2017 (**Fig. 4**).

Germany
In Germany, a population-based cohort study with a nested case–control design used ICD-10 codes from more than 80 German company statutory health insurance datasets for the years 2010 to 2011 to define 125 patients with NTM-PD and to calculate yearly incidence rates of 1.12/100,000 in 2010 and 1.48/100,000 in 2011.[26] Similarly, an anonymized German health claims database with an ICD-10 code 2011 to 2016 was analyzed to find 218 incident patients with NTM-PD; a prevalence of 3.79/100,000 was estimated. Using a prediction model, the prevalence of NTM-PD for both ICD-10-coded and noncoded individuals was 5-fold higher at 19.05/100,000.[71] A third German study based on the Health Risk Institute health services research database (subset of ≈7 million persons) used ICD-10 codes to identify patients with NTM-PD from 2009 to 2014. The data showed an increase in the annual overall prevalence rate from 2.3/100,000 to 3.3/100,000.[72] Using ICD-10 codes, it is probable that these studies underestimate the incidence and prevalence of NTM-PD because agreement of ICD-10 codes with the ATS diagnostic criteria has not been studied in Germany. The positive predictive value of ICD-9-CM codes ranged from 57% to 64%, and sensitivity for the diagnosis of NTM-PD to be low ranging from 21% to 26.9%.[83]

Greece
Adult inpatients and outpatients of the second largest tertiary referral hospital for patients with respiratory diseases in Athens were retrospectively assessed for the presence of NTM isolation and NTM-PD using the ATS criteria. The reported incidence of pulmonary isolation (18.9/100,000 patients) and disease (8.8/100,000 patients) during the study period (2007–2013) was calculated as the total number of patients with respective isolation and disease divided by the total number of patients who attended this hospital as inpatients or outpatients, for example, do not reflect the population of the area.[84]

Portugal
All 632 NTM patients treated at tuberculosis (TB) outpatient centers in Portugal (defined as patients with NTM-PD) that were recorded in the electronic database (structured questionnaire and stored in the Portugese National Tuberculosis Surveillance System [SVIG-TB], Lisbon, Portugal) between 2002 and 2012 were retrospectively analyzed. The estimated annual incidence of treated NTM-PD was 0.54/100,000, during the study period, an increase of NTM-PD, mostly due to an increase in MAC-PD, was described.[73] The inclusion of only treated patients with NTM-PD may have led to an underestimation; however, the fact that 41 of the treated patients had *M gordonae* isolates leaves questions regarding the accuracy of the classification of NTM-PD in the patient cohort.[85]

Serbia
In Serbia, a retrospective and noninterventional study was performed by the national TB laboratory network representative for the whole country. Overall, 565 patients with 777 pulmonary NTM isolates collected between 2010 and 2015 were analyzed for the presence of NTM-PD using the ATS microbiologic criteria. The annual isolation incidence of NTM increased from 0.9/100,000 to 1.6/100,000 without reaching statistical significance. In contrast, annual incidence rates of NTM-PD increased from 0.18/100,000 to 0.47/100,000. The most frequent NTM species in this country was *M xenopi* (with annual incidence rates

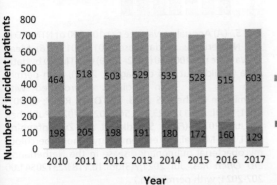

Fig. 4. Incidence of NTM-PD in France by treatment status from 2010 to 2017. (*From* Veziris N, Andréjak C, Bouée S, Emery C, Obradovic M, Chiron R. Non-tuberculous mycobacterial pulmonary diseases in France: an 8 years nationwide study. *BMC Infect Dis.* Nov 17 2021;21(1):1165. doi:10.1186/s12879-021-06825-x; with permission.(see Fig. 1 in original).)

of 0.04/100,000–0.11/100,000), the annual incidence rate for MAC-PD was low (between 0.01/100,000 and 0.07/100,000).[74]

Spain

In the Basque region in northern Spain, incidence rates of NTM-PD (as defined by ATS criteria) were calculated using the data from the Microbiology Laboratory and clinical records. Incidence of NTM-PD decreased from 1997 to 2016 significantly over the years from 10.6/100,000 and 8.8/100,000 in 2000 and 2001, respectively, to 1.8/100,000 in 2016. This decrease was solely explained by an annual decrease of 6.5% in *M kansasii*-PD, whereas *M avium*-PD had an annual increase of 3.3%.[78] In 13 municipalities in the Barcelona-South Health Region of Catalonia, a similar trend for the annual prevalence rates per 100,000 population for both *M kansasii* and MAC isolation and pulmonary disease has been calculated for the period between 1994 and 2014, with similar high decreases of 9% for isolation of, and 11% for disease due to *M kansasii* and increases of 10% for isolation of, and 13% for disease due to MAC. Here overall pulmonary disease prevalence was calculated at 42.8/100,000.[75] Rapid-growing mycobacteria isolated at a reference mycobacterial laboratory of the Catalan region similarly increased 5-fold from 2003 (0.34/100,000) to 2015 (1.73/100,000).[76] The 3 studies performed in Spain during 1997 and 2016 show an increase of the incidence of MAC-isolation, of MAC-PD and of isolation of rapid growing mycobacteria but a decrease in *M kansasii*-isolation and *M kansasii*–PD, supporting the conclusion that epidemiology of NTM should consider the different mycobacterial species separately.

The Netherlands

A study in the Netherlands used 4 separate databases, including 2 drug dispensing databases, an ICD-10 code database, and a hospitalization database to estimate the prevalence of NTM-PD for the whole country between 2012 and 2019 by assigning the patients to "probable" patients with NTM-PD and "possible" patients with NTM-PD depending on the drug regimen used in the drug prescription databases, and to "confirmed patients with NTM-PD" when the ICD-10 code A31.0 had been used. Prevalence estimates of the ICD-10 codes were corrected for the limited sensitivity (50%) for NTM-PD seen in previous studies and ranged in the different databases between 2.3/100,000 and 5.9/100,000 inhabitants, whereas a simultaneously performed survey among pulmonologists (likely overestimated) estimated the annual NTM-PD prevalence between

6.2/100,000 and 9.9/100,000. No increase was seen during the study period, in any of the study populations[70] (**Fig. 5**).

The United Kingdom

Primary care electronic health-care records (Clinical Practice Research Datalink) representing 6.8% of the UK population were used to extract data for patients with NTM isolates during 2006 and 2016 and to classify patients as highly likely to have NTM-PD ("strict cohort," 85% of these being treated) and possible NTM-PD ("expanded cohort"). A significant decrease in the incidence in the strict cohort from 2006 (3.85/100,000 person-years) to 2016 (1.28/100,000 person-years) was paralleled by a decrease of NTM-PD prevalence from 7.68/100,000 to 4.7/100,000 in primary care patients. This trend probably represents a shift of care of these (treated) patients toward secondary care.[79] This assessment is supported by a study from England, Wales, and Northern Ireland that included all culture positive NTM isolates between 2007 and 2012 reported to Public Health England by 5 mycobacterial reference laboratories. The NTM isolation incidence in people with pulmonary isolates rose significantly from 4.0/100,000 to 6.1/100,000, driven by the MAC isolation incidence increasing from 1.3/

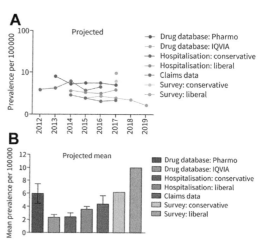

Fig. 5. (*A*) Annual prevalence per 100,000 of NTM-PD in the Netherlands by database (2012–2019). (*B*) Mean prevalence per 100,000 (2012–2019) of NTM-PD by database (Schildkraut and colleagues, 2021); with permission (see **Fig. 1** in original). Reproduced with permission of the ERS 2023. ERJ Open Res 7: 00,207-2021; DOI: 10.1183/23,120,541.00207-2021 Published 12 July 2021. (*From* Schildkraut JA, Zweijpfenning SMH, Nap M, et al. The epidemiology of nontuberculous mycobacterial pulmonary disease in the Netherlands. *ERJ Open Res.* Jul 2021;7(3)doi:10.1183/23120541.00207-2021; with permission.)

100,000 in 2007 to 2.2/100,000 in 2012.[77] Scottish isolates of NTM that had been submitted between 2000 and 2010 to the Scottish Mycobacteria Reference Laboratory were used to assign NTM-PD status to the respective patients using the ATS microbiologic criteria. A mean rate of 2.43 episodes of infection (that included extrapulmonary infections)/100,000 (range 2.06–2.71) was calculated, without significant trend during the study period. The incidence of NTM-PD was not calculated separately.[86]

African Region

Cohorts in African studies from 2014 to 2022 comprise patients with presumptive TB and/or patients with "chronic pulmonary TB" that were retrospectively analyzed. Data on NTM-PD were still rare and are mostly from studies from South Africa published before 2014[87] and thus not included in this review. Most of the studies have not performed chest imaging and seldom repetitive sputum isolation, so criteria for NTM-PD could not be applied. The data still suggest that a potentially significant proportion of African TB suspects may have NTM disease but may not be detected in routine care. The increasing availability of rapid TB-identification tests has decreased the number of studies reporting patients as being treated as MDR-TB while actually having NTM-PD. Good population-based studies to determine the incidence of NTM-PD in African countries are lacking; isolation prevalence in TB-suspects is reported here (**Table 5**). Similar to earlier studies summarized by Okoi,[87] most studies report an isolation prevalence of less than 10%. The ratio of growth of NTM to all mycobacterial growth varied significantly between 1% (Nigeria), 12% (Mali), 54% (Botswana), and 78% (Zambia), which may not be explained solely by different patient populations and detection methods (see **Table 5**). The species isolated from respiratory secretions differ significantly within the African continent with MAC being the most frequently isolated species in most studies (see **Table 3**). Maps of the continent with the distribution of the most frequent isolates from respiratory diseases and species causing NTM-PD have been published in a review covering African publications from 1940 to 2016.[87]

Sub-Saharan Africa

A systematic review published in 2017[87] retrieved 37 out of 373 articles published from 1940 to 2016 from which data on pulmonary NTM isolation in patient cohorts from sub-Saharan Africa were extracted. The calculated prevalence of pulmonary NTM isolation was 7.5% and 16.5% (512 of 3096) in those previously treated for TB. MAC was the most frequently isolated NTM in 19 of 37 studies with a large variation of MAC isolation prevalence from 15.0% in Tanzania to 57.8% in Mali. NTM-PD as defined in the ATS criteria was described in 7 of the 37 studies: 266 (27.7%) of 962 patients with sufficient data had NTM-PD. *M kansasii* (69.2%) was the most common species among the isolates.[87]

North Africa

A study during a long period (2002–2016) looked retrospectively at sputum collected from HIV-negative Tunisian patients with presumptive pulmonary TB. 60 of 1864 (3.2%) specimens grew NTM; from 30 isolates 7 were *M kansasii*, none belonged to the MAC group, possibly indicating problems in the selection and identification process. The estimated NTM isolation prevalence of 0.2/100,000 population calculated for the regions of Bizerte and Zaghouan during the period 2002 to 2011 should thus be quoted with caution.[88]

Southern Africa

In Botswana, a 2012 to 2014 substudy of the Xpert evaluation study for TB detection performed in 22 clinical sites (representing 12 out of the 28 districts and included HIV patients). A total of 228 out of 427 (53.4%) patients with mycobacterial growth had NTM (114 MAC, (109 *M intracellulare*), 16 *M gordonae*, 9 *M malmoense*, and 8 *M simiae*), only 8 of these (3.5%) had 2 positive sputum cultures and presumptive NTM disease.[89]

West Africa

Two studies from 2012 to 2014 were reported from Ghana looking at 1755 mycobacterial isolates from smear-positive sputum samples[90] in a HIV-positive cohort of 571 patients.[91] The NTM isolation rate in smear-positive sputum was 2.5%, identified by *hsp*65 gene PCR as *M avium* subs *paratuberculosis* (30.2%), *M intracellulare* (41.9), and *M abscessus* (11.3%).[90] In the HIV cohort, the NTM isolation rate was 51% (50 out of 98 patients with mycobacterial growth). Thirty-eight NTM isolates were speciated: 9 were MAC (23.7%), 3 were *M simiae* (7.9%), and 3 were *M chelonae* complex (7.9%). Sixty-five percent of the patients with NTM isolates had a CD4-count less than 100, 24% had died during the 6 months of follow-up, similar to 30% of patients with TB.[91] In a retrospective single-center study from Mali 2006 to 2013, NTM were detected in 41 out of 439 (9.34%) TB suspects and 41 out of 332 patients with mycobacterial isolations (12.3% isolation). Of the 20 species identified from patients, 50% were *M avium*.[92]

Table 5
Studies of rates of pulmonary nontuberculous mycobacterial isolates in Africa

Location (dates)	Patient Cohort	Isolation Method	Ratio NTM/Mycobacterial Growth (%)	Period Prevalence of NTM Isolation	
				Period Duration (years)	Prevalence
Prevalence of Sputum Isolates					
Botswana (Aug 2012–Nov 2014)[89]	228 of 1940 symptomatic HIV-infected patients with culture result	Negative SD-Bioline Ag MPT64 assay (Abbott); GenoType CM and AS assays (Hain Lifescience)	53.4 (3.5 with 2 positive sputum cultures)	3	53.4% among culture positive specimen
Mali (2006–2013)[92]	41 of 439 patients suspected of having TB	Negative MTBc Gen-Probe (AccuProbe); Nucleic acid probes for MAC, M gordonae, M kansasii (AccuProbe); gene sequencing	12.34	8	9.34% among individuals suspected of having TB
Nigeria, Cameroon, Ghana (Jan–Dec 2017)[153]	16 of 503 mycobacterial isolates from new and previously treated pulmonary TB patients	Negative IS6110 PCR; hsp65 PCR with sequencing	Nigeria: 1 Cameroon: 1.3 Ghana: 8.4	1	3.2% among isolates
Sub-Saharan Africa (1940–2016)[87]	ATS criteria (systematic review) in 37 relevant studies	Molecular techniques (n = 26), biochemical testing identification tools (n = 9); immunochromatographic assays (n = 2)		77	7.5% (isolation prevalence from all 37 articles reviewed)
Tunisia (2002–2016)[88]	60 of 1863 specimen from HIV-negative patients with presumptive clinical pulmonary TB with culture result	Biochemical tests: niacin, nitrate, heat-resistant catalase and para-nitro benzoic acid; PCR targeting the recA intein	3.2	15	Isolation prevalence of 0.2/100,000 population of northern Tunisia
Zambia (Aug 2013–July 2014)[96]	923 symptomatic patients with NTM-isolates among 6123 TB survey participants (1188 with mycobacterial growth)	Negative capilia (TAUNS) lateral flow assay	77.7	2	1477/100,000 symptomatic NTM-patients among TB survey participants aged 15 y and above

Location (dates)	N	Mean Age (years)	Female (%)	COPD (%)/Bronchiectasis (%)/TB (%)	Preexisting Pulmonary Disease (%)
Age and Sex Distribution and Preexisting Pulmonary Diseases					
Botswana (Aug 2012–Nov 2014)[89]	I: 228	NA; 45 patients >50 y	53.90	-/-/12.4	-
Ethiopia (2017)[93]	I: 51	32.4 (of all TB-aNA NTM-pts)	51	-/-/-	-
Gabon (2018–2020)[97]	I: 1363	40	38.70	-/-/23.3	-
Ghana (2012–2014)[90]	I: 43	39.4	37.2	-/-/-	-
Ghana (Jan 2013–Mar 2014)[91]	I: 473	39	68.4	-/-/-	-
Kenya (2020)[94]	I: 166	39	27	-/-/-	-
Mali (2006–2013)[92]	I: 41	35.8 y of all 439 pts	19.5	-/-/-	-
Nigeria, Cameroon, Ghana (Jan–Dec 2017)[153]	I: 503	45.14	35.30	-/-/-	-
Sub-Saharan Africa (1940–2016)[87]	D: 266 (from 37 studies)	35 y based on 17 of 37 studies with age data (isolation)	-	-/-/-	-
Tanzania (Nov 2019–Aug 2020)[154]	I: 24	47	33	-/-/-	Retreatment cases (60.9)
Tunisia (2002–2016)[88]	I: 60	-	30	-/-/-	-
Zambia (Aug 2013–July 2014)[96]	I: 923	NA; age groups 15–24 y: 8.7%; 65+: 28.6%	51.70	-/7.15/-	Chest x-ray: Nodules (22), Cavitation (13.8), Fibrosis (15)

East Africa

In Ethiopia, in 2017, 51 out of 697 (7.3%) patients with presumptive pulmonary TB had NTM isolates, 34 had been misclassified as TB (14 new cases, 12 relapses, and 7 treatment failures); species were identified in 35 isolates (42.9% *M simiae* and 14.3% *M abscessus*).[93] A study from Kenya in symptomatic patients detected 166 sputum isolates that were TB negative; of 146 identified, 122 were NTM, mostly MAC (31%), *M fortuitum* complex (20%), and *M abscessus* complex (14%).[94] In 2012 to 2013, in 744 sputum samples from 372 TB suspects in Tanzania, mycobacterial cultures were positive in 121 (32.5%) patients, 36 (9.7%) were NTM. The most frequent species of the 28 identified were *M gordonae* and *M interjectum* (each 6 out of 28).[95] Our search retrieved only one population-based Zambian study.[96] Nine hundred twenty-three participants in a one year period (Aug 2013–July 2014) national TB prevalence survey, NTM-positive sputum cultures and negative TB test were defined as NTM patients without further species differentiation. In this cohort, 923 out of 1188 (78%) of positive cultures were defined as NTM; 265 out of 1188 (12%) were MTB. Of the participants with NTM, 71% were symptomatic. The prevalence of symptomatic NTM was estimated at 1477/100,000.[96]

Central Africa

In 1363 sputum samples collected from presumptive patients with TB in Gabon (2018–2020) in a mixed retrospective and prospective cross-sectional study, 26.6% (137 out of 515) patients with mycobacterial isolates had NTM, most were MAC (61.4%, 81 out of 132) with *M intracellulare* dominating (74 out of 81). The next most common species were *M fortuitum* (21.9%) and *M abscessus* (6.6%).[97]

Asian Region

Population-based epidemiological data have been reported from Taiwan, Korea, and Japan, using primarily insurance claims data since 2014. These reports showed a consistent upward trend in these countries. Importantly, the incidence has surpassed that of TB in Japan, similar to Western countries, and the estimated prevalence reached approximately 150/100,000 in 2020. The species distribution shows *M intracellulare* predominance in China and Korea but *M avium* is common in Japan. Interestingly, the proportions of cases with *M abscessus* species are higher in the southern regions of China, Taiwan, and Japan. The proportion of NTM is also increasing in culture-positive specimens in China. Middle-aged female predominance is reported in most countries. However, patients with underlying lung diseases, such as COPD and previous TB, seem more common in Taiwan and other countries than in Korea and Japan. More epidemiological reports from Asian countries are warranted.

South Korea

During 2014 to 2022, population-based data on the incidence and prevalence of NTM-PD using the National Health Insurance Service (NHIS) database were reported in South Korea.[98,99] Park and colleagues reported that the incidence rate increased from 1.0/100,000 in 2002 to 17.9/100,000 in 2016; the prevalence rate was 1.2/100,000 in 2003 and increased to 33.3/100,000 in 2016[98] (**Fig. 6**). The 5-year mortality rate was 17.8% (2003–2016), higher among men than among women (28.3% vs 9.9%). Summarizing population-based and single-center studies, the proportion of patients with NTM-PD who were women in South Korea was 56.9% to 61.1%, with a mean age of 53.0 to 62.7 years.[98–100] Species in the *M avium* complex (63.6%–75%) were most commonly identified, followed by subspecies of *M abscessus* (10.8%–22%). *M intracellulare* (38.3%–50.6%) was isolated more frequently than *M avium* (17.5%–23.1%), in most regions, although there were exceptions.[100–104]

Japan

A nationwide laboratory data-based study analyzing 7167 NTM-PD using the ATS microbiologic criteria found a period prevalence of 24 during 2012 to 2013.[105] The most prevalent species was MAC (97.5%), followed by *M kansasii* and *M abscessus* (2%–3%). In contrast to South Korea, the proportion of *M avium* was higher than that of *M intracellulare* (65.1% vs 32.4%). Interestingly, the proportion of *M intracellulare* gradually increased from the eastern to the western part of Japan and further increased to South Korea[106](**Fig. 7**). Furthermore, the proportion of *M abscessus* was higher in the Kyushu-Okinawa regions close to Korea and Taiwan. An insurance claims data analysis showed that the incidence and prevalence rates were 8.6/100,000 treated individuals and 29.0/100,000 treated individuals, respectively.[107] Because this study used ICD codes to define disease, prevalence and incidence are likely underestimated. Patient characteristics were similar in South Korea, with an older female predominance[105,108,109] but lung disease complications were less common compared with South Korea. However, although bronchiectasis was common in women, COPD, sequelae of TB, and interstitial pneumonia were higher in men with age. Analysis of mortality data found that the crude mortality rate increased from 0.003/100,000 to.

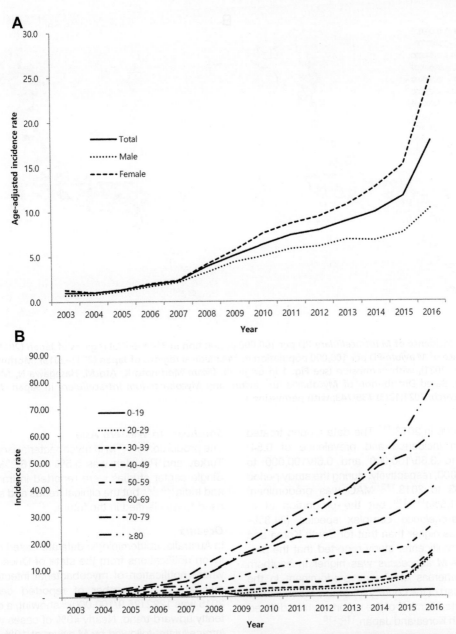

Fig. 6. (*A*) Age-adjusted incidence of NTM infection per 100,000 population by sex (2003–2016). (*B*) Incidence of NTM infection per 100,000 population by age group (2003–2016) (Park and colleagues, 2019); with permission (see **Fig. 2** in original). (*From* Park SC, Kang MJ, Han CH, et al. Prevalence, incidence, and mortality of nontuberculous mycobacterial infection in Korea: a nationwide population-based study. *BMC Pulm Med*. Aug 1 2019;19(1):140. doi:10.1186/s12890-019-0901-z; with permission.)

1.93/100,000 from 1970 to 2016.[23,110] In Japan, annual health examinations with regular chest imaging are optional for citizens aged older than 40 years and mandated for all workers aged older than 35 years. In South Korea, these examinations are biannual for persons aged older than 40 years, with high compliance rates. These annual examinations may lead to the detection of milder cases

but are unlikely to explain recent increasing trends because they have been in place for more than 30 years.[111]

Taiwan
Well-analyzed studies using several methodologies have been published.[112–116] The age-adjusted incidence rate increased from 5.3/100,000 in 2005 to

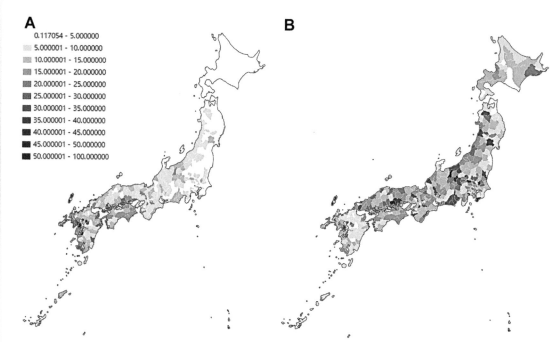

Fig. 7. (*A*) Incidence of *M intracellulare*-PD per 100,000 population in 344 medical regions of Japan (2011–2013). (*B*) Incidence of *M avium*-PD per 100,000 population in 344 medical regions of Japan (2011–2013) (Morimoto and colleagues, 2021); with permission (see **Fig. 1** in original). (*From* Morimoto K, Ato M, Hasegawa N, Mitarai S. Population-Based Distribution of *Mycobacterium avium* and *Mycobacterium intracellulare* in Japan. *Microbiology Research.* 2021;12(3):739-743; with permission.)

14.8/100,000 in 2013.[112] The data among treated cases, an incidence and prevalence of 0.54/100,000 to 3.35/100,000 and 0.68/100,000 to 7.17/100,000, respectively, during the study period from 2003 to 2018.[113] MAC was predominant (34.4%–41.5%)[114–116] but the proportion of *M abscessus-chelonae* complex species (24.3%–30.8%) was higher than that for South Korea and Japan. A multicenter study reported that the proportion of *M abscessus* was higher in southern Taiwan, whereas MAC was predominant in the northern part of the country.[116] Male predominance was reported in most of the reports, which differed from South Korea and Japan.[112–116]

China

No population-based data were found in China or other Asian regions. NTM represented between 4.8% and 8.5% of all mycobacteria isolated and between 6.6% and 15.5% of all pulmonary mycobacterial disease cases, with an upward trend.[117–119] The isolates and disease proportion were higher in the south coastal area. MAC was predominant, followed by *M abscessus* and *M kansasii*. The proportion of *M intracellulare* (28.2%–70.1%) was higher than that of *M avium* (2.8%–16.3%),[120] similar to South Korea. The proportion of RGM was higher in the southern region than in the other regions.

Southeast to Western Asia

The proportion of NTM in mycobacterial isolates in Turkey and Pakistan was 5.5% to 16.2%.[121,122] Single-center studies were reported in Iran[123,124] and India[125–127] but the clinical trends and species need to be clarified in the future.

Oceania

In Australia, epidemiologic data are based primarily on notifications from the state of Queensland, where notification of mycobacterial infections is mandated. The number of reported cases in 2015 was 1222 (25.9/100,000),[3] showing a consistently upward trend. Nearly 40% of cases were *M intracellulare*, followed by *M avium* at 10% and *M abscessus* at 8.5%. An isolated strain analysis was reported from French Polynesia and Papua New Guinea.[128,129]

SUMMARY AND RESEARCH GAPS

NTM-PD and NTM pulmonary isolation are increasing in most countries and regions globally. Isolate-based analysis in several countries indicates distinct trends by NTM species, highlighting the need for more species-specific analyses in NTM epidemiology. Available data regarding species indicates that MAC continues to predominate in most regions, although in Ontario, Canada, and distinct European countries *M kansasii*, *M xenopi*, and *M malmoense* are found with greater frequency. Variation in methods and case definitions limit comparisons across countries and regions. Population-based data including incidence and/or prevalence are available from North America, Europe, East Asia (Japan, South Korea, and Taiwan), and Queensland, Australia. Studies from Central and South America, Africa, China, the Middle East, and South Asia (India) among patients with suspected TB and MDR-TB are important to document the burden of undiagnosed NTM in this population and ensure appropriate treatment. This highlights the need for enhanced mycobacterial laboratory capacity to discriminate between cases of TB and NTM by routine speciation of mycobacterial isolates. Clinical data available from several regions have allowed better characterization of the affected populations. Across regions, the majority of cases occur among persons aged older than 50 years. In North America and East Asia, the proportion with COPD is typically less than 20%, whereas in Europe, the proportion with COPD is higher, above 30% in 9 of 13 studies with this information.

Implementation of surveillance systems with standard case definitions is needed to allow for global comparison of prevalence and trends. Current data where NTM-PD is a notifiable condition have shown the importance and utility of these surveillance data. In particular, timely notification data have allowed inference of the incubation period for infection and disease and have further allowed identification of specific high-risk environmental niches and environmental risk factors.

CLINICS CARE POINTS

- When physiicians or other health care providers suspect NTM pumonary infection or disease, they should collect appropriate samples including 3 samples for AFB culture, in addition to chest X rays or High Resolution CT (HRCT).

DISCLOSURE

D.R. Prevots, J. Marshall, and D. Wagner have no disclosures. K. Morimoto has received funding from INSMED, Japan Agency for Medical Research and Development (AMED), Japan Society for the Promotion of Science, KAKENHI, Boehringer Ingelheim, and Asahi Kasei Pharma Corp.

ACKNOWLEDGMENTS

This study was supported in part by the Division of Intramural Research, National Institute of Allergy and Infectious Diseases, National Institutes of Health, Bethesda, MD.

REFERENCES

1. Prevots DR, Marras TK. Epidemiology of human pulmonary infection with nontuberculous mycobacteria: a review. Clin Chest Med 2015;36(1):13–34.
2. Shih DC, Cassidy PM, Perkins KM, et al. Extrapulmonary nontuberculous mycobacterial disease surveillance - Oregon, 2014-2016. MMWR Morb Mortal Wkly Rep Aug 10 2018;67(31):854–7.
3. Thomson R, Donnan E, Konstantinos A. Notification of nontuberculous mycobacteria: an Australian perspective. Ann Am Thorac Soc 2017;14(3):318–23.
4. Winthrop KL, Henkle E, Walker A, et al. On the reportability of nontuberculous mycobacterial disease to public health authorities. Ann Am Thorac Soc 2017;14(3):314–7.
5. Vrijheid M. The exposome: a new paradigm to study the impact of environment on health. Thorax 2014;69(9):876–8.
6. Wild CP, Scalbert A, Herceg Z. Measuring the exposome: a powerful basis for evaluating environmental exposures and cancer risk. Environ Mol Mutagenesis 2013;54(7):480–99.
7. Griffith DE, Aksamit T, Brown-Elliott BA, et al. An official ATS/IDSA statement: diagnosis, treatment, and prevention of nontuberculous mycobacterial diseases. Am J Respir Crit Care Med 2007; 175(4):367–416.
8. Daley CL, Iaccarino JM, Lange C, et al. Treatment of nontuberculous mycobacterial pulmonary disease: an official ATS/ERS/ESCMID/IDSA clinical Practice guideline. Clin Infect Dis 2020;71(4):e1–36.
9. Dahl VN, Mølhave M, Fløe A, et al. Global trends of pulmonary infections with nontuberculous mycobacteria: a systematic review. Int J Infect Dis 2022;125:120–31.
10. Henkle E, Hedberg K, Schafer S, et al. Population-based incidence of pulmonary nontuberculous mycobacterial disease in Oregon 2007 to 2012. Ann Am Thorac Soc May 2015;12(5):642–7.
11. Lipner EM, Crooks JL, French J, et al. Nontuberculous mycobacterial infection and environmental molybdenum in persons with cystic fibrosis: a case-control study in Colorado. J Expo Sci Environ Epidemiol 2022;32(2):289–94.
12. Lipner EM, French JP, Falkinham JO 3rd, et al. Nontuberculous mycobacteria infection risk and trace metals in surface water: a population-based ecologic epidemiologic study in Oregon. Ann Am Thorac Soc 2022;19(4):543–50.

13. Andréjak C, Thomsen V, Johansen IS, et al. Nontuberculous pulmonary mycobacteriosis in Denmark: incidence and prognostic factors. Am J Respir Crit Care Med 2010;181(5):514–21.

14. Marras TK, Mehta M, Chedore P, et al. Nontuberculous mycobacterial lung infections in Ontario, Canada: clinical and microbiological characteristics. Lung Aug 2010;188(4):289–99.

15. Ghio AJ, Smith GS, DeFlorio-Barker S, et al. Application of diagnostic criteria for non-tuberculous mycobacterial disease to a case series of mycobacterial-positive isolates. J Clin Tuberc Other Mycobact Dis Dec 2019;17:100133.

16. Prevots DR, Shaw PA, Strickland D, et al. Nontuberculous mycobacterial lung disease prevalence at four integrated health care delivery systems. Am J Respir Crit Care Med Oct 1 2010;182(7): 970–6.

17. Winthrop KL, Baxter R, Liu L, et al. The reliability of diagnostic coding and laboratory data to identify tuberculosis and nontuberculous mycobacterial disease among rheumatoid arthritis patients using anti-tumor necrosis factor therapy. Pharmacoepidemiol Drug Saf 2011;20(3):229–35.

18. Ku JH, Henkle EM, Carlson KF, et al. Validity of diagnosis code-based claims to identify pulmonary NTM disease in bronchiectasis patients. Emerg Infect Dis 2021;27(3):982–5.

19. Winthrop KL, McNelley E, Kendall B, et al. Pulmonary nontuberculous mycobacterial disease prevalence and clinical features: an emerging public health disease. Am J Respir Crit Care Med Oct 1 2010;182(7):977–82.

20. Mercaldo RA, Marshall JE, Cangelosi GA, et al. Environmental risk of nontuberculous mycobacterial infection: strategies for advancing methodology. Tuberculosis 2023;102305. https://doi.org/10.1016/j.tube.2023.102305.

21. Grigg C, Jackson KA, Barter D, et al. Epidemiology of pulmonary and extrapulmonary nontuberculous mycobacteria infections in four U.S. Emerging infections program sites: a six-month pilot. Clin Infect Dis 2023. https://doi.org/10.1093/cid/ciad214.

22. Vinnard C, Longworth S, Mezochow A, et al. Deaths related to nontuberculous mycobacterial infections in the United States, 1999-2014. Ann Am Thorac Soc 2016;13(11):1951–5.

23. Morimoto K, Iwai K, Uchimura K, et al. A steady increase in nontuberculous mycobacteriosis mortality and estimated prevalence in Japan. Ann Am Thorac Soc 2014;11(1):1–8.

24. Marras TK, Vinnard C, Zhang Q, et al. Relative risk of all-cause mortality in patients with nontuberculous mycobacterial lung disease in a US managed care population. Respir Med 2018;145:80–8.

25. Mourad A, Baker AW, Stout JE. Reduction in expected survival associated with nontuberculous mycobacterial pulmonary disease. Clin Infect Dis May 18 2021;72(10):e552–7.

26. Diel R, Jacob J, Lampenius N, et al. Burden of nontuberculous mycobacterial pulmonary disease in Germany. Eur Respir J 2017;49(4). https://doi.org/10.1183/13993003.02109-2016.

27. Tzou CL, Dirac MA, Becker AL, et al. Association between Mycobacterium avium complex pulmonary disease and mycobacteria in home water and soil. Ann Am Thorac Soc 2020;17(1):57–62.

28. Thomson R, Tolson C, Carter R, et al. Isolation of nontuberculous mycobacteria (NTM) from household water and shower aerosols in patients with pulmonary disease caused by NTM. J Clin Microbiol 2013;51(9):3006–11.

29. Dirac MA, Horan KL, Doody DR, et al. Environment or host?: a case-control study of risk factors for Mycobacterium avium complex lung disease. Am J Respir Crit Care Med Oct 1 2012;186(7): 684–91.

30. Park Y, Kwak SH, Yong SH, et al. The association between behavioral risk factors and nontuberculous mycobacterial pulmonary disease. Yonsei Med J 2021;62(8):702–7.

31. Prevots DR, Adjemian J, Fernandez AG, et al. Environmental risks for nontuberculous mycobacteria. Individual exposures and climatic factors in the cystic fibrosis population. Ann Am Thorac Soc 2014;11(7):1032–8.

32. Bouso JM, Burns JJ, Amin R, et al. Household proximity to water and nontuberculous mycobacteria in children with cystic fibrosis. Pediatr Pulmonol Mar 2017;52(3):324–30.

33. Maekawa K, Ito Y, Hirai T, et al. Environmental risk factors for pulmonary Mycobacterium avium-intracellulare complex disease. Chest 2011;140(3): 723–9.

34. Reed C, von Reyn CF, Chamblee S, et al. Environmental risk factors for infection with Mycobacterium avium complex. Am J Epidemiol Jul 1 2006;164(1): 32–40.

35. Gebert MJ, Delgado-Baquerizo M, Oliverio AM, et al. Ecological analyses of mycobacteria in showerhead biofilms and their relevance to human health. mBio 2018;9(5):e01614–8.

36. Lipner EM, French JP, Nelson S, et al. Vanadium in groundwater aquifers increases the risk of MAC pulmonary infection in O'ahu, Hawai'i. Environ Epidemiol Oct 2022;6(5):e220.

37. Oh J, Shin SH, Choi R, et al. Assessment of 7 trace elements in serum of patients with nontuberculous mycobacterial lung disease. J Trace Elem Med Biol 2019;53:84–90.

38. DeFlorio-Barker S, Egorov A, Smith GS, et al. Environmental risk factors associated with pulmonary isolation of nontuberculous mycobacteria, a population-based study in the southeastern

United States. Sci Total Environ Apr 1 2021;763: 144552.

39. Adjemian J, Olivier KN, Seitz AE, et al. Spatial clusters of nontuberculous mycobacterial lung disease in the United States. Am J Respir Crit Care Med Sep 15 2012;186(6):553–8.

40. Adjemian J, Olivier KN, Prevots DR. Nontuberculous mycobacteria among patients with cystic fibrosis in the United States: screening practices and environmental risk. Am J Respir Crit Care Med 2014;190(5):581–6.

41. Thomson RM, Furuya-Kanamori L, Coffey C, et al. Influence of climate variables on the rising incidence of nontuberculous mycobacterial (NTM) infections in Queensland, Australia 2001-2016. Sci Total Environ Oct 20 2020;740:139796.

42. Chou MP, Clements ACA, Thomson RM. A spatial epidemiological analysis of nontuberculous mycobacterial infections in Queensland, Australia. BMC Infect Dis 2014;14(1):279.

43. Maki T, Noda J, Morimoto K, et al. Long-range transport of airborne bacteria over East Asia: Asian dust events carry potentially nontuberculous Mycobacterium populations. Environ Int 2022;168:107471.

44. Schildkraut JA, Gallagher J, Morimoto K, et al. Epidemiology of nontuberculous mycobacterial pulmonary disease in Europe and Japan by Delphi estimation. Respir Med 2020;173:106164.

45. Winthrop KL, Marras TK, Adjemian J, et al. Incidence and prevalence of nontuberculous mycobacterial lung disease in a large U.S. Managed care health plan, 2008-2015. Ann Am Thorac Soc 2020;17(2):178–85.

46. Strollo SE, Adjemian J, Adjemian MK, et al. The burden of pulmonary nontuberculous mycobacterial disease in the United States. Ann Am Thorac Soc Oct 2015;12(10):1458–64.

47. Pyarali FF, Schweitzer M, Bagley V, et al. Increasing non-tuberculous mycobacteria infections in veterans with COPD and association with increased risk of mortality. Front Med (Lausanne) 2018;5:311.

48. Spaulding AB, Lai YL, Zelazny AM, et al. Geographic distribution of nontuberculous mycobacterial species identified among clinical isolates in the United States, 2009-2013. Ann Am Thorac Soc 2017;14(11):1655–61.

49. Dean SG, Ricotta EE, Fintzi J, et al. Mycobacterial testing trends, United States, 2009-2015(1). Emerg Infect Dis 2020;26(9):2243–6.

50. Donohue MJ. Increasing nontuberculous mycobacteria reporting rates and species diversity identified in clinical laboratory reports. BMC Infect Dis 2018;18(1):163.

51. Donohue MJ, Wymer L. Increasing prevalence rate of nontuberculous mycobacteria infections in five states, 2008–2013. Ann Am Thorac Soc 2016; 13(12):2143–50.

52. Adjemian J, Frankland TB, Daida YG, et al. Epidemiology of nontuberculous mycobacterial lung disease and tuberculosis, Hawaii, USA. Emerg Infect Dis 2017;23(3):439–47.

53. Blakney RA, Ricotta EE, Frankland TB, et al. Incidence of nontuberculous mycobacterial pulmonary infection, by ethnic group, Hawaii, USA, 2005-2019. Emerg Infect Dis 2022;28(8):1543–50.

54. Lin C, Russell C, Soll B, et al. Increasing prevalence of nontuberculous mycobacteria in respiratory specimens from US-affiliated pacific island jurisdictions(1). Emerg Infect Disr 2018;24(3): 485–91.

55. Kambali S, Quinonez E, Sharifi A, et al. Pulmonary nontuberculous mycobacterial disease in Florida and association with large-scale natural disasters. BMC Public Health 2021;21(1):2058.

56. Garcia CV, Teo GE, Zeitler K, et al. The epidemiology, demographics, and comorbidities of pulmonary and extra-pulmonary non-tuberculous mycobacterial infections at a large central Florida Academic Hospital. J Clin Tuberc Other Mycobact Dis Dec 2021;25:100289.

57. Adjemian J, Olivier KN, Prevots DR. Epidemiology of pulmonary nontuberculous mycobacterial sputum positivity in patients with cystic fibrosis in the United States, 2010–2014. Ann Am Thorac Soc 2018/07/01 2018;15(7):817–26.

58. Smith GS, Ghio AJ, Stout JE, et al. Epidemiology of nontuberculous mycobacteria isolations among central North Carolina residents, 2006-2010. J Infect Jun 2016;72(6):678–86.

59. Marras TK, Mendelson D, Marchand-Austin A, et al. Pulmonary nontuberculous mycobacterial disease, Ontario, Canada, 1998-2010. Emerg Infect Dis 2013;19(11):1889–91.

60. Raats D, Brode SK, Mehrabi M, et al. Increasing and more commonly refractory Mycobacterium avium pulmonary disease, toronto, Ontario, Canada. Emerg Infect Dis 2022;28(8):1589–96.

61. Chaptal M, Andrejak C, Bonifay T, et al. Epidemiology of infection by pulmonary non-tuberculous mycobacteria in French Guiana 2008-2018. Plos Negl Trop Dis 2022;16(9):e0010693.

62. Lopez-Luis BA, Sifuentes-Osornio J, Pérez-Gutiérrez MT, et al. Nontuberculous mycobacterial infection in a tertiary care center in Mexico, 2001-2017. Braz J Infect Dis May-Jun 2020;24(3): 213–20.

63. Carneiro MDS, Nunes LS, David SMM, et al. Nontuberculous mycobacterial lung disease in a high tuberculosis incidence setting in Brazil. J Bras Pneumol 2018;44(2):106–11.

64. Marques LRM, Ferrazoli L, Chimara É. Pulmonary nontuberculous mycobacterial infections: presumptive diagnosis based on the international microbiological criteria adopted in the state of

São Paulo, Brazil, 2011-2014. J Bras Pneumol Apr 25 2019;45(2):e20180278.

65. De Lima Mota MA, De Melo DM, Christyan Nunes Beserra FL, et al. Clinical-epidemiological profile and factors related to the mortality of patients with nontuberculous mycobacteria isolated at a reference hospital in Ceará, Northeastern Brazil. Int J Mycobacteriol 2020;9(1):83–90.

66. López A, Acosta F, Sambrano D, et al. Direct molecular characterization of acid-fast bacilli smear of nontuberculosis Mycobacterium species causing pulmonary tuberculosis in guna yala region, Panama. Am J Trop Med Hyg 2021;105(3):633–7.

67. Greif G, Coitinho C, van Ingen J, et al. Species distribution and isolation frequency of nontuberculous mycobacteria, Uruguay. Emerg Infect Dis 2020; 26(5):1014–8.

68. Hermansen TS, Ravn P, Svensson E, et al. Nontuberculous mycobacteria in Denmark, incidence and clinical importance during the last quarter-century. Scientific Rep 2017;7(1):6696.

69. Veziris N, Andréjak C, Bouée S, et al. Non-tuberculous mycobacterial pulmonary diseases in France: an 8 years nationwide study. BMC Infect Dis 2021; 21(1):1165.

70. Schildkraut JA, Zweijpfenning SMH, Nap M, et al. The epidemiology of nontuberculous mycobacterial pulmonary disease in The Netherlands. ERJ Open Res 2021;7(3). https://doi.org/10.1183/23120 541.00207-2021.

71. Ringshausen FC, Ewen R, Multmeier J, et al. Predictive modeling of nontuberculous mycobacterial pulmonary disease epidemiology using German health claims data. Int J Infect Dis 2021;104: 398–406.

72. Ringshausen FC, Wagner D, de Roux A, et al. Prevalence of nontuberculous mycobacterial pulmonary disease, Germany, 2009-2014. Emerg Infect Dis 2016;22(6):1102–5.

73. Oliveira MJ, Gaio AR, Gomes M, et al. Mycobacterium avium infection in Portugal. Int J Tuberc Lung Dis 2017;21(2):218–22.

74. Dakić I, Arandjelović I, Savić B, et al. Pulmonary isolation and clinical relevance of nontuberculous mycobacteria during nationwide survey in Serbia, 2010-2015. PLoS One 2018;13(11):e0207751.

75. Santin M, Barrabeig I, Malchair P, et al. Pulmonary infections with nontuberculous mycobacteria, Catalonia, Spain, 1994-2014. Emerg Infect Dis 2018; 24(6):1091–4.

76. Alcaide F, Peña MJ, Pérez-Risco D, et al. Increasing isolation of rapidly growing mycobacteria in a low-incidence setting of environmental mycobacteria, 1994-2015. Eur J Clin Microbiol Infect Dis Aug 2017;36(8):1425–32.

77. Shah NM, Davidson JA, Anderson LF, et al. Pulmonary Mycobacterium avium-intracellulare is the main driver of the rise in non-tuberculous mycobacteria incidence in England, Wales and Northern Ireland, 2007-2012. BMC Infect Dis May 6 2016;16: 195.

78. Pedrero S, Tabernero E, Arana-Arri E, et al. Changing epidemiology of nontuberculous mycobacterial lung disease over the last two decades in a region of the Basque country. ERJ Open Res Oct 2019;5(4). https://doi.org/10.1183/23120541.00110-2018.

79. Axson EL, Bloom CI, Quint JK. Nontuberculous mycobacterial disease managed within UK primary care, 2006-2016. Eur J Clin Microbiol Infect Dis 2018;37(9):1795–803.

80. Hoefsloot W, van Ingen J, Andrejak C, et al. The geographic diversity of nontuberculous mycobacteria isolated from pulmonary samples: an NTM-NET collaborative study. Eur Respir J 2013;42(6):1604.

81. Modrá H, Ulmann V, Caha J, et al. Socio-economic and environmental factors related to spatial differences in human non-tuberculous mycobacterial diseases in the Czech republic. Int J Environ Res Public Health 2019;16(20). https://doi.org/10. 3390/ijerph16203969.

82. Dahl VN, Fløe A, Wejse C. Nontuberculous mycobacterial infections in a Danish region between 2011 and 2021: evaluation of trends in diagnostic codes. Infect Dis (Lond) 2023;30:1–5.

83. Mejia-Chew C, Yaeger L, Montes K, et al. Diagnostic accuracy of health care administrative diagnosis codes to identify nontuberculous mycobacteria disease: a systematic review. Open Forum Infect Dis 2021;8(5):ofab035. http://europepmc. org/abstract/MED/34041304.

84. Panagiotou M, Papaioannou AI, Kostikas K, et al. The epidemiology of pulmonary nontuberculous mycobacteria: data from a general hospital in Athens, Greece, 2007-2013. Pulm Med 2014; 2014:894976.

85. Lange C, Böttger EC, Cambau E, et al. Consensus management recommendations for less common non-tuberculous mycobacterial pulmonary diseases. Lancet Infect Dis 2022;22(7):e178–90.

86. Russell CD, Claxton P, Doig C, et al. Non-tuberculous mycobacteria: a retrospective review of Scottish isolates from 2000 to 2010. Thorax 2014; 69(6):593–5.

87. Okoi C, Anderson STB, Antonio M, et al. Non-tuberculous mycobacteria isolated from pulmonary samples in sub-saharan Africa - a systematic review and meta analyses. Sci Rep 2017;7(1):12002.

88. Gharbi R, Mhenni B, Ben Fraj S, et al. Nontuberculous mycobacteria isolated from specimens of pulmonary tuberculosis suspects, Northern Tunisia: 2002-2016. BMC Infect Dis 2019;19(1):819.

89. Agizew T, Basotli J, Alexander H, et al. Higher-than-expected prevalence of non-tuberculous mycobacteria in HIV setting in Botswana: implications

for diagnostic algorithms using Xpert MTB/RIF assay. PLoS One 2017;12(12):e0189981.

90. Otchere ID, Asante-Poku A, Osei-Wusu S, et al. Isolation and characterization of nontuberculous mycobacteria from patients with pulmonary tuberculosis in Ghana. Int J Mycobacteriol 2017;6(1): 70–5.

91. Bjerrum S, Oliver-Commey J, Kenu E, et al. Tuberculosis and non-tuberculous mycobacteria among HIV-infected individuals in Ghana. Trop Med Int Health 2016;21(9):1181–90.

92. Kone B, Sarro YS, Maiga M, et al. Clinical characteristics of non-tuberculous mycobacterial pulmonary infections in Bamako, Mali. Epidemiol Infect 2018;146(3):354–8.

93. Alemayehu A, Kebede A, Neway S, et al. A glimpse into the genotype and clinical importance of non tuberculous mycobacteria among pulmonary tuberculosis patients: the case of Ethiopia. PLoS One 2022;17(9):e0275159.

94. Mwangi ZM, Mukiri NN, Onyambu FG, et al. Genetic diversity of nontuberculous mycobacteria among symptomatic tuberculosis negative patients in Kenya. Int J Mycobacteriol 2022;11(1):60–9.

95. Hoza AS, Mfinanga SG, Rodloff AC, et al. Increased isolation of nontuberculous mycobacteria among TB suspects in Northeastern, Tanzania: public health and diagnostic implications for control programmes. BMC Res Notes 2016;9:109.

96. Chanda-Kapata P, Kapata N, Klinkenberg E, et al. Non-tuberculous mycobacteria (NTM) in Zambia: prevalence, clinical, radiological and microbiological characteristics. BMC Infect Dis 2015;15:500.

97. Epola Dibamba Ndanga M, Agbo Abdul JBP Achimi, Edoa JR, et al. Non-tuberculous mycobacteria isolation from presumptive tuberculosis patients in Lambaréné. Gabon Trop Med Int Health 2022; 27(4):438–44.

98. Park SC, Kang MJ, Han CH, et al. Prevalence, incidence, and mortality of nontuberculous mycobacterial infection in Korea: a nationwide population-based study. BMC Pulm Med 2019;19(1):140.

99. Park JH, Shin S, Kim TS, et al. Clinically refined epidemiology of nontuberculous mycobacterial pulmonary disease in South Korea: overestimation when relying only on diagnostic codes. BMC Pulm Med 2022;22(1):195.

100. Park Y, Kim CY, Park MS, et al. Age- and sex-related characteristics of the increasing trend of nontuberculous mycobacteria pulmonary disease in a tertiary hospital in South Korea from 2006 to 2016. Korean J Intern Med 2020;35(6):1424–31.

101. Lee YM, Kim MJ, Kim YJ. Increasing trend of non-tuberculous mycobacteria isolation in a referral clinical laboratory in South Korea. Medicina (Kaunas) 2021;57(7). https://doi.org/10.3390/medicina 57070720.

102. Ahn K, Kim YK, Hwang GY, et al. Continued upward trend in non-tuberculous mycobacteria isolation over 13 Years in a tertiary care hospital in Korea. Yonsei Med J 2021;62(10):903–10.

103. Kim N, Yi J, Chang CL. Recovery rates of non-tuberculous mycobacteria from clinical specimens are increasing in Korean tertiary-care hospitals. J Korean Med Sci 2017;32(8):1263–7.

104. Ko RE, Moon SM, Ahn S, et al. Changing epidemiology of nontuberculous mycobacterial lung diseases in a tertiary referral hospital in Korea between 2001 and 2015. J Korean Med Sci 2018; 33(8):e65.

105. Morimoto K, Hasegawa N, Izumi K, et al. A laboratory-based analysis of nontuberculous mycobacterial lung disease in Japan from 2012 to 2013. Ann Am Thorac Soc 2017;14(1):49–56.

106. Morimoto K, Ato M, Hasegawa N, et al. Population-based distribution of Mycobacterium avium and Mycobacterium intracellulare in Japan. Microbiol Res 2021;12(3):739–43.

107. Izumi K, Morimoto K, Hasegawa N, et al. Epidemiology of adults and children treated for nontuberculous mycobacterial pulmonary disease in Japan. Ann Am Thorac Soc 2019;16(3):341–7.

108. Ito Y, Hirai T, Fujita K, et al. Increasing patients with pulmonary Mycobacterium avium complex disease and associated underlying diseases in Japan. J Infect Chemother 2015;21(5):352–6.

109. Furuuchi K, Morimoto K, Yoshiyama T, et al. Interrelational changes in the epidemiology and clinical features of nontuberculous mycobacterial pulmonary disease and tuberculosis in a referral hospital in Japan. Respir Med 2019;152:74–80.

110. Harada K, Hagiya H, Funahashi T, et al. Trends in the nontuberculous mycobacterial disease mortality rate in Japan: a nationwide observational study, 1997-2016. Clin Infect Dis 2021;73(2):e321–6.

111. Hagiwara E, Katano T, Isomoto K, et al. Clinical characteristics and early outcomes of patients newly diagnosed with pulmonary Mycobacterium avium complex disease. Respir Investig 2019;57(1):54–9.

112. Lin CK, Yang YH, Lu ML, et al. Incidence of nontuberculous mycobacterial disease and coinfection with tuberculosis in a tuberculosis-endemic region: a population-based retrospective cohort study. Medicine (Baltimore) 2020;99(52):e23775.

113. Chen HH, Lin CH, Chao WC. Mortality association of nontuberculous mycobacterial infection requiring treatment in Taiwan: a population-based study. Ther Adv Respir Dis 2022;16. https://doi.org/10.1177/17534666221103213. 17534666221103213.

114. Chiang CY, Yu MC, Yang SL, et al. Surveillance of tuberculosis in taipei: the influence of nontuberculous mycobacteria. PLoS One 2015;10(11): e0142324.

115. Chien JY, Lai CC, Sheng WH, et al. Pulmonary infection and colonization with nontuberculous mycobacteria, Taiwan, 2000-2012. Emerg Infect Dis 2014;20(8):1382–5.

116. Huang HL, Cheng MH, Lu PL, et al. Epidemiology and predictors of NTM pulmonary infection in taiwan - a retrospective, five-year multicenter study. Sci Rep 2017;7(1):16300.

117. Tan Y, Deng Y, Yan X, et al. Nontuberculous mycobacterial pulmonary disease and associated risk factors in China: a prospective surveillance study. J Infect 2021;83(1):46–53.

118. Ji LC, Chen S, Piao W, et al. Increasing trends and species diversity of nontuberculous mycobacteria in A coastal migrant city-shenzhen, China. Biomed Environ Sci 2022;35(2):146–50.

119. Sun Q, Yan J, Liao X, et al. Trends and species diversity of non-tuberculous mycobacteria isolated from respiratory samples in northern China, 2014-2021. Front Public Health 2022;10:923968.

120. Duan H, Han X, Wang Q, et al. Clinical significance of nontuberculous mycobacteria isolated from respiratory specimens in a Chinese tuberculosis tertiary care center. Sci Rep 2016;6:36299.

121. Sumbul B, Doymaz MZ. A current microbiological picture of Mycobacterium isolates from istanbul, Turkey. Pol J Microbiol 2020;69(2):1–7.

122. Karamat A, Ambreen A, Ishtiaq A, et al. Isolation of non-tuberculous mycobacteria among tuberculosis patients, a study from a tertiary care hospital in Lahore, Pakistan. BMC Infect Dis 2021;21(1):381.

123. Khosravi AD, Mirsaeidi M, Farahani A, et al. Prevalence of nontuberculous mycobacteria and high efficacy of d-cycloserine and its synergistic effect with clarithromycin against Mycobacterium fortuitum and Mycobacterium abscessus. Infect Drug Resist 2018;11:2521–32.

124. Ayoubi S, Aghajani J, Farnia P, et al. Prevalence of Mycobacterium abscessus among the patients with nontuberculous mycobacteria. Arch Iran Med 2020;23(3):163–8.

125. Suresh P, Kumar A, Biswas R, et al. Epidemiology of nontuberculous mycobacterial infection in tuberculosis suspects. Am J Trop Med Hyg 2021;105(5):1335–8.

126. Umrao J, Singh D, Zia A, et al. Prevalence and species spectrum of both pulmonary and extrapulmonary nontuberculous mycobacteria isolates at a tertiary care center. Int J Mycobacteriol 2016;5(3):288–93.

127. Sebastian G, Nagaraja SB, Vishwanatha T, et al. Non-tuberculosis mycobacterium speciation using HPLC under revised national TB control programme (RNTCP) in India. J Appl Microbiol 2018;124(1):267–73.

128. Phelippeau M, Osman DA, Musso D, et al. Epidemiology of nontuberculous mycobacteria in French Polynesia. J Clin Microbiol 2015;53(12):3798–804.

129. Ley S, Carter R, Millan K, et al. Non-tuberculous mycobacteria: baseline data from three sites in Papua New Guinea, 2010-2012. West. Pac Surveill Response J 2015;6(4):24–9.

130. Foote SL, Lipner EM, Prevots DR, et al. Environmental predictors of pulmonary nontuberculous mycobacteria (NTM) sputum positivity among persons with cystic fibrosis in the state of Florida. PLoS One 2021;16(12):e0259964.

131. Brode SK, Marchand-Austin A, Jamieson FB, et al. Pulmonary versus nonpulmonary nontuberculous mycobacteria, Ontario, Canada. Emerg Infect Dis 2017;23(11):1898–901.

132. Ide S, Nakamura S, Yamamoto Y, et al. Epidemiology and clinical features of pulmonary nontuberculous mycobacteriosis in Nagasaki, Japan. PLoS One 2015;10(5):e0128304.

133. Kim HO, Lee K, Choi HK, et al. Incidence, comorbidities, and treatment patterns of nontuberculous mycobacterial infection in South Korea. Medicine (Baltimore) 2019;98(45):e17869.

134. Nasiri MJ, Dabiri H, Darban-Sarokhalil D, et al. Prevalence of non-tuberculosis mycobacterial infections among tuberculosis suspects in Iran: systematic review and meta-analysis. PLoS One 2015;10(6):e0129073.

135. Boyle DP, Zembower TR, Reddy S, et al. Comparison of clinical features, virulence, and relapse among Mycobacterium avium complex species. Am J Respir Crit Care Med 2015;191(11):1310–7.

136. Hannah CE, Ford BA, Chung J, et al. Characteristics of nontuberculous mycobacterial infections at a midwestern tertiary hospital: a retrospective study of 365 patients. Open Forum Infect Dis 2020;7(6):ofaa173.

137. Martin A, Colmant A, Verroken A, et al. Laboratory diagnosis of nontuberculous mycobacteria in a Belgium Hospital. Int J Mycobacteriol Apr-Jun 2019;8(2):157–61.

138. Vande Weygaerde Y, Cardinaels N, Bomans P, et al. Clinical relevance of pulmonary non-tuberculous mycobacterial isolates in three reference centres in Belgium: a multicentre retrospective analysis. BMC Infect Dis 2019;19(1):1061.

139. Glodić G, Samaržija M, Sabol I, et al. Risk factors for nontuberculous mycobacterial pulmonary disease (NTM-PD) in Croatia. Wien Klin Wochenschr 2021;133(21–22):1195–200.

140. Blanc P, Dutronc H, Peuchant O, et al. Nontuberculous mycobacterial infections in a French hospital: a 12-year retrospective study. PLoS One 2016;11(12):e0168290.

141. Bemer P, Peuchant O, Guet-Revillet H, et al. Management of patients with pulmonary mycobacteriosis in France: a multicenter retrospective cohort study. BMC Pulm Med 2021;21(1):333.

142. Wetzstein N, Hügel C, Wichelhaus TA, et al. Species distribution and clinical features of infection

and colonisation with non-tuberculous mycobacteria in a tertiary care centre, central Germany, 2006-2016. Infection 2019;47(5):817–25.

143. Chong SG, Kent BD, Fitzgerald S, et al. Pulmonary non-tuberculous mycobacteria in a general respiratory population. Ir Med J Jul-Aug 2014;107(7):207–9.

144. Zweijpfenning S, Kops S, Magis-Escurra C, et al. Treatment and outcome of non-tuberculous mycobacterial pulmonary disease in a predominantly fibro-cavitary disease cohort. Respir Med Oct 2017;131:220–4.

145. Szturmowicz M, Siemion-Szcześniak I, Wyrostkiewicz D, et al. Factors predisposing to non-tuberculous mycobacterial lung disease in the patients with respiratory isolates of non-tuberculous mycobacteria. Adv Respir Med 2018. https://doi.org/10.5603/ARM.a2018.0043.

146. Kwiatkowska S, Augustynowicz-Kopeć E, Korzeniewska-Kosela M, et al. Nontuberculous mycobacteria strains isolated from patients between 2013 and 2017 in Poland. Our data with respect to the global trends. Adv Respir Med 2018. https://doi.org/10.5603/ARM.a2018.0047.

147. Ramos AL, Carvalho T, Guimarães JT. The importance of multiple samples in mycobacterial recovery: a 10-year retrospective study. Int J Mycobacteriol Apr-Jun 2019;8(2):175–9.

148. Adzic-Vukicevic T, Barac A, Blanka-Protic A, et al. Clinical features of infection caused by non-tuberculous mycobacteria: 7 years' experience. Infection 2018;46(3):357–63.

149. Blanco Pérez JJ, Pérez González A, Morano Amado LE, et al. Clinical significance of environmental mycobacteria isolated from respiratory specimens of patients with and without silicosis. Arch Bronconeumol 2016;52(3):145–50.

150. Matesanz López C, Loras Gallego C, Cacho Calvo J, et al. Patients with non-tuberculous mycobacteria in respiratory samples: a 5-year epidemiological study. Rev Esp Quimioter Apr 2021;34(2):120–5.

151. Vongthilath-Moeung R, Plojoux J, Poncet A, et al. Nontuberculous mycobacteria under scrutiny in the geneva area (2015-2020). Respiration 2022;101(4):367–75.

152. Schiff HF, Jones S, Achaiah A, et al. Clinical relevance of non-tuberculous mycobacteria isolated from respiratory specimens: seven year experience in a UK hospital. Sci Rep 2019;9(1):1730.

153. Pokam BDT, Yeboah-Manu D, Ofori S, et al. Prevalence of non-tuberculous mycobacteria among previously treated TB patients in the Gulf of Guinea, Africa. IJID Reg 2022;3:287–92.

154. Maya TG, Komba EV, Mensah GI, et al. Drug susceptibility profiles and factors associated with non-tuberculous mycobacteria species circulating among patients diagnosed with pulmonary tuberculosis in Tanzania. PLoS One 2022;17(3):e0265358.

155. Wu J, Zhang Y, Li J, et al. Increase in nontuberculous mycobacteria isolated in Shanghai, China: results from a population-based study. PLoS One 2014;9(10):e109736.

156. Zhu Y, Hua W, Liu Z, et al. Identification and characterization of nontuberculous mycobacteria isolated from suspected pulmonary tuberculosis patients in eastern China from 2009 to 2019 using an identification array system. Braz J Infect Dis 2022;26(2):102346.

157. Tan Y, Su B, Shu W, et al. Epidemiology of pulmonary disease due to nontuberculous mycobacteria in Southern China, 2013-2016. BMC Pulm Med 2018;18(1):168.

158. Hu C, Huang L, Cai M, et al. Characterization of non-tuberculous mycobacterial pulmonary disease in Nanjing district of China. BMC Infect Dis 2019;19(1):764.

159. Xu J, Li P, Zheng S, et al. Prevalence and risk factors of pulmonary nontuberculous mycobacterial infections in the Zhejiang Province of China. Epidemiol Infect Sep 11 2019;147:e269.

160. Nagano H, Kinjo T, Nei Y, et al. Causative species of nontuberculous mycobacterial lung disease and comparative investigation on clinical features of Mycobacterium abscessus complex disease: a retrospective analysis for two major hospitals in a subtropical region of Japan. PLoS One 2017;12(10):e0186826.

161. Sharma SK, Upadhyay V. Non-tuberculous mycobacteria: a disease beyond TB and preparedness in India. Expert Rev Respir Med 2021;15(7):949–58.

162. Lim AYH, Chotirmall SH, Fok ETK, et al. Profiling non-tuberculous mycobacteria in an Asian setting: characteristics and clinical outcomes of hospitalized patients in Singapore. BMC Pulm Med 2018;18(1):85.

163. Zhang ZX, Cherng BPZ, Sng LH, et al. Clinical and microbiological characteristics of non-tuberculous mycobacteria diseases in Singapore with a focus on pulmonary disease, 2012-2016. BMC Infect Dis May 17 2019;19(1):436.

164. Al-Harbi A, Al-Jahdali H, Al-Johani S, et al. Frequency and clinical significance of respiratory isolates of non-tuberculous mycobacteria in Riyadh, Saudi Arabia. Clin Respir J 2016;10(2):198–203.

165. Gochi M, Takayanagi N, Kanauchi T, et al. Retrospective study of the predictors of mortality and radiographic deterioration in 782 patients with nodular/bronchiectatic Mycobacterium avium complex lung disease. BMJ Open Aug 5 2015;5(8):e008058.

166. Uno S, Asakura T, Morimoto K, et al. Comorbidities associated with nontuberculous mycobacterial disease in Japanese adults: a claims-data analysis. BMC Pulm Med Oct 9 2020;20(1):262.

Host Susceptibility to Nontuberculous Mycobacterial Pulmonary Disease

Ho Namkoong, MD, PhD, MPH[a],*, Steven M. Holland, MD[b]

KEYWORDS

• NTM • MAC • Host susceptibility • WES • GWAS

KEY POINTS

- Nontuberculous Mycobacteria (NTM) now contains more than 200 distinct species of mycobacteria excluding *Mycobacterium tuberculosis* and *Mycobacterium leprae*.
- The number of NTM is growing due to better cultivation and markedly improved sequence-based identification.
- In parallel, the worldwide prevalence of NTM infections has also risen over the last several decades, reflecting improved awareness, improved diagnosis, and reduced prevalence of competing and confounding diseases, such as tuberculosis.

INTRODUCTION

Nontuberculous Mycobacteria (NTM) now contains more than 200 distinct species of mycobacteria excluding *Mycobacterium tuberculosis* and *Mycobacterium leprae*,[1] and the number of NTM is growing due to better cultivation and markedly improved sequence-based identification.[2] In parallel, the worldwide prevalence of NTM infections has also risen over the last several decades, reflecting improved awareness, improved diagnosis, and reduced prevalence of competing and confounding diseases, such as tuberculosis.[3] The existence of host susceptibility to NTM infection has been recognized since early in the appreciation of these infections, since NTM are low virulent bacteria that are ubiquitous in the environment, such as water and soil, and affect only a very few patients compared to those exposed.[4,5] This hypothesis is supported by multiple epidemiological observations, including a high incidence among Asians compared to other populations in the United States, a high incidence among slender, middle-aged women, and the presence of familial clusters.[6–11]

In recent years, new findings in the field of NTM have been obtained through new analyses, including next generation sequencing (NGS), which will be summarized in this review.[12]

CLINICAL FEATURES OF NONTUBERCULOUS MYCOBACTERIA INFECTIONS

NTM disease manifests with heterogeneous clinical presentations, each potentially exhibiting distinct pathophysiological mechanisms. Consequently, understanding the clinical characteristics of NTM disease is crucial for examining disease susceptibility genes. NTM disease is mainly categorized into four types based on pathological findings and radiological imaging: (1) nodular bronchiectatic disease (NB type), (2) fibrocavitary

[a] Department of Infectious Diseases, Keio University School of Medicine, 35 Shinanomachi Shinjyuku-ku, Tokyo 160-8582, Japan; [b] Division of Intramural Research, Laboratory of Clinical Immunology and Microbiology, National Institute of Allergy and Infectious Diseases (NIAID), National Institutes of Health (NIH), 10/11N248, MSC 1960, Bethesda, MD 20892-1960, USA
* Corresponding author.
E-mail address: hounamugun@keio.jp

Clin Chest Med 44 (2023) 723–730
https://doi.org/10.1016/j.ccm.2023.07.002
0272-5231/23/© 2023 Elsevier Inc. All rights reserved.

disease (FC type), (3) hot tub lung (hypersensitivity-like disease), and (4) systemic dissemination (disseminated disease).[13]

The nodular bronchiectatic type is the most prevalent form predominantly afflicting middle-aged nonsmoking women, with a predilection for the right middle lobe and the left lingula. The fibrocavitary type was initially observed in those who had pre-existing lung destruction, such as due to pulmonary tuberculosis and smoking. Both prior tuberculosis and COPD are more frequent in males, heavy smokers, and the elderly, and in this setting the fibrocavitary disease progresses more rapidly than the nodular bronchiectatic type, and is associated with a poorer prognosis.[14] On the other hand, it appears that the nodular bronchiectatic type is thought to be more affected by intrinsic host susceptibility. The presence of different mycobacterial strains recovered over time in many of the relapsed nodular bronchiectatic type patients in the pre- and post-treatment phases indicates that the redevelopment of MAC in these patients reflects patient-specific vulnerability to infection rather than the relapse of a latent pathogen.[15]

Both scenarios are considered distinct from hot tub lung and systemically disseminated forms. Hot tub lung is characterized by acute to subacute fever and dyspnea, resulting from the inhalation of aerosols containing MAC.[16] Chest CT imaging reveals findings similar to those of hypersensitivity pneumonitis. The systemically disseminated form occurs most frequently in children and adults with inborn cellular immunodeficiencies affecting macrophage/T cell interactions, those with advanced HIV/AIDS, those with anti-IFN-γ neutralizing autoantibodies, or following hematopoietic stem cell or organ transplantation.[4,17–19]

Clinical observations suggest that NTM-related bronchiectasis without underlying conditions such as cystic fibrosis (CF) or primary ciliary dyskinesia (PCD) is more frequent in postmenopausal thin women.[20] Several studies have reported an association between female hormones and the pathogenesis of NTM.[21–23] While low serum estradiol levels are reported to be associated with *Mycobacterium avium* complex infection,[23] Choi and colleagues[22] reported that that hormone replacement therapy is associated with an increased risk of NTM infection in postmenopausal women. The pathogenesis of female hormones and NTM infection needs to be further studied. Other risk factors include vitamin D deficiency, immunoglobulin deficiency, rheumatoid arthritis and other connective tissue disorders, silicosis, aspiration and gastro-esophageal reflux disease(-GERD). Tobacco and marijuana smoking, and

the use of immunosuppressive drugs and inhaled steroids, have also been identified as risk factors.[1,4]

RARE VARIANTS VERSUS COMMON VARIANTS

It is important to understand the concept of rare variants and common variants when considering host susceptibility to disease including infectious diseases.[24] Rare variants exhibit a low allele frequency within the population but exert a substantial effect on disease manifestations. Often including mutations in exonic regions (missense mutations, nonsense mutations, insertion-deletion mutations), these variants result in functional alterations of proteins, leading to disease development. Exonic mutations are frequently detected through whole-exome sequencing (WES) or whole-genome sequencing (WGS). Such mutations often contribute to monogenic diseases and adhere to Mendelian inheritance patterns (although rare variants inside of introns can also cause monogenic disorders) (**Fig. 1**).

Conversely, common variants display a relatively high allele frequency within the population, yet each variant's impact on disease may be minimal. Although common variants may reside in exonic regions, the majority are situated in intronic or intergenic regions. These variants are typically identified through genome-wide association studies (GWAS) (see **Fig. 1**).

PATHOPHYSIOLOGY OF NONTUBERCULOUS MYCOBACTERIA DISEASE

The pathophysiology of NTM disease has multiple components ranging from bacteriological and immunological aspects to genes implicated in NTM disease as part of congenital and acquired immunodeficiencies. Over 40% of the acid-fast bacillus' cell body consists of lipid components, predominantly mycolic acid, a unique long-chain branched fatty acid featuring 60 to 90 carbon chains.[25] Mycolic acid is uncommon in nature and absent in other pathogenic microorganisms. These lipid components reside in the outermost layers of the antimicrobe, serving as crucial molecules in host interactions.

Various lipid molecules present in *Mycobacterium tuberculosis*, including glycolipids and phospholipids, are expressed in several NTMs such as *Mycobacterium avium* complex (MAC), which display glycopeptidolipid (GPL) antigens absent in *Mycobacterium tuberculosis*.[26] Differences in pathogenicity and infectivity have been observed among serotypes of MAC. Moreover, anti-GPL-

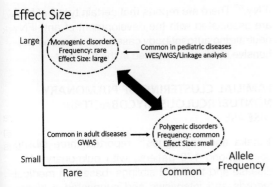

Fig. 1. Rare variants vs common variants. Monogenic disorders are common in pediatric diseases. Their allele frequency is rare. Whole exome sequencing, whole genome sequencing and linkage analysis is effective, and its effect size is large. Polygenic disorders are common in adult diseases. Their allele frequency is common. Genome-wide association study is effective. WES: Whole exome sequencing, WGS: whole genome sequencing, GWAS: genome-wide association study.

core-IgA antibodies in patient sera can be employed as auxiliary diagnostic tools for MAC disease.[27]

When *Mycobacterium smegmatis*, the representative NTM laboratory strain, was mutated to become non-GPL-producing through transposon insertion, not only did colony morphology change from smooth to rough, but the bacteria's virulence factors, including sliding ability and biofilm formation, also disappeared. This suggested the potential role of GPL as critical virulence factors.[28,29]

Other known glycolipid molecules in MAC include phosphatidylinositol mannoside (PIM), lipoarabinomannan (LAM), and lipomannan (LM), all of which may serve as Toll-like receptor (TLR) ligands leading to the activation of macrophages and dendritic cells through their pattern-recognition receptors (PRRs).[30]

Additional pattern-recognition receptors recognizing antimicrobial bacterial components include TLR9, C-type receptors such as the mannose receptor, Dectin-1, Mincle, and DC-SIGN, scavenger receptors SR-A1, SA-A2, MARCO, SR-B1, and CD36, as well as RIG-I and NOD2. These receptors have been thoroughly investigated in tuberculosis research, and warrant further examination of their possible roles in NTM diseases.[31]

Antigen-presenting cells (APCs), including macrophages and dendritic cells that phagocytose NTM and other antimicrobial agents, express MHC (HLA) class II molecules on their cell surfaces. These APCs also secrete cytokines such as IL-12, stimulating NK cells and antigen-presenting CD4$^+$ cells. IL-12 activates STAT4 phosphorylation via TYK2 and JAK2 signaling, leading to IFN-γ secretion. In APCs stimulated by IFN-γ, STAT1 is phosphorylated via JAK1 and JAK2, promoting bactericidal activity against microbes in activated APCs.[4] Phosphorylated STAT1 forms dimers that translocate to the nucleus, binding to IFN-γ activated sites (GAS) and further activating APCs.[32] Through these pathways cellular immunity, primarily Th1, plays a significant role in NTM disease.

GENES RESPONSIBLE FOR MENDELIAN SUSCEPTIBILITY TO MYCOBACTERIAL DISEASE

Mendelian susceptibility to mycobacterial disease (MSMD) encompasses a group of congenital abnormalities characterized by familial clustering due to a Mendelian mode of inheritance.[17] In these disorders the aforementioned aspects of cellular immune signaling, primarily Th1, is impaired. **Table 1** identifies the genes implicated in MSMD, which comprise molecules related to IFN-γ-IL-12 signaling and function (see **Table 1**). These genes are indeed involved in many cases of mycobacterial susceptibility, they are more accurately seen as predisposing to intramacrophagic infection and underlie many other infections, such as Salmonella. IFNGR1 and IFNGR2 encode IFN-γ receptors 1 and 2, respectively. Downstream, STAT1, interferon regulatory factor 8 (IRF8), and other interferon-stimulated genes are also involved.[33] Mutations in IL12B, which encodes the subunit IL-12p40, and IL12RB1, which encodes the IL-12 receptor β1 chain, have been observed.[34] Additionally, mutations in IKBKG, which encodes the NFkB essential modulator (NEMO), and cytochrome b(558) subunit beta (CYBB), which encodes gp91phox, a component of the NADPH oxidase complex, have also been described.[35,36] Abnormalities in GATA2, a hematopoietic transcription factor, may also result in disseminated NTM disease. MonoMAC syndrome, initially reported in 2010, is a primary immunodeficiency disorder typified by monocytopenia and susceptibility to intracellular parasites such as NTM.[37] Disseminated NTM disease may complicate other conditions as well, including STAT1 dominant negative deficiency, and IL23R deficiencies.[38,39] A congenital deficiency of the RORC gene, a master transcription factor of Th17 cells, leading to susceptibility to Candida and NTM is also reported.[40]

Table 1
Genetic etiologies of mendelian susceptibility to mycobacterial disease

Gene	Inheritance Pattern
IFNGR1	AR, AD
IFNGR2	AR, AD
STAT1	AR, AD
IL12B	AR
IL12RB1	AR
IL12RB2	AR
IL23R	AR
TYK2	AR
IRF8	AR, AD
GATA2	AD
ISG15	AR
IKBKG	XR
NFKBIA	AD
CYBB	XR
SPPL2A	AR
RORC	AR
JAK1	AR
TBX21	AR
ZNFX1	AR
PDCD1	AR
USP18	AR

Abbreviations: AD, autosomal dominant; AR, autosomal recessive; XR, x-linked recessive.

DISSEMINATED NONTUBERCULOUS MYCOBACTERIA DUE TO NEUTRALIZING ANTI-IFNγ AUTOANTIBODIES

Since the 1980s, the majority of disseminated NTM disease developing in adults occurred in those with advanced HIV/AIDS.[18] However, more recently reports have identified neutralizing anti-IFNγ autoantibodies in some patients who developed disseminated NTM disease without previously recognized immunodeficiency.[41] This condition has gained attention because it is due to acquired autoantibodies against cytokines and is characterized by numerous lesions in bones and lymph nodes, in addition to the lungs. The majority of anti-IFNγ neutralizing autoantibody cases have been reported in East Asian patients.[42] HLA class II alleles, and the primary epitope to which anti-IFNγ neutralizing autoantibodies bind, have been identified, revealing an amino acid sequence in IFNγ that is highly homologous to a portion of the Aspergillus *Noc2* protein, which is thought to induce autoantibodies that cross-react with endogenous IFNγ.[43] There are reports that certain types of HLA are associated with the development of anti-IFNγ neutralizing autoantibody cases, but more comprehensive studies are needed in the future.[44]

FAMILIAL CLUSTERING OF PULMONARY NONTUBERCULOUS MYCOBACTERIA DISEASE

Tanaka and colleagues[45] reported three sibling pairs among 170 patients with pulmonary MAC disease and their 622 siblings, based on medical records and interviews and suggested a higher prevalence among siblings compared to the general population. Kuwabara and colleagues[46] also documented cases of pulmonary MAC disease in siblings, and their Restriction Fragment Length Polymorphism (RFLP) analysis demonstrated that the bacteria detected in sibling cases were distinct strains. From the United States, the National Institutes of Health (NIH) reported 120 cases of pulmonary NTM disease in six families, in which a parent and child or siblings had pulmonary NTM disease. Five of these families had three or more cases of pulmonary MAC within the same family, suggesting the presence of a disease susceptibility gene.[11] Given that MAC is an environmental bacterium not believed to be transmitted from human to human in the majority of cases (suspected *M. abscessus* transmission within cystic fibrosis units has been reported[47]), these epidemiological findings reveal the likely involvement of important host factors in infection and the subsequent development of disease. The epidemiology of NTM in cystic fibrosis remains complex with both host and environmental aspects mutually confounding.

WHOLE-EXOME SEQUENCING OF NONTUBERCULOUS MYCOBACTERIA-PULMONARY DISEASE

A comprehensive whole exome sequencing (WES) study for pulmonary NTM disease was conducted.[48] Whole exome sequencing was performed on 69 Caucasian patients with pulmonary NTM and 18 unaffected family members. The researchers carried out candidate gene analysis using immune, CFTR, cilia, and connective tissue gene sets. As these genes were presumed to be associated with pulmonary NTM disease, the WES analysis revealed that, compared to unaffected family members and controls, patients with pulmonary NTM harbored more variants in immune, CFTR, cilia, and connective tissue genes that impacted proteins at low frequencies. Whereas in disseminated MSMD NTM disease, a single genetic variant alone was sufficient to cause disseminated NTM disease, numerous factors may be implicated in isolated pulmonary disease.[48]

GENOME WIDE ASSOCIATION STUDIES OF NONTUBERCULOUS MYCOBACTERIA-PULMONARY DISEASE

Focusing on pulmonary MAC disease, which constitutes over 90% of the clinical frequency of pulmonary NTM disease, a genome-wide association study(GWAS) was conducted on 1,066 patients with pulmonary MAC disease and identified a disease susceptibility SNP (rs109592) that met the genome-wide significance threshold (P < 5.0 × 10⁻⁸).[49] In rs109592, situated on chromosome 16, the proportion of homozygotes for the Minor Allele was markedly lower in the pulmonary MAC disease group (odds ratio: 0.54), p = 1.6 × 10⁻¹³. This SNP is located in the intronic region of CHP2 and was identified in the GTEX database as having an expression-regulating expression quantitative trait locus (eQTL) effect. CHP2 regulates pH via NHE (Na⁺-H⁺ exchanger) expressed in epithelial cells, suggesting that airway epithelial cells may play a crucial role in pulmonary MAC disease.[50,51] Immunostaining of resected lungs from patients with pulmonary MAC disease indeed demonstrated the expression of CHP2 in airway epithelial cells. Moreover, this SNP was discovered to be a risk for pulmonary MAC disease not only in the Japanese population but also in Korean and American populations.[49] By evaluating our Asian TB cohort (686 Asian TB cases and 771 controls), this association was not observed in patients with TB (p = 0.361, odds ratio = 1.09, 95% confidence interval = 0.91–1.29). These findings suggest rs109592 is specific to pulmonary NTM disease.

GWAS analysis was also conducted on 403 Korean patients with pulmonary NTM disease and 306 healthy controls from the Healthy Twin Study, Korea cohort.[52] The results identified rs849177 on chromosome 7p13 as a genetic polymorphism associated with disease susceptibility to pulmonary NTM disease. Moreover, this risk allele (rs849177) was shown to be linked to diminished expression of STK17A, a pro-apoptotic gene. Additionally, STK17A expression was observed to be significantly elevated in both *M. abscessus* and *M. avium*-infected macrophages compared to uninfected macrophages, utilizing two published datasets. Consequently, genetic variants on 7p13 may be associated with susceptibility to pulmonary NTM disease in the Korean population by modulating STK17A expression levels in macrophages.

Host Susceptibility and Radiological Findings

Our GWAS study showed that the rs109592 risk genotype was more common in patients with the NB type than the FC type.[49] The FC type is more common in older males with underlying diseases such as chronic obstructive pulmonary disease and previous pulmonary tuberculosis. The NB type is more common in females with no history of smoking. The global increase in pulmonary NTM disease arises mainly from an increase in the NB type. Previous studies reported that the NB type showed a higher redevelopment rate than the FC type after standard antimicrobial treatment, although patients with the FC type had a poorer long-term prognosis.[15] Interestingly, different mycobacterial strains were present at the pre- and post-treatment stages in most patients with relapsed NB-type, indicating that the redevelopment of MAC in these patients reflected their intrinsic susceptibility to infection rather than a recurrence of a latent pathogen. Based on these previous studies, the NB subtype may be more influenced by host genetic factors, while the FC subtype may be more influenced by other factors such as smoking or previous pulmonary tuberculosis.

Cystic Fibrosis Transmembrane Conductance Regulator

Mutations in the CFTR gene, which is responsible for cystic fibrosis (CF) and encodes a protein that functions as a Cl-channel in epithelial cells, is more prevalent in Europe and the United States than Asia.[53,54] Kim and colleagues[20] analyzed the CFTR gene in 63 pulmonary NTM disease cases in the United States, finding that 23 cases exhibited one or more CFTR mutations, a higher rate than the general population. The mutation group had normal sweat Cl-test results, suggesting a pathogenic involvement of genetic mutations in CFTR that may be distinct from CF (29). Mai and colleagues[54] examined three CFTR polymorphisms (TG repeat, polyT, and M470V) in 300 Japanese pulmonary MAC disease cases and identified an association of pulmonary NTM disease with the ISV8-T5 allele.[55]

Recently, the results of a GWAS using whole genome data from 7,840 patients with CF to search for gene modifiers that define CF severity were reported.[56] Interestingly, the CHP2 region at chromosome 16, which we identified in our GWAS for pulmonary MAC disease, was associated with CF severity. This genetic overlap may be the key to elucidating the disease susceptibility genes and pathogenesis of NTM. Indeed, the incidence of NTM infection in persons with CF, has reportedly declined after the introduction of CF modulators, supporting the potential of host-directed therapies for patients with NTM.[57]

FUTURE DIRECTIONS

Pulmonary nontuberculous mycobacteria (NTM) disease is a chronic progressive pulmonary infectious disease caused by low virulence pathogens. Despite the dramatic global increase of NTM disease, issues such as ineffective antimicrobial agents, challenges in the development of novel antimicrobial drugs, and the risk of emergence of drug-resistant bacteria following long-term use of antimicrobial agents persist. Therefore, new strategies are warranted for better therapeutic options. In addition to thinking about drug discovery strategies from the pathogen, elucidation of individual host susceptibility may enable solutions for novel treatment development.

Genetic studies of NTM infection to date have revealed disease susceptibility genes in moderate sample sizes compared to other fields. This means that while NTM is an infectious disease, it is strongly influenced by the host factors. If genetic studies are conducted with larger sample sizes, it is likely that additional genetic factors and pathological pathways are likely to be revealed. In order to analyze large sample sizes and reveal scientific findings, many groups need to collaborate internationally and perform trans-population meta-analysis of GWAS.

Also, it is essential to perform the functional validation of the identified regions to better understand the pathogenesis of pulmonary NTM disease. Genetic-based translational research in the area of pulmonary NTM disease will contribute to elucidate pathogenesis and explore the potential for novel treatment strategies.

FUNDING SOURCE

This study was supported by AMED, Japan (JP20nk0101612, JP20fk0108415, JP21jk0210034), JSPS(23H02952, 21K15667).

CLINICS CARE POINTS

- Host susceptibility is presumed to exist in NTM-PD and it is expected to recur due to reinfection from the environment.

- It is hoped that host factors will be elucidated and adapted to therapeutic strategies for NTM-PD in the future.

DISCLOSURE

None.

REFERENCES

1. Daley CL, Iaccarino JM, Lange C, et al. Treatment of nontuberculous mycobacterial pulmonary disease: an official ats/ers/escmid/idsa clinical practice guideline. Clin Infect Dis 2020;71(4):E1–36.
2. Schildkraut JA, Coolen JPM, Severin H, et al. MGIT enriched shotgun metagenomics for routine identification of nontuberculous mycobacteria: a route to personalized health care. J Clin Microbiol 2023; 61(3):e0131822.
3. Dahl VN, Mølhave M, Fløe A, et al. Global trends of pulmonary infections with nontuberculous mycobacteria: a systematic review. Int J Infect Dis 2022;125: 120–31.
4. Wu UI, Holland SM. Host susceptibility to nontuberculous mycobacterial infections. Lancet Infect Dis 2015;15(8):968–80.
5. Honda JR, Alper S, Bai X, et al. Acquired and genetic host susceptibility factors and microbial pathogenic factors that predispose to nontuberculous mycobacterial infections. Curr Opin Immunol 2018; 54:66–73.
6. Prevots DR, Marras TK. Epidemiology of human pulmonary infection with nontuberculous mycobacteria a review. Clin Chest Med 2015;36(1):13–34.
7. Blakney RA, Ricotta EE, Frankland TB, et al. Incidence of nontuberculous mycobacterial pulmonary infection, by ethnic group, Hawaii, USA, 2005–2019. Emerg Infect Dis 2022;28(8):1543–50.
8. Adjemian J, Frankland TB, Daida YG, et al. Epidemiology of nontuberculous mycobacterial lung disease and Tuberculosis, Hawaii, USA. Emerg Infect Dis 2017;23(3):439–47.
9. Adjemian J, Olivier KN, Seitz AE, et al. Prevalence of nontuberculous mycobacterial lung disease in U.S. medicare beneficiaries. Am J Respir Crit Care Med 2012;185(8):881–6.
10. Adjemian J, Olivier KN, Seitz AE, et al. Spatial clusters of nontuberculous mycobacterial lung disease in the United States. Am J Respir Crit Care Med 2012;186(6):553–8.
11. Colombo RE, Hill SC, Claypool RJ, et al. Familial clustering of pulmonary nontuberculous mycobacterial disease. Chest 2010;137(3):629–34.
12. Kwok AJ, Mentzer A, Knight JC. Host genetics and infectious disease: new tools, insights and translational opportunities. Nat Rev Genet 2021;22(3): 137–53.
13. Lee Y, Song JW, Chae EJ, et al. CT findings of pulmonary non-tuberculous mycobacterial infection in non-AIDS immunocompromised patients: a case-controlled comparison with immunocompetent

patients. Br J Radiol 2013;86(1024). https://doi.org/10.1259/bjr.20120209.

14. Hayashi M, Takayanagi N, Kanauchi T, et al. Prognostic factors of 634 HIV-negative patients with Mycobacterium avium complex lung disease. Am J Respir Crit Care Med 2012;185(5):575–83.

15. Koh WJ, Moon SM, Kim SY, et al. Outcomes of Mycobacterium avium complex lung disease based on clinical phenotype. Eur Respir J 2017;50(3). https://doi.org/10.1183/13993003.02503-2016.

16. Aksamit TR. Hot tub lung: infection, inflammation, or both? Semin Respir Infect 2003;18(1):33–9.

17. Noma K, Mizoguchi Y, Tsumura M, et al. Mendelian susceptibility to mycobacterial diseases: state of the art. Clin Microbiol Infect 2022;28(11):1429–34.

18. Varley CD, Ku JH, Henkle E, et al. Disseminated nontuberculous mycobacteria in HIV-infected patients, Oregon, USA, 2007–2012. Emerg Infect Dis 2017;23(3):533–5.

19. Al-Anazi KA, Al-Jasser AM, Al-Anazi WK. Infections caused by non-tuberculous mycobacteria in recipients of hematopoietic stem cell transplantation. Front Oncol 2014;4(NOV). https://doi.org/10.3389/fonc.2014.00311.

20. Kim RD, Greenberg DE, Ehrmantraut ME, et al. Pulmonary nontuberculous mycobacterial disease: prospective study of a distinct preexisting syndrome. Am J Respir Crit Care Med 2008;178(10):1066–74.

21. Chan ED, Iseman MD. Slender, older women appear to be more susceptible to nontuberculous mycobacterial lung disease. Gend Med 2010;7(1):5–18.

22. Choi H, Han K, Yang B, et al. Female reproductive factors and incidence of nontuberculous mycobacterial pulmonary disease among postmenopausal women in Korea. Clin Infect Dis 2022;75(8):1397–404.

23. Uwamino Y, Nishimura T, Sato Y, et al. Low serum estradiol levels are related to Mycobacterium avium complex lung disease: a cross-sectional study. BMC Infect Dis 2019;19(1). https://doi.org/10.1186/s12879-019-4668-x.

24. Manolio TA, Collins FS, Cox NJ, et al. Finding the missing heritability of complex diseases. Nature 2009;461(7265):747–53.

25. Tran T, Bonham AJ, Chan ED, et al. A paucity of knowledge regarding nontuberculous mycobacterial lipids compared to the tubercle bacillus. Tuberculosis 2019;115:96–107.

26. Kitada S, Kobayashi K, Ichiyama S, et al. Serodiagnosis of Mycobacterium avium-complex pulmonary disease using an enzyme immunoassay kit. Am J Respir Crit Care Med 2008;177(7):793–7.

27. Hernandez AG, Brunton AE, Ato M, et al. Use of anti-glycopeptidolipid-core antibodies serology for diagnosis and monitoring of Mycobacterium avium complex pulmonary disease in the United States. Open Forum Infect Dis 2022;9(11). https://doi.org/10.1093/ofid/ofac528.

28. Johansen MD, Herrmann JL, Kremer L. Non-tuberculous mycobacteria and the rise of Mycobacterium abscessus. Nat Rev Microbiol 2020;18(7):392–407.

29. Recht J, Asunció A, Martínez A, et al. Genetic analysis of sliding motility in mycobacterium smegmatis. J Bacteriol 2000;182. Available at: http://gasp.med.har-.

30. Ishikawa E, Mori D, Yamasaki S. Recognition of mycobacterial lipids by immune receptors. Trends Immunol 2017;38(1):66–76.

31. Ravesloot-Chávez MM, Dis E Van, Stanley SA. The innate immune response to mycobacterium tuberculosis infection. Annu Rev Immunol 2021;39:611–37.

32. Ahn J, Barber GN. STING signaling and host defense against microbial infection. Exp Mol Med 2019;51(12). https://doi.org/10.1038/s12276-019-0333-0.

33. Hambleton S, Salem S, Bustamante J, et al. IRF8 mutations and human dendritic-cell immunodeficiency. N Engl J Med 2011;365(2):127–38.

34. Teng MWL, Bowman EP, McElwee JJ, et al. IL-12 and IL-23 cytokines: from discovery to targeted therapies for immune-mediated inflammatory diseases. Nat Med 2015;21(7):719–29.

35. Filipe-Santos O, Bustamante J, Haverkamp MH, et al. X-linked susceptibility to mycobacteria is caused by mutations in NEMO impairing CD40-dependent IL-12 production. J Exp Med 2006;203(7):1745–59.

36. Bustamante J, Arias AA, Vogt G, et al. Germline CYBB mutations that selectively affect macrophages in kindreds with X-linked predisposition to tuberculous mycobacterial disease. Nat Immunol 2011;12(3):213–21.

37. Hsu AP, Johnson KD, Falcone EL, et al. GATA2 haploinsufficiency caused by mutations in a conserved intronic element leads to MonoMAC syndrome Key Points. Blood 2013;121:3830–7.

38. Martínez-Barricarte R, Markle JG, Ma CS, et al. Human IFN-γ immunity to mycobacteria is governed by both IL-12 and IL-23. Sci Immunol 2018;3: eaau6759. Available at: http://gnomad.

39. Mizoguchi Y, Okada S. Inborn errors of STAT1 immunity. Curr Opin Immunol 2021;72:59–64.

40. Okada S, Markle JG, Deenick EK, et al. Impairment of immunity to Candida and Mycobacterium in humans with bi-allelic RORC mutations. Science (1979) 2015;349(6248):606–13.

41. Browne SK, Burbelo PD, Chetchotisakd P, et al. Adult-onset immunodeficiency in Thailand and taiwan. N Engl J Med 2012;367(8):725–34.

42. Aoki A, Sakagami T, Yoshizawa K, et al. Clinical significance of interferon-γ neutralizing autoantibodies against disseminated nontuberculous mycobacterial disease. Clin Infect Dis 2018;66(8):1239–45.

43. Lin CH, Chi CY, Shih HP, et al. Identification of a major epitope by anti-interferon-γ autoantibodies in patients with mycobacterial disease. Nat Med 2016;22(9):994–1001.

44. Chi CY, Chu CC, Liu JP, et al. Anti-IFN-autoantibodies in adults with disseminated nontuberculous mycobacterial infections are associated with HLA-DRB1*16:02 and HLA-DQB1*05:02 and the reactivation of latent varicella-zoster virus infection. Blood. 2013;121(8):1357-1366.

45. Tanaka E, Kimoto T, Matsumoto H, et al. Familial pulmonary mycobacterium avium complex disease. Am J Respir Crit Care Med 2000;161:1643–7. Available at: www.atsjournals.org.

46. Kuwabara K, Watanabe Y, Wada K, et al. [Molecular epidemiological analysis by IS1245-based restriction fragment length polymorphism typing on cases with pulmonary Mycobacterium avium disease observed in the same family]. Kekkaku 2004;79(9): 519–23.

47. Bryant JM, Grogono DM, Rodriguez-Rincon D, et al. Emergence and Spread of a Human-Transmissible Multidrug-Resistant Nontuberculous Mycobacterium. Available at: https://www.science.org

48. Szymanski EP, Leung JM, Fowler CJ, et al. Pulmonary nontuberculous mycobacterial infection a multisystem, multigenic disease. Am J Respir Crit Care Med 2015;192(5):618–28.

49. Namkoong H, Omae Y, Asakura T, et al. Genome-wide association study in patients with pulmonary Mycobacterium avium complex disease. Eur Respir J 2021;58(2). https://doi.org/10.1183/13993003.02269-2019.

50. Ammar Y Ben, Takeda S, Hisamitsu T, et al. Crystal structure of CHP2 complexed with NHE1-cytosolic region and an implication for pH regulation. EMBO J 2006;25(11):2315–25.

51. Bartoszewski R, Matalon S, Collawn JF. Ion channels of the lung and their role in disease pathogenesis. REVIEW Ion Channels and Transporters in Lung Function and Disease Am J Physiol Lung Cell Mol Physiol 2017;313:859–72.

52. Cho J, Park K, Choi SM, et al. Genome-wide association study of non-tuberculous mycobacterial pulmonary disease. Thorax 2021;76(2):169–77.

53. Ratjen F, Bell SC, Rowe SM, et al. Cystic fibrosis. Nat Rev Dis Primers 2015;1(1). https://doi.org/10.1038/NRDP.2015.10.

54. Mai HN, Hijikata M, Inoue Y, et al. Pulmonary Mycobacterium avium complex infection associated with the IVS8-T5 allele of the CFTR gene. Int J Tuberc Lung Dis 2007;11(7):808–13.

55. Zhou YH, Gallins PJ, Pace RG, et al. Genetic modifiers of cystic fibrosis lung disease severity: whole genome analysis of 7,840 patients. Am J Respir Crit Care Med 2023;207(10):1324–33. https://doi.org/10.1164/rccm.202209-1653oc.

56. Ricotta EE, Rebecca Prevots D, Olivier KN. CFTR modulator use and risk of nontuberculous mycobacteria positivity in cystic fibrosis, 2011–2018. ERJ Open Res 2022;8(2). https://doi.org/10.1183/23120541.00724-2021.

57. Miller AC, Harris LM, Cavanaugh JE, et al. The Rapid Reduction of Infection-Related Visits and Antibiotic Use Among People With Cystic Fibrosis After Starting Elexacaftor-Tezacaftor-Ivacaftor. Clin Infect Dis 2022;75(7):1115–22.

Investigation and Management of Bronchiectasis in Nontuberculous Mycobacterial Pulmonary Disease

Pamela J. McShane, MD

KEYWORDS

• Bronchiectasis • Airway clearance • *Pseudomonas aeruginosa* • Pulmonary rehabilitation

KEY POINTS

• Bronchiectasis management is integral to the success in caring for a patient with nontuberculous mycobacterial pulmonary disease.
• Investigation into the underlying cause of bronchiectasis is important for all patients, as it may alter the management strategy.
• Airway clearance is a comprehensive management strategy that includes multiple breathing techniques, devices, and mucoactive agents. The exact airway clearance regimen should be customized to each individual patient.
• Chronic pathogenic airway bacteria, such as Pseudomonas *aeruginosa*, may warrant consideration of eradication therapy and/or chronic use of maintenance inhaled antibiotics.
• Bronchiectasis exacerbations should be recognized and treated according to available bacterial culture data.
• Pulmonary rehabilitation improves quality of life, exercise capacity, and respiratory symptoms.

INTRODUCTION

The official ATS/ERS/ESCMID/IDSA clinical practice guideline for the treatment of nontuberculous mycobacterial (NTM) pulmonary disease sets forth specific criteria for the diagnosis of NTM pulmonary disease. These criteria include radiographic features that are consistent with or show bronchiectasis.[1] As such, managing a patient with pulmonary NTM disease is, by definition, managing a patient with bronchiectasis. Furthermore, although culture conversion rates for NTM lung disease range from 50% to 80%,[2–4] bronchiectasis is a permanent condition.[5] Patients with NTM lung infection will require life-long attention to their bronchiectasis, whether or not their NTM infection has been cured. These principles are also true for a patient with emphysema and NTM lung disease, but this chapter is dedicated to bronchiectasis and will focus on investigation and management of bronchiectasis in the NTM-infected patient.

Practice guidelines for the management of bronchiectasis have been developed by multiple national and international organizations: Thoracic Society of Australia and New Zealand (TSANZ 2023), the European Respiratory Society (ERS 2017), British Thoracic Society (BTS 2019), Spanish Society of Pulmonology and Thoracic Surgery (SEPAR 2018), Brazilian Thoracic Association (BTA 2019), and Saudi Thoracic Society (STS 2017). Currently, there are no guidelines published by a US organization.

Department of Medicine, University of Texas Health Science Center at Tyler, 11937 Hwy 271, Tyler, TX 75708, USA
E-mail address: pamela.mcshane@uttyler.edu

Clin Chest Med 44 (2023) 731–742
https://doi.org/10.1016/j.ccm.2023.07.005
0272-5231/23/© 2023 Elsevier Inc. All rights reserved.

DEFINITION OF BRONCHIECTASIS

Bronchiectasis is defined as a constellation of respiratory symptoms and radiographic criteria.[6] The clinic symptoms include chronic cough, sputum production, and/or frequent respiratory exacerbations. Radiographic criteria of bronchiectasis are airway to vessel ratio of greater than 1.5, a lack of the normal tapering of the airway, and visibility of airways at the periphery of the chest.[6] Examples of the radiographic criteria for the diagnosis of bronchiectasis are shown in **Fig. 1**. An important feature of bronchiectasis is its underlying heterogeneity. Bronchiectasis can be present as the sole diagnosis, or it can be accompanied by a diagnosis of immunodeficiency, autoimmunity, or other systemic diseases. This heterogeneity inherent to bronchiectasis has stymied progress of clinical trials directed toward therapeutic interventions.

INVESTIGATION INTO ETIOLOGY

The existence of NTM lung disease should not preclude the search for additional etiologic or associated conditions in bronchiectasis. Nor should the age of the patient foster an assumption that an undiagnosed childhood disease is not present. In one study of cystic fibrosis patients diagnosed after age 18 years, the time of diagnosis ranged from 19 to 71 years of age.[7] Whether coexisting conditions are the cause of the bronchiectasis or whether they share an underlying pathogenesis is yet to be determined. Accordingly, the importance of identifying such abnormalities cannot be overestimated. Prior studies of etiologic testing have shown that identifying an underlying cause of bronchiectasis changed management in 13% to 37% of cases.[8,9] Furthermore, identification and treatment of certain conditions may reduce NTM infection. For example, patients with cystic fibrosis who receive cystic fibrosis transmembrane conductance regulator (CFTR) modulators have a lower risk of NTM

infection.[10] Similarly, there is scientific evidence that patients who are alpha-1 antitrypsin (A1AT)-deficient will be better able to control NTM infection with A1AT replacement therapy.[11]

Three practice guidelines (ERS 2017, BTS 2019, TSANZ 2019) recommend a minimum bundle of diagnostic tests for all patients.[12–14] Further diagnostic testing should be expanded based on the unique clinical history and features of the patient.[15–18] **Table 1**[12–14,19–26] shows minimum bundle and other diagnostic tests that may be appropriate for patients with bronchiectasis.

MANAGEMENT
Airway Clearance

The basis for airway clearance lies in the fundamental pathologic properties of the sputum in patients with bronchiectasis. Compared with healthy control subjects, sputum from patients with bronchiectasis has a higher percentage of solid content, higher mucin content, and is less hydrated.[27] This alteration in the property of the sputum causes a "gel-on-brush" phenomenon in which the cilia are compressed, their action is slowed, and eventually, sputum clearance is halted. The result is a nidus of inflammation and infection.[28] The official ATS/ERS/ESCMID/IDSA clinical practice guideline for NTM pulmonary disease does not provide a specific recommendation for or against the use of airway clearance, but airway clearance is considered an undeniable mainstay of bronchiectasis management. All 6 practice guidelines for the management of bronchiectasis include a recommendation for some form of airway clearance.[12–17]

Airway Clearance Encompasses Two Main Components

1. Airway clearance techniques (maneuvers and devices)
2. Mucoactive agents

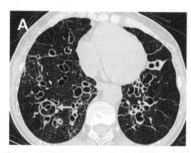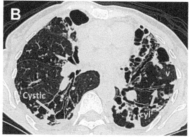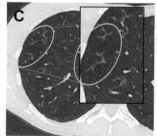

Fig. 1. Radiographic criteria for bronchiectasis. (*A*) Signet ring sign demonstrating the cross-sectional diameter of the airway is larger than the accompanying vessel. (*B*) Three different descriptions of bronchiectactic airways: cystic; cylindrical (cyl); varicose (V). (*C*) "Tree-in-bud" opacities often present in patients with nontuberculosis pulmonary disease. Note, "tree-in-bud" opacities are not included in the radiographic criteria to diagnose bronchiectasis but are included here because they are so frequently associated with nontuberculous pulmonary disease.

Table 1
Diagnostic evaluation for patients with bronchiectasis[6,12–14]

Test	Indication	Clinical Features to Support Testing
Historical review of possible coexisting conditions: • Asthma • COPD • Gastroesophageal reflux • Connective tissue disease • Inflammatory bowel disease • Cystic fibrosis • Primary ciliary dyskinesia • Human immunodeficiency virus syndrome • Family history of immune deficiency	All patients with bronchiectasis	All patients with bronchiectasis
Sputum culture for regular bacteria[a,b,e] and acid-fast bacteria[a,b,e]	All patients with bronchiectasis	All patients with bronchiectasis
Complete blood count (CBC)[a,b,e]	Primary or secondary immunodeficiency and hematologic malignancy	All patients with bronchiectasis
Serum immunoglobulins (total IgG, IgA, IgM)[a,b,e,19,20]	Common variable immune deficiency and other defects in antibody production	• Frequent bronchiectasis exacerbations • Frequent sinus infections • Ther significant infections (osteomyelitis, septic arthritis, meningitis, septicemia) • Recurrent abscesses of the skin, lymph nodes, or internal organs • Chronic diarrhea • Persistent thrush
Baseline levels of specific antibodies against capsular polysaccharides of *Streptococcus pneumoniae* If low, recheck levels 4 wk after immunization with pneumococcal polysaccharide vaccine 23[19]	Immune deficiency in the context of normal IgG, A, or M levels	• Frequent bronchiectasis exacerbations • Frequent sinus infections
Total serum IgE[b], and specific IgE & IgG, or skin prick test to *Aspergillus fumigatus*[e,21]	Allergic bronchopulmonary aspergillosis	• Concomitant asthma • Central bronchiectasis
Sweat chloride[b], followed by genetic panel testing, if indicated[22]	Cystic fibrosis	• Upper lobe bronchiectasis • Family history of cystic fibrosis bronchiectasis • Chronic gastrointestinal symptoms • Malabsorption • Pancreatitis • Male infertility
Nasal nitric oxide, cilia biopsy, genetic panel testing, if indicated[23,24]	Primary ciliary dyskinesia	• Lower lobe bronchiectasis • Neonatal distress • History of frequent sinus infections • History of ear infections • Infertility • Childhood sinopulmonary symptoms

(continued on next page)

Table 1
(continued)

Test	Indication	Clinical Features to Support Testing
Alpha-1 antitrypsin level and phenotype[b,25]	Alpha-1 antitrypsin deficiency	• Family history of lung or liver disease • Airflow obstruction at a younger than expected age • Emphysema in lung bases
pH monitoring, barium swallow, esophagogastroduodenoscopy[26]	Gastroesophageal reflux	• Coughing after eating • Evidence of chronic aspiration (tree-in-bud opacities in the right middle lobe, right lower lobe)

Abbreviations: COPD, chronic obstructive pulmonary disease; Ig, immunoglobulin.
 [a] Minimum investigations recommended by Thoracic Society of Australia and New Zealand.[13]
 [b] Recommended investigation by Brazilian Consensus on noncystic fibrosis bronchiectasis.
 [e] Recommended for all patients by the European Respiratory Society[14] and British Thoracic Society.[12]

Airway Clearance Techniques

Airway clearance techniques include various breathing maneuvers and devices that range from simple independent passive maneuvers to complex, expensive assist devices (**Table 2**).[29,30] Videos of airway clearance techniques and devices can be viewed at the "Bronchiectasis Toolbox" Web site, www.bronchiectasis.com.au. All practice guidelines recommend at least some form of airway clearance techniques. The techniques improve the sputum clearance by the following mechanisms:[31]

1. Increased airway surface liquid
2. Decreased sputum rigidity
3. Movement of the dynamic compression (equal pressure point) of the airway toward the periphery that targets sputum in the small airways
4. Shearing of mucus from the airway wall (by accelerating expiratory airflow and creating high linear velocity)
5. Improved ventilation of obstructed lung units
6. Reexpansion of collapsed alveoli

Mucoactive Agents

Mucoactive agents with some evidence to support their use in bronchiectasis are hypertonic saline solutions (7% sodium chloride) and mannitol (not available in the United States). Hypertonic saline (HS) and mannitol are hyperosmolar agents that hydrate the airway and reduce mucin connections, thereby reducing sputum viscosity and easing expectoration.[32] Trials of HS and mannitol in patients with noncystic fibrosis (CF) bronchiectasis are relatively small and not without limitations. Nevertheless, beneficial effects seen in such trials are improved quality of life as measured by the St. George Respiratory Questionnaire (HS and mannitol),[33,34] reduced time to exacerbation in patients with greater than or equal to 2 exacerbations per year (mannitol),[34] reduced health care utilization (HS),[33] and improvement in forced expiratory volume in the first second (FEV1) and forced vital capacity at 3 months (HS).[33] Based on these findings, national and international recommend the use of either nebulized HS or mannitol if symptoms are present after airway clearance techniques have failed to optimize sputum production (**Box 1**).

Both mannitol and HS can induce airway reactivity. Clinical observation in the outpatient setting is recommended, and pretreatment with a short-acting beta-agonist may be necessary for some patients. DNase is a mucoactive agent that has been shown to increase exacerbations and reduce FEV1 in the patient with non-CF bronchiectasis[35] and is therefore universally not recommended by bronchiectasis practice guidelines.

Clinically, the goal of airway clearance is to reduce the sputum volume, reduce exacerbations, improve quality of life, and preserve lung function. Unfortunately, despite the scientific and physiologic basis for airway clearance, there is a near absence of large, high-quality clinical trial evidence to support specific strategies.[36,37] This relatively stagnant area in bronchiectasis has led to a call to action to researchers, clinicians, funding bodies, and respiratory societies to prioritize research in airway clearance.[38] Moving forward, determination of the proper outcomes and balancing population heterogeneity are critical goals. In the meantime, airway clearance is, nevertheless, standard care in patients with bronchiectasis.[37] According to practice guidelines, a comprehensive approach to airway clearance

Table 2
Airway clearance techniques and devices

Modality	Specific Maneuver or Device	Comments
Passive maneuvers	Postural positioning/postural drainage	May worsen GERD; modifies ventilation to perfusion ratio in dependent regions of the lung
Active maneuvers without devices	3-s breath-hold/thoracic expansion	Allows air to move from unobstructed to obstructed regions
	Huff/huff coughing	Exhalation of various tidal volumes with an open glottis. When performed correctly, moves the point of dynamic compression on the airways toward the periphery, targeting secretions in the small airways
	Active cycle of breathing Autogenic drainage	Requires instruction, patience, and practice. The technique is adapted to the unique patient needs. Begins with controlled breaths, followed by thoracic expansion (3-s breath-hold), followed by forced exhalation with an open glottis (huff). Using sequentially increasing volumes of huffs (small, medium, and large) can aid in unsticking, collecting, and evacuating phases of mucus.
	Total slow expiration with open glottis and infralateral position (L'Expiration Lente Totale Glotte Ouverte en decubitus Lateral, ELTGOL)[29,30]	Combination of postural positioning, 3-s breath-hold, and active cycle of breathing. Optimizes airflow velocity to cross-sectional airway area. Results in a shear force that overcomes resistive forces of mucous layer.
	Percussion/chest clapping	Requires partner/caregiver Augments the volume of expectorated sputum
Devices		
Small, portable, hand-held PEP at the mouth *without* oscillation	PEP mask, Thera-PEP	Temporarily increases functional residual capacity. Should be combined with huffing and or active cycle of breathing.
Small, portable, hand-held PEP at the mouth *with* oscillation	Acapella, Flutter, Aerobika	Oscillation modifies rheological properties (viscosity, elasticity, and spinnability) of mucus to make expectoration easier

(continued on next page)

Table 2
(continued)

Modality	Specific Maneuver or Device	Comments
External pressure and oscillation Around the chest	High-frequency chest wall oscillation	Modifies rheologic properties of mucus and creates an expiratory flow bias
Oscillation and lung expansion	Volara	Expense is likely to limit use. Provides continuous positive expiratory pressure with oscillation. Can administer nebulized treatments.
Exercise	Walking, cycling, weightlifting	Increases mucus/sputum clearance. Improves overall respiratory muscle fitness.
	Pulmonary rehabilitation	Formal customized program that includes disease specific education and supervised exercise training.
Mucoactive agents	Hypertonic saline (3%, 7%)	Can induce bronchospasm. Consider first trial in clinic and/or use of bronchodilator before use.
	Mannitol	Not available in the United States
	rhDNase—for use in cystic fibrosis (CF) patients; not recommended in non-CF bronchiectasis)	Shown to increase exacerbation frequency and decrease FEV1 in non-CF bronchiectasis

*Videos of airway clearance techniques and devices can be viewed at the Bronchiectasis Toolbox Web site, www.bronchiectasis.com.au.

Caution is advised for patients who have or are at risk for gastroesophageal reflux.

Abbreviations: GERD, gastroesophageal reflux disease; PEP, positive expiratory device.

Adapted from McIlwaine M, Bradley J, Elborn JS, et al. Personalizing airway clearance in chronic lung disease. *Eur Respir Rev* 2017; 26: 160086 and the *Bronchiectasis Toolbox* Web site, www.bronchiectasis.com.au.

includes the following steps, which can be done concurrently or sequentially.

1. Allow the patient to trial available techniques and customize which technique or combination of techniques provides most benefit as

Box 1
Details of mucoactive agent and their recommending organizations

Indication to add mucoactive agent	Recommending organizations
Difficulty expectorating sputum	ERS 2017; BTS2019; STS 2017
Persistent/uncontrolled sputum	BTA 2019; SEPAR 2018
Poor quality of life or uncontrolled symptoms	ERS 2017
Frequent/≥ 2 exacerbations per year	SEPAR 2018; TSANZ 2023

perceived by the patient. Refer to the patient's computed tomography imaging to guide techniques and postural positioning toward affected areas.
2. Trial of mucoactive agent to hydrate the airway and aid in sputum clearance.
3. Add devices (eg, positive expiratory pressure device with oscillation) to further alter sputum properties and enhance clearance.
4. If available, refer to a respiratory therapist for one-on-one coaching.
5. Increase airway clearance during exacerbations.

A phase 2a, 28-day investigational use of ARINA-1 (88 mg/mL ascorbic acid and 150 mg/mL reduced glutathione) inhaled twice daily via nebulization in patients with bronchiectasis has begun enrollment. The study sponsored by Renovion, Inc. is randomized, double-blind, placebo-controlled (isotonic saline, 0.9%) and will include quality of life, use of airway clearance techniques, lung function, sputum rheology, and blood inflammatory markers as secondary endpoints. A separate but similarly designed upcoming Renovion study of ARINA-1 will focus exclusively on patients with NTM disease. Key secondary endpoints will additionally include change from baseline bacterial counts.

Pulmonary Rehabilitation

Pulmonary rehabilitation is a comprehensive intervention that includes patient education and supervised physical exercise (treadmill walking, cycle ergometry, upper arm ergometry, and weightlifting).[39] A pulmonary rehabilitation program is designed to improve the physical and psychological condition of patients with chronic respiratory diseases. It requires a baseline assessment of the patient and implements a regimen tailored to the individual patient. Traditionally, pulmonary rehabilitation existed within the domain of chronic obstructive pulmonary disease (COPD). Thus, these programs tend to be geared toward the patient with COPD. There is now recognition of the benefit of pulmonary rehabilitation in other chronic pulmonary diseases[40] that has led to the modification of pulmonary rehabilitation programs toward other chronic lung diseases. All bronchiectasis practice guidelines include pulmonary rehabilitation or exercise training in the overall management of these patients.[13–17] Several clinical trials have shown that pulmonary rehabilitation can improve exercise capacity and health-related quality of life in patients with bronchiectasis.[41] For example, in a study of patients with limited exercise tolerance who were already using airway clearance, subjects were randomized to receive either an 8-week pulmonary rehabilitation program plus airway clearance or airway clearance alone. All subjects were encouraged to continue the assigned exercise regimen after the study period. The group randomized to pulmonary rehabilitation plus airway clearance had significantly improved quality-of-life symptoms (mean 8 unit improvement in St. George Respiratory Questionnaire), cough symptoms (mean 2.6 unit improvement in the Leicester Cough Questionnaire), and exercise capacity (mean 193.3 m improvement in the endurance walk test).[42] This study was notable because the measured benefits persisted 12 weeks after the end of the 8-week program.

Some investigators have studied the effect of pulmonary rehabilitation on exacerbation frequency. Lee and colleagues performed a multicenter, randomized, single-blinded, controlled study of the effects of exercise training in 85 patients with bronchiectasis who were also already on airway clearance therapy.[43] Inclusion criteria

included a modified medical research council dyspnea score greater than or equal to 1 (correlates with shortness of breath with hurrying on level ground or walking up a slight hill). The intervention was an 8-week program of twice weekly exercise sessions of walking, cycling, and extremity strengthening exercises. Similar to other studies, the pulmonary rehabilitation group improved exercise capacity and reduced respiratory symptoms. The mean improvement in the incremental shuttle walk test was 62 m (95% confidence interval, 24–101 m), and the chronic respiratory disease questionnaire showed reduction in dyspnea ($P = .009$) and fatigue ($P = .01$) in patients who underwent pulmonary rehabilitation compared with controls. This study was notable because it also demonstrated a reduction in exacerbation frequency in patients with bronchiectasis who take part in pulmonary rehabilitation. There were fewer exacerbations over 12 months in the exercise group (1, range 0–2) compared with the control group (1, range 1–3), $P = .012$.

Based on the available evidence, patients with bronchiectasis can reduce respiratory symptoms and improve quality of life and exercise capacity by taking part in pulmonary rehabilitation. More recently, investigators have begun to analyze if pulmonary rehabilitation can affect the underlying inflammation associated with pulmonary disease. In a study of 74 clinically stable patients with bronchiectasis compared with 42 controls subjects without cardiopulmonary disease and matched by age, sex, and body mass index,[44] the investigators explored the relationship between markers of inflammation and oxidative stress with functional status. Although consistent correlations were not identified between all measurements of inflammation and functional status, the investigators did identify some correlation with absolute values of oxygen consumption (Vo_2) and certain inflammatory markers (interleukin-1 [IL-1] β, r = -0.408; IL-6, r = -0.308), suggesting that higher inflammation was associated with lower Vo_2. There is more work to be done in this area, but the study suggests a therapeutic role of exercise in bronchiectasis pathophysiology.

Management of Chronic Pathogenic Bacteria

Chronic infection with pathogenic bacteria during the stable, nonexacerbation state is characteristic of patients with bronchiectasis, including those who also have NTM pulmonary disease.[45] Bacterial infection is key in the pathogenesis of bronchiectasis because it incites inflammation, which causes sputum accumulation and results in airway damage and remodeling.[46] The presence of

Pseudomonas, Enterobacteriaceae, and *Stenotrophomonas* is associated with more severe bronchiectasis and more frequent exacerbations.[47,48] *Pseudomonas aeruginosa,* specifically, has been shown to correlate with higher mortality rate in patients with bronchiectasis.[49] Given the impact of this organism on outcomes of patients with bronchiectasis, most practice guidelines outline a strategy for attempting eradication when the bacteria is first or newly identified. BTA 2019, BTS 2019, ERS 2017, and SEPAR 2018 all specifically outline eradication protocols, which typically include a 2- to 3-week course of systemic anti-Pseudomonal antibiotic followed by 3 months of inhaled antibiotics. TSANZ 2023 recommends an eradication attempt when *P aeruginosa* is newly identified in the lower airways.[18] STS 2017 makes no recommendation for eradication and instead highlights the need for more studies to show efficacy of this strategy in the Saudi population.

For many patients, eradication of pathogenic bacteria is not successful. In this setting, inhaled antibiotics deliver high antibiotic concentrations directly to the lung with minimal systemic exposure and toxicity. A meta-analysis of 16 randomized controlled trials of inhaled antibiotics in patients with bronchiectasis and chronic respiratory tract infections included 2597 subjects and showed a reduction of bacteria colony forming units, an increase in bacterial eradication, and reduction in exacerbation frequency. The analysis did not identify treatment-emergent or adverse effects, but emergence of bacterial resistance at the end of treatment was noted.[50] BTA 2019, BTS 2019, ERS 2017, and TSANZ 2023 recommend consideration of long-term inhaled antibiotics in patients experiencing frequent ($\geq$3) exacerbations. SEPAR 2018 recommends inhaled antibiotics for all patients with chronic *P aeruginosa* infection and in patients with other pathogenic organisms who have had 2 exacerbations or 1 hospitalization in the previous year, or manifest a decline in lung function, or deterioration of quality of life. STS 2017 withholds this recommendation in favor of waiting for more definitive data to support inhaled antibiotic use in their specific population.

BRONCHIECTASIS EXACERBATIONS
Definition of Bronchiectasis Exacerbation

In the last decade, there has been a surge in the number of clinical trials available to patients with bronchiectasis. Most trials use exacerbations as key inclusion criteria and adhere to an expert consensus definition of a bronchiectasis exacerbation (**Box 2**). Thus, it is appropriate to incorporate this definition into clinical practice. Although

---

> **Box 2**
> **Definition of bronchiectasis exacerbation for clinical trials by exert consensus[51]**
>
> Deterioration in 3 or more of the following key symptoms over a period of
>
> 48 hours or more[a] with other potential causes excluded.
>
> 1. Cough
> 2. Increase in sputum volume and/or change in consistency
> 3. Sputum purulence
> 4. Breathlessness and/or exercise intolerance
> 5. Fatigue and/or malaise
> 6. Hemoptysis
>
> In addition, a clinician determines that a change in treatment is required (prescription of antibiotic or modification of therapy, such as an increase in airway clearance).
>
> [a]This does not mean that symptoms must persist for 48 hours or more before an exacerbation is diagnosed. This means that collectively, the symptoms may occur over a 48-hour period.

---

clinical trials for bronchiectasis typically exclude patients who are receiving treatment of NTM pulmonary disease, it is likely that at various points in the life of these patients, they will not be on NTM antibiotics, and may thus be eligible for a bronchiectasis trial. But beyond trial enrollment, use of the consensus definition will help to define the severity of disease and support systematic and reproducible prescription of new drugs. The expert consensus definition of a bronchiectasis exacerbation for clinical trials is given in **Box 2**.

Educating the patient on the definition of an exacerbation is an important part of optimally managing bronchiectasis. Patients need to be able to recognize what is (and is not) an exacerbation so they can notify their clinician promptly when symptoms occur and/or avoid overuse of antibiotics.

Management of Exacerbations

The theory that bronchiectasis exacerbations are caused by an increase in bacterial load or acquisition of a new virus is becoming an outdated notion because integrative microbiomics have revealed a more complex relationship within the respiratory biome. Exacerbations are now believed to be related to an antagonistic relationship between resident microbes rather than a simple change in proportion of organisms.[52] Unfortunately, therapeutic options lag behind scientific discovery of pathophysiologic mechanisms. Until specific therapies are available to undermine antagonistic relationships between microbes, antibiotics remain the main therapeutic intervention. All practice guidelines recommend antibiotics for bronchiectasis exacerbations. Duration of therapy varies slightly between societies (see later discussion) but generally is for between 10 and 14 days (**Box 3**).

Management of exacerbations can be problematic in the NTM pulmonary disease patient who may already be on several antibiotics. For example, a patient with bronchiectasis with *Mycobacterium avium* complex pulmonary disease may experience an acute exacerbation thought to be related to coexisting *P aeruginosa*. Addition of fluoroquinolones can increase the risk of QTc prolongation in a patient already receiving azithromycin. Unfortunately, there are no data to guide how to manage the cumulative risk in these specific scenarios, and each case is likely to be slightly different. Options include holding azithromycin during treatment of the exacerbation, adding the fluoroquinolone to the azithromycin regimen and checking frequent electrocardiograms, or using alternate anti-*Pseudomonas* drug (intravenous) to treat the exacerbation.

Chronic macrolide therapy is a strategy to reduce exacerbation frequency (**Box 4**). Three placebo-controlled trials have demonstrated reduced exacerbation frequency and improved quality of life from chronic macrolide therapy in patients with bronchiectasis who experience frequent exacerbations (3 or more exacerbations per year).

Although the reduction of exacerbations in bronchiectasis is an important goal, the risk to benefit ratio must be considered extremely carefully,[56] especially in the patient with NTM infection.[57] During long-term macrolide use, monitoring for hearing and vestibular toxicity is a must. It is important to keep in mind that these potential adverse effects may be compounded by concomitant medications such as amikacin liposome inhalation suspension. The importance of ruling out NTM infection before initiation of macrolide monotherapy and continual surveillance for such organisms cannot be overstated as the development of macrolide resistant organisms complicates therapy, results in lower conversion rates, and increases mortality.[57]

Vaccination

Bronchiectasis practice guidelines recommend annual influenza immunization to all patients with bronchiectasis.[12,13,15–18] Likewise, pneumococcal vaccination should be offered to patients with bronchiectasis according to local guidelines. Pneumococcal vaccines are either polysaccharide (partially purified pneumococcal capsular polysaccharide, PPSV23) or conjugate vaccines (polysaccharides conjugated to a protein, PCV 10, PVC13, PCV15, and PCV 20). Specific recommendations for their administration (in combination vs PPSV23 alone and timing) are guided by local or national immunization program schedules.

Box 3
Management of a bronchiectasis exacerbation

1. Use existing culture data, if present, to guide empirical antibiotic coverage.

2. Whenever possible, at the beginning of the exacerbation, obtain a sputum sample for culture before antibiotics have been initiated.

3. Modify antibiotic therapy as new culture data become available.

4. Duration of therapy: [a]

   - 14 days (ERS 2017; BTS 2019; STS 2017; TSANZ 2023)

   - 10 to 21 days (SEPAR 2018)

5. For known *P aeruginosa*–related exacerbations, dual intravenous therapy can be considered using an extended spectrum penicillin (ie, ceftazidime) and an aminoglycoside (ie, tobramycin) with caution and vigilance toward adverse events (eg, nephrotoxicity, vestibular toxicity) (TSANZ 2023, STS 2017, SEPAR 2018, BTS 2019, BTA 2019).

6. If the patient fails to improve, consider repeat cultures, intravenous antibiotics, or hospitalization.

[a]Can be shortened for mild bronchiectasis exacerbations.

Box 4
Three placebo-controlled trials that reduced exacerbation frequency

The Bronchiectasis and Low-dose Erythromycin Study (BLESS)[53]	Erythromycin ethylsuccinate, 400 mg, daily
EMBRACE[54]	Azithromycin, 500 mg, thrice weekly
The Bronchiectasis and Long-term Azithromycin Treatment (BAT)[55]	Azithromycin, 250 mg, daily

Emerging Therapies

In bronchiectasis, neutrophils behave in an aberrant manner. Compared with healthy controls, neutrophils from patients with bronchiectasis demonstrate delayed apoptosis and impaired bacterial phagocytosis.[58] At the same time, neutrophil serine proteases are elevated in the sputum of these patients,[59] and the level of elevation correlates with markers of severe disease.[60] Neutrophil serine protease activity has been the recent focus of therapeutic intervention. Brensocatib is a reversible inhibitor of dipeptidyl peptidase, an enzyme responsible for the activation of neutrophil serine proteases.[61] In a randomized, double-blind, placebo-controlled, phase 2 clinical trial, the oral drug reduced neutrophil elastase activity and prolonged time to first exacerbation. A 52-week, international, double-blind, placebo-controlled, phase 3 clinical trial of Brensocatib is currently underway (The ASPEN Study, clinicaltrials.gov identifier NCT04594369). In addition, BI 1291583, another oral drug that blocks activation of neutrophil serine proteases, is currently being studied in an international, randomized, double-blind, placebo-controlled, phase 2 trial for efficacy, safety, and dosing (Airleaf, clincialtrials.gov identifier NCT05238675). Both trials have an estimated completion date of March 2024.

CLINICS CARE POINTS

- A thorough and thoughtful investigation into the cause of bronchiectasis and coexisting diseases is important in patients with bronchiectasis with NTM pulmonary disease, as it may change management and clinical course.

- Airway clearance is a comprehensive collection of breathing techniques, devices, and mucoactive agents. It is a mainstay of bronchiectasis management and should be customized to each patient.

- In patients with bronchiectasis, pulmonary rehabilitation has been shown to reduce respiratory symptoms and improve quality of life. All practice guidelines recommend pulmonary rehabilitation for patients with bronchiectasis with reduced exercise capacity.

- Patients with NTM pulmonary disease may also have chronic infection with other pathogenic bacteria. Consideration should be given to eradication and/or maintenance inhaled antibiotic therapy to ameliorate the effects of this chronic infection.

- Exacerbations are an important marker of disease in patients with bronchiectasis and dictate a change in therapy. Patients with bronchiectasis should be educated on what an exacerbation is to optimize prudent overall management.

- New therapies that target the underlying inflammation of bronchiectasis are being studied in clinical trials.

DISCLOSURE

Dr P.J. McShane is primary investigator for clinical trials sponsored by AN2 Therapeutics, Armata, Boehringer Ingelheim, Electromed, Insmed, MannKind, Paratek, Renovian, and Spero. She participates in trial steering committees for Boehringer Ingelheim, Insmed, and Spero.

REFERENCES

1. Daley CL, Iaccarino JM, Lange C, et al. Treatment of nontuberculous mycobacterial pulmonary disease: an official ATS/ERS/ESCMID/IDSA clinical practice guideline. Clin Infect Dis 2020;71(4):e1–36.
2. Koh WJ, Moon SM, Kim SY, et al. Outcomes of Mycobacterium avium complex lung disease based on clinical phenotype. Eur Respir J 2017;50(3).
3. Wallace RJ Jr, Brown-Elliott BA, McNulty S, et al. Macrolide/Azalide therapy for nodular/bronchiectatic mycobacterium avium complex lung disease. Chest 2014;146(2):276–82.
4. Jeong BH, Jeon K, Park HY, et al. Intermittent antibiotic therapy for nodular bronchiectatic Mycobacterium avium complex lung disease. Am J Respir Crit Care Med 2015;191(1):96–103.
5. Chalmers JD, Chang AB, Chotirmall SH, et al. Bronchiectasis. Nat Rev Dis Primers. 2018;4(1):45.
6. Aliberti S, Goeminne PC, O'Donnell AE, et al. Criteria and definitions for the radiological and clinical diagnosis of bronchiectasis in adults for use in clinical trials: international consensus recommendations. Lancet Respir Med 2022;10(3):298–306.
7. Farley H, Poole S, Chapman S, et al. Diagnosis of cystic fibrosis in adulthood and eligibility for novel CFTR modulator therapy. Postgrad Med J 2022;98(1159):341–5.
8. Lonni S, Chalmers JD, Goeminne PC, et al. Etiology of non-cystic fibrosis bronchiectasis in adults and its correlation to disease severity. Ann Am Thorac Soc 2015;12(12):1764–70.
9. Shoemark A, Ozerovitch L, Wilson R. Aetiology in adult patients with bronchiectasis. Respir Med 2007;101(6):1163–70.
10. Ricotta EE, Prevots DR, Olivier KN. CFTR modulator use and risk of nontuberculous mycobacteria positivity in cystic fibrosis, 2011-2018. ERJ Open Res 2022;8(2).

11. Bai X, Bai A, Honda JR, et al. Alpha-1-Antitrypsin enhances primary human macrophage immunity against non-tuberculous mycobacteria. Front Immunol 2019;10:1417.

12. Hill AT, Sullivan AL, Chalmers JD, et al. British thoracic society guideline for bronchiectasis in adults. Thorax 2019;74(Suppl 1):1–69.

13. Chang AB, Bell SC, Torzillo PJ, et al. Chronic suppurative lung disease and bronchiectasis in children and adults in Australia and New Zealand Thoracic Society of Australia and New Zealand guidelines. Med J Aust 2015;202(1):21–3.

14. Polverino E, Goeminne PC, McDonnell MJ, et al. European Respiratory Society guidelines for the management of adult bronchiectasis. Eur Respir J 2017;50(3).

15. Martinez-Garcia MA, Maiz L, Olveira C, et al. Spanish guidelines on treatment of bronchiectasis in adults. Arch Bronconeumol 2018;54(2):88–98.

16. Pereira MC, Athanazio RA, Dalcin PTR, et al. Brazilian consensus on non-cystic fibrosis bronchiectasis. J Bras Pneumol 2019;45(4):e20190122.

17. Al-Jahdali H, Alshimemeri A, Mobeireek A, et al. The Saudi Thoracic Society guidelines for diagnosis and management of noncystic fibrosis bronchiectasis. Ann Thorac Med 2017;12(3):135–61.

18. Chang AB, Bell SC, Byrnes CA, et al. Thoracic Society of Australia and New Zealand (TSANZ) position statement on chronic suppurative lung disease and bronchiectasis in children, adolescents and adults in Australia and New Zealand. Respirology 2023;28(4):339–49.

19. Bonilla FA, Barlan I, Chapel H, et al. International consensus document (ICON): common variable immunodeficiency disorders. J Allergy Clin Immunol Pract 2016;4(1):38–59.

20. Seidel MG, Kindle G, Gathmann B, et al. The European society for immunodeficiencies (ESID) registry working definitions for the clinical diagnosis of inborn errors of immunity. J Allergy Clin Immunol Pract 2019;7(6):1763–70.

21. Agarwal R, Sehgal IS, Dhooria S, et al. Developments in the diagnosis and treatment of allergic bronchopulmonary aspergillosis. Expert Rev Respir Med 2016;10(12):1317–34.

22. Farrell PM, White TB, Ren CL, et al. Diagnosis of cystic fibrosis: consensus guidelines from the cystic fibrosis foundation. J Pediatr 2017;181S:S4–15 e11.

23. Lucas JS, Barbato A, Collins SA, et al. European Respiratory Society guidelines for the diagnosis of primary ciliary dyskinesia. Eur Respir J 2017;49(1).

24. Shapiro AJ, Davis SD, Polineni D, et al. Diagnosis of primary ciliary dyskinesia. An official American thoracic society clinical practice guideline. Am J Respir Crit Care Med 2018;197(12):e24–39.

25. Miravitlles M, Dirksen A, Ferrarotti I, et al. European Respiratory Society statement: diagnosis and treatment of pulmonary disease in alpha(1)-antitrypsin deficiency. Eur Respir J 2017;50(5).

26. Gyawali CP, Kahrilas PJ, Savarino E, et al. Modern diagnosis of GERD: the lyon consensus. Gut 2018;67(7):1351–62.

27. Ramsey KA, Chen ACH, Radicioni G, et al. Airway mucus hyperconcentration in non-cystic fibrosis bronchiectasis. Am J Respir Crit Care Med 2020;201(6):661–70.

28. Button B, Cai LH, Ehre C, et al. A periciliary brush promotes the lung health by separating the mucus layer from airway epithelia. Science 2012;337(6097):937–41.

29. Wong C, Sullivan C, Jayaram L. ELTGOL airway clearance in bronchiectasis: laying the bricks of evidence. Eur Respir J 2018;51:1702232.

30. Munoz G, de Gracia J, Buxo M, et al. Long-term benefits of airway clearance in bronchiectasis: a randomized placebo-controlled trial. Eur Respir J 2017;51:1701926.

31. McIlwaine M, Bradley J, Elborn JS, et al. Personalising airway clearance in chronic lung disease. Eur Respir Rev 2017;26(143).

32. Daviskas E, Anderson SD. Hyperosmolar agents and clearance of mucus in the diseased airway. J Aerosol Med 2006;19(1):100–9.

33. Kellett F, Robert NM. Nebulised 7% hypertonic saline improves lung function and quality of life in bronchiectasis. Respir Med 2011;105(12):1831–5.

34. Bilton D, Tino G, Barker AF, et al. Inhaled mannitol for non-cystic fibrosis bronchiectasis: a randomised, controlled trial. Thorax 2014;69(12):1073–9.

35. O'Donnell AE, Barker AF, Ilowite JS, et al. Treatment of idiopathic bronchiectasis with aerosolized recombinant human DNase I. rhDNase Study Group. Chest 1998;113(5):1329–34.

36. Franks LJ, Walsh JR, Hall K, et al. Measuring airway clearance outcomes in bronchiectasis: a review. Eur Respir Rev 2020;29(156).

37. Hill AT, Barker AF, Bolser DC, et al. Treating cough due to non-CF and CF bronchiectasis with nonpharmacological airway clearance: CHEST expert panel report. Chest 2018;153(4):986–93.

38. Spinou A, Chalmers JD. Respiratory physiotherapy in the bronchiectasis guidelines: is there a loud voice we are yet to hear? Eur Respir J 2019;54(3).

39. Spruit MA, Singh SJ, Garvey C, et al. An official American Thoracic Society/European Respiratory Society statement: key concepts and advances in pulmonary rehabilitation. Am J Respir Crit Care Med 2013;188(8):e13–64.

40. Holland AE, Wadell K, Spruit MA. How to adapt the pulmonary rehabilitation programme to patients with chronic respiratory disease other than COPD. Eur Respir Rev 2013;22(130):577–86.

41. Lee AL, Hill CJ, McDonald CF, et al. Pulmonary rehabilitation in individuals with non-cystic fibrosis

bronchiectasis: a systematic review. Arch Phys Med Rehabil 2017;98(4):774–782 e771.

42. Mandal P, Sidhu MK, Kope L, et al. A pilot study of pulmonary rehabilitation and chest physiotherapy versus chest physiotherapy alone in bronchiectasis. Respir Med 2012;106(12):1647–54.

43. Lee AL, Hill CJ, Cecins N, et al. The short and long term effects of exercise training in non-cystic fibrosis bronchiectasis–a randomised controlled trial. Respir Res 2014;15:44.

44. de Camargo AA, de Castro RAS, Vieira RP, et al. Systemic inflammation and oxidative stress in adults with bronchiectasis: association with clinical and functional features. Clinics 2021;76:e2474.

45. Tunney MM, Einarsson GG, Wei L, et al. Lung microbiota and bacterial abundance in patients with bronchiectasis when clinically stable and during exacerbation. Am J Respir Crit Care Med 2013; 187(10):1118–26.

46. Flume PA, Chalmers JD, Olivier KN. Advances in bronchiectasis: endotyping, genetics, microbiome, and disease heterogeneity. Lancet 2018; 392(10150):880–90.

47. Dicker AJ, Lonergan M, Keir HR, et al. The sputum microbiome and clinical outcomes in patients with bronchiectasis: a prospective observational study. Lancet Respir Med 2021;9(8):885–96.

48. Metersky ML, Choate R, Aksamit TR, et al. Stenotrophomonas maltophilia in patients with bronchiectasis: an analysis of the US bronchiectasis and NTM Research Registry. Respir Med 2022;193: 106746.

49. Finch S, McDonnell MJ, Abo-Leyah H, et al. A comprehensive analysis of the impact of Pseudomonas aeruginosa colonization on prognosis in adult bronchiectasis. Ann Am Thorac Soc 2015; 12(11):1602–11.

50. Laska IF, Crichton ML, Shoemark A, et al. The efficacy and safety of inhaled antibiotics for the treatment of bronchiectasis in adults: a systematic review and meta-analysis. Lancet Respir Med 2019;7(10):855–69.

51. Hill AT, Haworth CS, Aliberti S, et al. Pulmonary exacerbation in adults with bronchiectasis: a consensus definition for clinical research. Eur Respir J 2017;49(6).

52. Mac Aogain M, Narayana JK, Tiew PY, et al. Integrative microbiomics in bronchiectasis exacerbations. Nat Med 2021;27(4):688–99.

53. Serisier DJ, Martin ML, McGuckin MA, et al. Effect of long-term, low-dose erythromycin on pulmonary exacerbations among patients with non-cystic fibrosis bronchiectasis: the BLESS randomized controlled trial. JAMA 2013;309(12):1260–7.

54. Wong C, Jayaram L, Karalus N, et al. Azithromycin for prevention of exacerbations in non-cystic fibrosis bronchiectasis (EMBRACE): a randomised, double-blind, placebo-controlled trial. Lancet 2012; 380(9842):660–7.

55. Altenburg J, de Graaff CS, Stienstra Y, et al. Effect of azithromycin maintenance treatment on infectious exacerbations among patients with non-cystic fibrosis bronchiectasis: the BAT randomized controlled trial. JAMA 2013;309(12):1251–9.

56. Hill AT. Macrolides for clinically significant bronchiectasis in adults: who should receive this treatment? Chest 2016;150(6):1187–93.

57. Griffith DE, Brown-Elliott BA, Langsjoen B, et al. Clinical and molecular analysis of macrolide resistance in Mycobacterium avium complex lung disease. Am J Respir Crit Care Med 2006;174(8):928–34.

58. Bedi P, Davidson DJ, McHugh BJ, et al. Blood neutrophils are reprogrammed in bronchiectasis. Am J Respir Crit Care Med 2018;198(7):880–90.

59. Oriano M, Amati F, Gramegna A, et al. Protease-antiprotease imbalance in bronchiectasis. Int J Mol Sci 2021;22(11).

60. Chalmers JD, Moffitt KL, Suarez-Cuartin G, et al. Neutrophil elastase activity is associated with exacerbations and lung function decline in bronchiectasis. Am J Respir Crit Care Med 2017;195(10): 1384–93.

61. Chalmers JD, Haworth CS, Metersky ML, et al. Phase 2 trial of the DPP-1 inhibitor Brensocatib in bronchiectasis. N Engl J Med 2020;383(22): 2127–37.

Culture, Identification, and Antimicrobial Susceptibility Testing of Pulmonary Nontuberculous Mycobacteria

Reeti Khare, PhD, D(ABMM)[a],*, Barbara A. Brown-Elliott, MS, MT(ASCP) SM[b]

KEYWORDS

- Nontuberculous mycobacteria • Laboratory methods • Culture • Identification
- Antimicrobial susceptibility testing

KEY POINTS

- Molecular methods of identification of NTM should be used in place of older, less definitive phenotypic methods and should be performed at the species and subspecies level where possible.
- *In vitro* antimicrobial susceptibility testing of NTM is an important adjunctive test although MICs do not always correlate with clinical response.
- Molecular detection of antimicrobial resistance mechanisms, including current single and multiple gene sequencing and genomic sequencing technologies, provide useful clinical data associated with patients and NTM organisms.

BACKGROUND

Nontuberculous mycobacterial (NTM) pulmonary disease is increasing globally.[1] Pulmonary infections are typically opportunistic and associated with immune-compromise and underlying comorbidities such as chronic obstructive pulmonary disease, Sjogren's syndrome, cystic fibrosis, asthma, interstitial pneumonia, and other lung abnormalities.[2,3]

NTM are common environmental organisms that can be found in soil, natural and municipal water sources, urban dust, and environmental ameba.[4] They have also been found as part of normal oral flora in 26% to 33% of people without disease.[5,6] NTM may be transmitted to people via aerosolized water sources, such as showerheads, hot tubs, and humidifiers.[7–9] Medical equipment such as endoscopes, dental waterlines, and heater-coolers used in surgery have also been associated with patient infections.[10]

One of the key factors for diagnosis is culture-positive specimens, which highlights the need for reliable laboratory results.[11] This publication will review the important laboratory techniques used to culture, identify and perform antimicrobial susceptibility testing (AST) for NTM.

SAMPLE COLLECTION AND PROCESSING

For pulmonary disease, sputum is the most common specimen type, though positive cultures from this source may reflect NTM from the oral cavity. Therefore, current guidelines by the American Thoracic Society/European Respiratory Society/European Society of Clinical Microbiology and Infectious Diseases/Infectious Disease Society of America indicate that at least two positive

[a] Mycobacteriology Laboratory, 1400 Jackson Street, National Jewish Health, Denver, CO 80238, USA; [b] The University of TX Health Science Center at Tyler, Mycobacteria/Nocardia Laboratory, 11937 US Highway 271, Tyler, TX 75708, USA
* Corresponding author.
E-mail address: kharer@njhealth.org

Clin Chest Med 44 (2023) 743–755
https://doi.org/10.1016/j.ccm.2023.06.001

specimens from sputa are needed to support a diagnosis of disease, while one positive bronchoalveolar lavage (BAL), transbronchial or lung biopsy specimen may be sufficient.[11]

BAL and bronchial washes with large volumes can be concentrated by centrifugation.[12] Sputum samples are first digested with mucolytic agents such as n-acetyl-L-cysteine, and then decontaminated with chemicals such as sodium hydroxide. This decreases the amount of routine bacteria present in the sample, so that they do not overgrow during culture.[12] Certain organisms, such as *Pseudomonas aeruginosa*, may form protective capsules that protect them from decontamination. Therefore, providers should specify if their patient samples may contain *Pseudomonas* sp. since additional decontamination reagents, such as oxalic acid, may be added.[12] However, despite their hardy cell wall, NTM may also be damaged by decontamination reagents. In order to prevent both under and over decontamination, it is expected that routine bacterial contamination rate is between 2% and 5% for solid cultures and 7% to 8% for liquid cultures.[13]

MICROSCOPY

NTM contain mycolic acids in their cell walls that allows them to retain dyes even in the presence of low concentrations of acid, thus giving them the moniker of "acid-fast" (**Fig. 1**).

Carbolfuchsin-based smears apply a primary red stain to a sample on a microscope slide. Then, either phenols are added (Kinyoun) or the slide is heated (Ziehl-Neelsen) to allow the dye to penetrate into the mycobacterial cell walls. A decolorizer, such as 3% acid-alcohol, is used to wash the stain from nonmycobacterial cells, which are then counterstained with methylene blue. The acid-fast bacilli (AFB) are seen with a light microscope as reddish-pink bacilli, while the non-acid-fast organisms stain blue. In fluorescent (eg, auramine O) smears, dyes bind mycolic acids and cause mycobacterial cells to fluoresce yellow-green.

Some NTM species may produce a cording phenotype when viewed microscopically. Cords are long serpentine bundles of AFB in parallel and are typically associated with *Mycobacterium tuberculosis*, though in rare instances some variants of *Mycobacterium abscessus*, *Mycobacterium marinum* and other NTM may also demonstrate cording.[14]

AFB smears have relatively poor sensitivity. Carbolfuchsin-based smears require as much as 10^4-10^5 acid-fast bacilli (AFB)/ml of specimen to be seen, which corresponds to a sensitivity of ~20 to 80%.[15,16] Fluorescent smears are slightly more sensitive, and can detect ~10% more AFB.[17,18] Despite their poor sensitivity, AFB smears are typically reportable within 24 hours,[13] are low cost, and require minimal equipment. They are also reported semi-quantitatively (eg, 4+ vs 1+), which may estimate the burden of disease. Patient samples with positive AFB smear results and negative rapid nucleic acid amplification results for *M tuberculosis* should increase clinical suspicion for NTM disease.

CLASSIFICATION OF NONTUBERCULOUS MYCOBACTERIA

NTM are divided into two main groups: rapidly growing mycobacteria (RGM), which form visible, mature colonies on solid media within 7 days, and slowly growing mycobacteria (SGM), which grow on solid media after 7 days.[19]

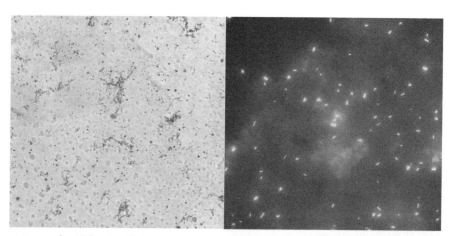

Fig. 1. Appearance of acid fast bacilli (AFB) on Ziehl Neelsen (left) and fluorescent (right) stains. Images taken under 400x with oil.

Newer classification methods take advantage of whole genome sequencing (WGS) methods to classify organisms.[20,21] According to these types of studies, new groupings of NTM have been proposed, although there is a division within the community about whether the five new genera (*Mycobacteroides*, *Mycolicibacterium*, *Mycolicibacter*, and *Mycolicibacillus*, and *Mycobacterium*), are still similar enough to be combined under the current genus *Mycobacterium*.[22,23] For the purposes of this publication, the NTM species will continue to be referred to as *Mycobacterium*.[24]

CULTURE

In order to grow NTM, processed specimens are inoculated in both liquid and solid media. Liquid culture is typically performed in Middlebrook 7H9-based broth supplemented with additives such as oleic acid, albumin, dextrose, and catalase (OADC).[25] A cocktail of broad-spectrum antibiotics and antifungals is added to help suppress the growth of routine bacteria and fungi.[25]

Liquid growth is typically measured in real-time using instruments such as the MGIT (BD) or the Versatrek (Thermo Fisher Scientific). The VersaTREK system measures bacterial growth and respiration by detecting the changing partial pressures of CO_2 and O_2.[26] MGIT instruments detect growth by reading the fluorescent indicator in MGIT tubes which fluoresce as bacterial respiration occurs and O_2 is depleted.[26]

Liquid cultures produce growth approximately 12 to 15 days earlier than solid culture.[27,28] Monitoring the time it takes for organisms to grow in liquid culture, or time to positivity (TTP), may assist providers in predicting clinical outcomes. For instance, a longer TTP is associated with patients who achieve negative cultures after the treatment of *Mycobacterium avium* complex (MAC), compared to those who continue to have positive cultures, presumably because of lower bioburden.[29]

The limitation of liquid cultures is the greater rate of bacterial contamination compared to solid culture, and the inability to determine whether multiple mycobacteria are growing in culture.[13] On the other hand, while solid cultures may yield slower growth, they can help distinguish potentially mixed cultures. Another benefit of solid agar is the ability to determine colony counts, and values are typically reported as specific counts up to 200 colonies or as greater than 200 colonies, or 1+ to 4+. Mean semiquantitative culture scores have been shown to be inversely correlated with sputum culture conversion.[30]

Solid culture can be performed using egg-based media (such as Lowenstein-Jensen media) which contain malachite green, a dye that suppresses the growth of other bacterial organisms.[25] Agar-based media, such as Middlebrook 7H10 or 7H11, is also commonly used. Agar media must be stored and incubated in the dark to prevent deterioration, but colonies may grow several days sooner compared to egg-based media.[25] Additionally, the agar-based media may make the detection of pigmentation easier.

When used together, the sensitivity of solid and liquid culture is greater than 90% and the specificity is greater than 99%.[28] Both solid and liquid cultures are incubated for up to 6 to 8 weeks following inoculation. Cultures are typically incubated at 35 to 37°C, although additional replicates of media may be incubated at higher or lower temperatures in order to support the growth of different mycobacteria. For instance, *Mycobacterium xenopi* may grow best at 42 to 45°C.[31] Similarly, some fastidious mycobacteria may require additional supplements. For instance, *M avium* subsp. *paratuberculosis* requires mycobactin J.[31] Note that growth supplements and different temperatures are not used routinely in all laboratories so it is helpful for providers to alert the laboratory when additional conditions should be applied.

METHODS OF IDENTIFICATION

Following growth in solid or liquid culture, NTM are identified. In North America, the most commonly identified NTM are MAC organisms (52%-76% of NTM identified), followed by RGM (16%–20%).[32,33] Assays used vary based on multiple factors such as availability, performance, complexity, cost, turnaround-time, and labor-intensiveness (**Table 1**).

Nucleic acid hybridization is a relatively low-cost, low-complexity technique. It uses oligonucleotide probes to bind directly to ribosomal RNA in target organisms. When bound, light is released and read with a luminometer.[34] However, because probes bind directly to DNA without a prior nucleic acid amplification step, resolution is low and the assay must be performed on cultured organisms from liquid or solid media. Five hybridization probes currently exist for the detection of mycobacteria (see **Table 1**). However, the manufacturer announced their discontinuation at the end of 2022.[35]

Matrix-assisted laser desorption ionization-time of flight mass spectrometry (MALDI-TOF MS) is an increasingly utilized platform for mycobacterial identification. In this method, the protein spectrum from pure mycobacterial culture is interrogated against a database of reference spectra to get a final identification. Advantages of the MALDI-TOF MS

Table 1
Commercial assays available for testing of nontuberculous mycobacteria

Name of Assay	Method	ID for MTBC	ID of NTM	# of NTM Species or Subspecies Identified	Manufacturer
Intended for samples (eg, sputum) only					
GenoType CMdirect VER 1.0[76]	NAAT (Line probe)	Y	Y	20	Hain Lifescience, Germany
AdvanSure TB/NTM real time PCR[77]	NAAT (Real-time PCR)	Y	Y	0; (generic NTM detection)	LG Life Science, Korea
NTM from sputum and isolates					
MolecuTech Real MTB-ID[78]	NAAT (Real-time PCR)	Y	Y	6	YD Diagnostics, Korea
MolecuTech TB-Tag Two[78]	NAAT (nested, conventional PCR)	Y	Y	8	YD Diagnostics, Korea
MolecuTech REBA Myco-ID[78]	NAAT (Reverse Blot Hybridization)	Y	Y	19	YD Diagnostics, Korea
MolecuTech Real MTB-ID[78]	NAAT (Real-time PCR)	Y	Y	6	YD Diagnostics, Korea
Genoscholar NTM + MDRTB II (Previously called NTM + MDRTB Detection Kit 2)[79]	NAAT (Line probe)	Y	Y	3	Nipro, Japan
Anyplex MTB/NTM Real-time PCR[80]	NAAT (Real-time PCR)	Y	Y	0; generic NTM detection	Seegene, Korea
PowerChek MTB/NTM Real time PCR Kit[81]	NAAT (Real-time PCR)	Y	Y		Kogene Biotech, Korea
Deeplex Myc-TB[82]	Targeted NGS	Y	Y	>100	Genoscreen, France
TB/NTM PCR[83]	NAAT (Conventional PCR, 2 reactions)	Y	Y	0; generic NTM detection	Biocore, Korea
TB/NTM PCR (one tube)[84]	NAAT (Conventional PCR, single reaction)	Y	Y	0; generic NTM detection	Biocore, Korea
TB/NTM Real Time PCR[85]	NAAT (Real-time PCR)	Y	Y	0; generic NTM detection	Biocore, Korea
NTM from isolates only					
Accuprobe *Mycobacterium avium* Culture Identification Test[a,86]	Hybridization probe	N	Y	1	Hologic, US
Accuprobe *M avium* complex Culture Identification Test[a,86]	Hybridization probe	N	Y	1	Hologic, US
Accuprobe *Mycobacterium intracellulare* Culture Identification Test[a,86]	Hybridization probe	N	Y	1	Hologic, US

(continued on next page)

Table 1
(continued)

Name of Assay	Method	ID for MTBC	ID of NTM	# of NTM Species or Subspecies Identified	Manufacturer
Accuprobe *Mycobacterium gordonae* Culture Identification Test[a],[86]	Hybridization probe	N	Y	1	Hologic, US
Accuprobe *Mycobacterium kansasii* Culture Identification Test[a],[86]	Hybridization probes	N	Y	1	Hologic, US
GenoType NTM-DR VER 1.0[76],[87]	NAAT (Line probe)	N	Y	7	Hain Lifescience, Germany
GenoType Mycobacterium AS[76]	NAAT (Line probe)	N	Y	19	Hain Lifescience, Germany
GenoType Mycobacterium CM VER 2.0[76]	NAAT (Line probe)	Y	Y	20	Hain Lifescience, Germany
FluoroType Mycobacteria VER 1.0[88]	NAAT (Asymmetrical FRET PCR)	N	Y	32	Hain Lifescience, Germany
MolecuTech MTB-ID V3[78]	NAAT (Nested, conventional PCR)	Y	Y	11	YD Diagnostics, Korea
Speed-Oligo Mycobacteria[89]	NAAT (Line probe)	Y	Y	14	Vircell, Spain
INNO-LiPA Mycobacteria v2[90]	NAAT (Line probe)	Y	Y	16	Fujirebio, Japan
Vitek MS[91]	MALDI-TOF MS	Y	Y	18	bioMerieux, France
Bruker Mycobacteria RUO[92]	MALDI-TOF MS	Y	Y	182	Bruker Daltonics GmbH & Co. KG, Germany

[a] To be discontinued. FRET, fluorescence resonance energy transfer; MALDI-TOF MS, matrix-assisted laser desorption ionization time of flight mass spectrometry; MTBC, mycobacterium tuberculosis; NAAT, nucleic acid amplification test; NGS: next-generation sequencing; NTM, nontuberculous mycobacteria; PCR, polymerase chain reaction; US, USA.

platform include rapid turnaround time (<1 hour), low operational cost (although the initial instrument expenditure is high), and is its broad coverage of many mycobacterial species. For instance, 67 species could be identified in one study.[36] The sensitivity reported from most studies is between 80% and 98%, though the protein extraction method and cut-off thresholds can significantly affect the performance of NTM identification.[37]

While MALDI-TOF MS has acceptable performance on plated isolates, it shows relatively poor performance for NTM identification from primary specimens or growth of newly positive liquid cultures.[38],[39] Another limitation is that highly similar NTM, such as *subsp. intracellulare, M intracellulare*

subsp. *chimaera*, and *M intracellulare* subsp. *yongonense*, *Mycobacterium mucogenicum* and *Mycobacterium phocaicum*, and *M. abscessus* subspecies, cannot be discriminated by MALDI-TOF MS.[40] Furthermore, the robustness of the reference database is essential for breadth and accuracy of identification; for example, *Mycobacterium gastri* may be misidentified as *Mycobacterium kansasii* by the bioMérieux SA Vitek MS V3.0 (Marcy L'Étoile, France).[41] Importantly, the Bruker database for mycobacteria is not cleared by the FDA, while the Vitek MS V3.0 is FDA cleared.[41]

Line probe assays (LPAs) are PCR-based, reverse hybridization assays that can be used to identify specific bacterial species with high accuracy. First, a multiplex PCR is performed to amplify various mycobacterial targets using biotinylated primers. Amplicons are then applied to a membrane containing capture probes. A substrate is added, and if the amplicons of interest have been captured, the enzymes will break down the substrate to cause a color change at a specific location on the membrane.[42] The resulting bands of color that appear on the membrane are correlated with specific organism identifications. Evaluations of the most common line probe assays have been shown to have high sensitivity for NTM from liquid culture (>98%).[43]

LPAs can also, simultaneously, identify markers of drug resistance (see later in discussion). Alternately, these assays can be subjective to read, labor-intensive, and will not identify organisms beyond those on the membrane. Furthermore, none of these assays are FDA approved and must be validated as a laboratory-developed test (LDT), which can be a barrier for laboratories in the United States (USA).

Other LDTs for NTM may be developed and evaluated by laboratories. For instance, the PCR/MALDI-TOF MS uses a combination of methods in order to maintain high sensitivity and specificity but also provide high throughput capabilities at lower cost. In this method, a multiplex PCR is performed to amplify many mycobacterial targets prior to the addition of detection probes. In the presence of their target amplicons, the detection probes will be extended by a single base, which increases their molecular weight by a known amount. MALDI-TOF MS is then used to determine which probes have increased mass, and this is converted into an organism identification.[44] Despite the high accuracy of the assay, it can currently only be performed on cultured isolates.

Sequencing assays are considered the gold standard for the identification of most mycobacterial organisms. Whole genome sequencing (WGS) interrogates the sequence of the entire NTM isolate, and can be used for multiple purposes, including identification, mutations associated with resistance, and phylogenetic-relatedness studies.[45] Sanger sequencing of single, conserved genes is a more commonly available methodology and typically used for the identification of cultured isolates. With this methodology, genes such as rpoB (encodes the β-subunit of bacterial RNA polymerase), hsp65 (encodes a bacterial heatshock protein), 16S (encodes ribosomal RNA used in the 30S subunit of bacterial ribosomes), and 16S-23S ITS (the intergenic spacer region between ribosomal RNA genes) are sequenced.[46] The resulting sequences are compared to curated or public (eg, National Center for Biotechnology Institute) databases. High levels of sequence homology with reliable reference sequences (typically >97%) may be used for final identification.

Sequencing assays may have variable performance depending upon the species and gene target sequenced.[47] For example, rpoβ gene sequencing is able to distinguish the M. abscessus subspecies and M intracellulare subsp. chimaera unlike 16S sequencing.[45] In addition, the quality of the database used can markedly affect the results, and in-house databases are often needed to supplement public databases, which may be of lesser quality.[48] WGS and Sanger sequencing are not typically performed in most laboratories for routine identification purposes because of high cost and high complexity.

Identification to the relevant species or subspecies is considered preferable to "complex," "group," or generic classification (eg, Mycobacterium chelonae-abscessus), for two main reasons. Differentiation of individual species can help resolve whether prolonged patient positivity is due to refractory disease or because of an infection with a similar but distinct organism.[11] Secondly, even highly related organisms may have significantly different treatment options, and accurate identification can ensure appropriate treatment. For example, M chelonae typically has lower MICs to tobramycin, which is the preferred aminoglycoside for that species, while M. abscessus subspecies generally have high tobramycin MICs and are preferentially treated with amikacin.[49,50] Similarly, most M. abscessus subsp. abscessus and subsp. bolletii exhibit inducible resistance to clarithromycin due to a functional erm(41) gene. In contrast, M. abscessus subsp. massiliense typically has a truncated erm(41) gene, and should be susceptible to clarithromycin by this mechanism.[51]

STRAIN TYPING

Determining the similarity between NTM isolates can be useful for identifying sources of exposure, tracing transmission during outbreaks, understanding how patient isolates are changing in vivo, or in differentiating isolates associated with new infection versus those from relapse. Strain typing has been used frequently for M tuberculosis, but in some instances, it has been important to understand similarities in NTM species. For example, WGS was used to trace an international outbreak of invasive M intracellulare subsp. chimaera to heater-cooler devices used during cardiothoracic surgery.[52]

Pulsed field gel electrophoresis was the first molecular method to determine the "DNA fingerprint" of NTM and has been most often used with MAC and the *M. abscessus* species. However, few laboratories perform the test as it is time consuming, and expensive, and instrumentation was recently discontinued.[53–56]

Strain-relatedness can be most comprehensively determined with WGS performed using next generation sequencing methods. Another useful method is multilocus sequence typing (MLST), which focuses on strain similarities based on a limited number of genes.[57]

PHENOTYPIC ANTIMICROBIAL SUSCEPTIBILITY TESTING

Currently, only broth microdilution methods have been recommended by the Clinical Laboratory Standards Institute (CLSI) for AST of NTM.[58]

Briefly, broth microdilution methods use 2-fold concentrations of antimicrobials to determine the lowest concentration, or minimum inhibitory concentration (MIC), at which growth of the mycobacteria are inhibited. The reproducibility of MICs is generally acceptable within one 2-fold dilution of the actual end point of the inhibition of growth.[58]

In order to assure accurate MICs, the test organism is confirmed as a pure culture macroscopically or optimally using a stereoscope to determine colony appearance (eg, rough, smooth, and so forth).[13] The colonies are then inoculated into a suitable diluent. For the RGM, the use of sterile glass beads added to sterile water is recommended to assure more adequate homogenization of the suspension especially with rough colonies.

Standardization of inoculum is important to help to ensure the quality of the test results. For example, a heavy inoculum may result in falsely elevated (resistant) MIC readings whereas a light inoculum may cause MICs to appear falsely susceptible. To avoid these types of errors, the inoculum should be standardized using a nephelometer or other similar turbidity meter to prepare a suspension that is equivalent to a 0.5 McFarland standard. The suspension is then inoculated into a 96-well microtiter microdilution panel that contains 2-fold dilutions of antimicrobials.[58]

Importantly, cation-adjusted Mueller Hinton broth (CAMHB) for RGM and CAMHB +5% oleic acid-albumin-dextrose-catalase (OADC) for slowly growing mycobacteria (SGM) should be used as all current MIC breakpoints were developed using these alkaline media rather than acidic Middlebrook 7H9 broth.[58,59]

Time and temperature of incubation should also be standardized, since it is also based on previous data indicating that most RGM grow best at $30° \pm 2°C$ while SGM grow more optimally at $36 \pm 2°C$. A few exceptions do exist such as *M xenopi* (which may grow better at $42 \pm 2°C$) and the rare pulmonary pathogen, *Mycobacterium haemophilum* (which optimally grows at $30 \pm 2°C$).[58,59]

The CLSI has recommended batteries of antimicrobials for the AST of RGM and SGM (**Table 2**). Special conditions apply for some species of SGM including the MAC. Currently, testing of rifampin, rifabutin, and ethambutol is not currently recommended since data suggests no correlation of *in vitro* MICs and clinical response with these antimicrobials.[58] However, MICs for clarithromycin (chosen over azithromycin as the class macrolide) and amikacin should be reported. In some cases, MICs for antimicrobials for which no studies of clinical correlation have been done may be reported. These would include linezolid and moxifloxacin along with some of the newer antimicrobials which have shown limited *in vitro* activity against the MAC.[59] Although these MICs may be performed, they should not be considered as substitutes for the primary agents which should be used in combination with a macrolide (clarithromycin or azithromycin) with or without amikacin or streptomycin for treatment regimens.[55,60]

Recently definitions of amikacin have been modified to include the inhaled formulation of amikacin. Resistance to amikacin liposome inhalation suspension has been defined as ≥ 128 µg/mL while resistance to IV amikacin has been defined as ≥ 64 µg/mL.[61] These definitions were based on patient outcomes including with intravenous and liposomal inhaled amikacin.[60,62] In the former study of 462 clinical isolates of MAC, five isolates, for which clinical data was available, had amikacin MICs greater than 64 µg/mL; four of these patients were known to be treated with amikacin and contained the 16S rRNA gene mutation whereas the mutation was not detected in isolates with amikacin MICs ≤ 64 µg/mL.[60] Similarly, 26/336 (7.7%) patients in the amikacin liposome inhalation suspension study had amikacin MICs greater than 64 µg/mL with no sustained conversion.[62]

Generally, all untreated strains of MAC are macrolide susceptible, and this definition also applies to azithromycin although there are no breakpoints for azithromycin.[59,63] Macrolide resistance has been defined as a clarithromycin MIC ≥ 32 µg/mL.[58,59] It should also be noted that MAC isolates with intermediate (16 µg/mL) clarithromycin MICs are rare and may be a harbinger of impending macrolide resistance.[59]

The other SGM species for which special conditions may apply is *M kansasii*. The CLSI recommends routine AST of rifampin and clarithromycin only. If the isolate is resistant to one of these agents, the full SGM battery of antimicrobials

Table 2
Recommended antimicrobials and breakpoints for antimicrobial susceptibility testing of nontuberculous mycobacteria, as recommended by the Clinical and Laboratory Standards Institute (CLSI)[61]

Antimicrobial	MIC (µg/mL) Susceptible	Intermediate	Resistant
Rapidly growing mycobacteria			
Amikacin	≤16	32	≥64
Cefoxitin	16	32–64	≥128
Clarithromycin	≤2	4	≥8
Ciprofloxacin	≤1	2	≥4
Doxycycline	≤1	2–4	≥8
Imipenem	≤4	8–16	≥32
Linezolid	≤8	16	≥32
Minocycline	≤1	2–4	≥8
Meropenem	≤4	8–16	≥32
Moxifloxacin	≤1	2	≥4
Linezolid	≤8	16	≥32
Tigecycline[a]	-	-	-
Tobramycin[b]	≤2	4	≥8
Trimethoprim/sulfamethoxazole	≤2/38	-	≥4/76
Slowly growing mycobacteria[c]			
Amikacin (Intravenous)	≤16	32	≥64
Amikacin (Inhaled, liposomal, MAC only)	≤64	-	≥128
Clarithromycin	≤8	16	≥32
Ciprofloxacin	≤1	2	≥4
Doxycycline	≤1	2–4	≥8
Linezolid	≤8	16	≥32
Minocycline	≤1	2–4	≥8
Moxifloxacin	≤1	2	≥4
Rifabutin	≤2	-	≥4
Rifampin	≤1	-	≥2
Trimethoprim/sulfamethoxazole	≤2/38	-	≥4/76

[a] The CLSI has not addressed breakpoints for tigecycline. Therefore, MICs should be reported without interpretation.
[b] Tobramycin MIC is recommended to be reported only against isolates of M. chelonae complex.
[c] For the M. avium complex (MAC), only clarithromycin and amikacin should be reported routinely.

should be tested and reported.[58] Rifabutin should be substituted for HIV-infected patients on protease inhibitors.[64] Isolates that are susceptible to rifampin should be susceptible to rifabutin. Treatment failure of patients with M kansasii is rare but is usually associated with rifampin resistance and occasionally one or more companion agents including a macrolide (clarithromycin or azithromycin).[64] There are no standardized breakpoints for isoniazid (INH). Generally, MICs for M kansasii are 0.5-5 µg/mL so that INH breakpoint determination has been difficult. An MIC value for INH may be reported without interpretation if needed.[58] It should be noted that modifications of the CLSI guidelines

omitted testing of ethambutol against any NTM due to technical difficulty in testing and non-reproducible MICs. However, this antimicrobial can and should continue to be used in combination treatment regimens of NTM including M kansasii and MAC.[58]

Limitations of phenotypic antimicrobial susceptibility testing of nontuberculous mycobacteria

The following caveats are summarized from the current CLSI M24, 3rd Edition.[58]

- The only standardized and recommended AST method is the broth microdilution method. No agar-based methods have been standardized or recommended by the CLSI.
- Except for clarithromycin, for which extended incubation for the determination of inducible macrolide resistance conferred by the erm(41) gene is required, incubations beyond 4 to 5 days for RGM and beyond 14 days for SGM, should be carefully interpreted especially with less stable antimicrobials such as carbapenems and tetracyclines (doxycycline, minocycline and tigecycline). Stability of the newer tetracyclines (omadacycline and eravacycline) has not been evaluated. MICs of isolates that require longer incubation should be repeated and/or the isolate should be sent to an experienced reference laboratory. If increased incubation times are necessary, a comment that extended incubation may be detrimental to the stability of these agents and may result in falsely resistant MIC values, is recommended.
- Amikacin MICs ≥64 μg/mL should be repeated and/or the isolate should be sent to an experienced reference laboratory. This type of resistance is often associated with prior treatment with tobramycin or amikacin (but not streptomycin) (See Gene-based AST for details).[59,65] TMP-SMX MICs should be read at 80% inhibition.[66]
- Clarithromycin MICs ≥16 μg/mL in RGM after initial (3–4 days) and 7 days for SGM (eg, MAC) incubation generally suggests mutational macrolide resistance. Clarithromycin MICs should be repeated and/or the isolate should be sent to an experienced reference laboratory. (See Gene-based AST for details).
- Trailing endpoints have been observed with some antimicrobials including the tetracyclines and this problem may be due to heavy inoculum. If, however, after repeat testing, trailing is not resolved, for newer antimicrobials such as omadacycline and eravacycline investigation by a qualified reference laboratory may be warranted. MICs have previously been reported with 80% and 100% inhibition endpoints. Currently, the CLSI has not yet addressed this issue and further study of this phenomenon is necessary to attempt to resolve the problem and determine how to interpret these endpoints.[67,68]

GENE-BASED ANTIMICROBIAL SUSCEPTIBILITY TESTING

Molecular assays to detect genetic markers of resistance are more rapid than standard phenotypic AST and may be helpful in defining antimicrobial resistance in NTM including those isolates that grow poorly. Additionally, they may also be valuable investigative tools to confirm unusual or unexpected phenotypic susceptibility results. PCR-based assays, such as line probes, as well as single gene sequencing assays can be used to detect these antimicrobial resistance mutations. Recent whole genomic characterization has uncovered previously undescribed resistance determinants and classes of virulence factors, which may replace current single target sequencing methods.[69–72] However, at this time, gene sequencing and especially whole genomic sequencing platforms are not feasible in many laboratories (see discussion in Methods of Identification).

Macrolide resistance by the methylation of the 23S rRNA gene, which prevents binding of the macrolide antibiotic to the ribosomes, has been described in M tuberculosis [(erm(37)] and several NTM. Inducible clarithromycin resistance is seen in isolates with functional erm genes such as Mycobacterium smegmatis and Mycobacterium goodii [erm(38)], Mycobacterium fortuitum [erm(39)], Mycobacterium mageritense and Mycobacterium wolinskyi [erm(40)], 80% of M. abscessus subsp. abscessus and most subsp. bolletii [erm(41)]. The former five taxa are not typical pulmonary pathogens. Isolates of M. abscessus subsp. massiliense and 20% of subsp. abscessus typically have nonfunctional erm(41) genes.[59,69,70,73]

Other RGM, such as the pigmented RGM, have been less well evaluated for the presence of an erm gene as the species/subspecies listed here. Genotypic determination of the erm gene can be substituted for phenotype clarithromycin MICs which require extended (up to 14 days) incubation, as long as species identification has been confirmed by molecular methods.[58,71–73]

Acquired (mutational) clarithromycin resistance is associated with a single base pair mutation in the 23SrRNA (rrl) gene at the adenine 2058 or 2059 position. Unlike the inducible (erm gene) resistance, which requires extended incubation, this macrolide resistance is usually seen at the initial (3–5 days in RGM and 7 days with SGM) MIC reading as previously noted.[74,75]

Amikacin mutational resistance in MAC, the M. abscessus species, and M chelonae has been associated with a point mutation at the adenine 1408 position in the 16SrRNA (rrs) gene. Prolonged exposure to amikacin is generally related to a to G (adenine to guanine) mutation as demonstrated in previous studies of NTM isolates with amikacin MICs greater than 64 μg/mL.[60,65]

As the recognition of NTM increases globally, clinicians and laboratorians should be aware of the need for appropriate laboratory identification and susceptibility testing to guide in the selection of optimal treatment regimens. As newer technologies become available, especially in the areas of antimicrobial resistance mechanisms, the hope is for improved treatment strategies.

DISCLOSURE

RK has lab contracted research with Insmed and Paratek Pharmaceuticals. BBE has had lab contracted research with Paratek Pharmaceuticals, Insmed and Tetraphase Pharmaceuticals.

REFERENCES

1. Winthrop KL, Marras TK, Adjemian J, et al. Incidence and prevalence of nontuberculous mycobacterial lung disease in a large U.S. managed care health plan, 2008-2015. Ann Am Thorac Soc 2020; 17(2):178–85.
2. Uno S, Asakura T, Morimoto K, et al. Comorbidities associated with nontuberculous mycobacterial disease in Japanese adults: a claims-data analysis. BMC Pulm Med 2020;20(1):262.
3. Skolnik K, Kirkpatrick G, Quon BS. Nontuberculous mycobacteria in cystic fibrosis. Curr Treat Options Infect Dis 2016;8(4):259–74.
4. Honda JR, Virdi R, Chan ED. Global environmental nontuberculous mycobacteria and their contemporaneous man-made and natural niches. Front Microbiol 2018;9:2029.
5. Thornton CS, Mellett M, Jarand J. The respiratory microbiome and nontuberculous mycobacteria: an emerging concern in human health. Eur Respir Rev 2021;30(160).
6. Wali SO, Abdelaziz MM, Krayem AB, et al. The presence of atypical mycobacteria in the mouthwashes of normal subjects: role of tap water and oral hygiene. Ann Thorac Med 2008;3(1):5–8.
7. Gebert MJ, Delgado-Baquerizo M, Oliverio AM, et al. Ecological analyses of mycobacteria in showerhead biofilms and their relevance to human health. mBio 2018;9(5).
8. Utsugi H, Usui Y, Nishihara F. *Mycobacterium gordonae*-induced humidifier lung. BMC Pulm Med 2015; 15:108.
9. Fjallbrant H, Akerstrom M, Svensson E, et al. Hot tub lung: an occupational hazard. Eur Respir Rev 2013; 22(127):88–90.
10. Weeks JW, Segars K, Guha S. The research gap in non-tuberculous Mycobacterium (NTM) and reusable medical devices. Front Public Health 2020;8:399.
11. Daley CL, Iaccarino JM, Lange C, et al. Treatment of nontuberculous mycobacterial pulmonary disease: an official ATS/ERS/ESCMID/IDSA clinical practice guideline. Clin Infect Dis 2020;71(4):905–13.
12. Wengenack N. 7.2 general mycobacterial procedures. In: Leber AL, editor. Clinical Microbiology procedures handbook. 4th edition. Washington, DC: ASM Press; 2016.
13. Laboratory CLSI. Detection and identification of mycobacteria M48. 2nd edition. USA: Clinical and Laboratory Standards Institute; 2018.
14. Sanchez-Chardi A, Olivares F, Byrd TF, et al. Demonstration of cord formation by rough Mycobacterium abscessus variants: implications for the clinical microbiology laboratory. J Clin Microbiol 2011;49(6):2293–5.
15. Azadi D, Motallebirad T, Ghaffari K, et al. Mycobacteriosis and tuberculosis: laboratory diagnosis. Open Microbiol J 2018;12:41–58.
16. Ghiasi M, Pande T, Pai M. Advances in tuberculosis diagnostics. Current Tropical Medicine Reports 2015;2(2):54–61.
17. Cattamanchi A, Davis JL, Worodria W, et al. Sensitivity and specificity of fluorescence microscopy for diagnosing pulmonary tuberculosis in a high HIV prevalence setting. Int J Tuberc Lung Dis 2009; 13(9):1130–6.
18. Somoskovi A, Hotaling JE, Fitzgerald M, et al. Lessons from a proficiency testing event for acid-fast microscopy. Chest 2001;120(1):250–7.
19. Runyon EH. Pathogenic mycobacteria. Bibl Tuberc 1965;21:235–87.
20. Gupta RS, Lo B, Son J. Phylogenomics and comparative genomic studies robustly support division of the genus *Mycobacterium* into an emended genus *Mycobacterium* and four novel genera. Front Microbiol 2018;9:67.
21. Gupta RS, Lo B, Son J. Corrigendum: phylogenomics and comparative genomic studies robustly support division of the genus Mycobacterium into an emended genus Mycobacterium and four novel genera. Front Microbiol 2019;10:714.
22. Tortoli E, Brown-Elliott BA, Chalmers JD, et al. Same meat, different gravy: ignore the new names of mycobacteria. Eur Respir J 2019;54(1).
23. Oren A, Trujillo ME. On the valid publication of names of mycobacteria. Eur Respir J 2019;54(4).
24. Meehan CJ, Barco RA, Loh Y-HE, et al. Reconstituting the genus Mycobacterium. Int J Syst Evol Microbiol 2021;71(9):004922.
25. Martin I, Pfyffer GE, Parrish N. Mycobacterium: general characteristics, laboratory detection, and staining procedures. 12th Ed. ed. Washington, DC: ASM Press; 2019.
26. Pfeltz RF, Wengenack N. 7.4 liquid media used for isolation. In: Leber AL, editor. Clinical Microbiology procedures handbook. 4th Edition ed. Washington, DC: ASM Press; 2021.
27. Zhao P, Yu Q, Chen L, et al. Evaluation of a liquid culture system in the detection of mycobacteria at

an antituberculosis institution in China; A retrospective study. J Int Med Res 2016;44(5):1055–60.

28. Sorlozano A, Soria I, Roman J, et al. Comparative evaluation of three culture methods for the isolation of mycobacteria from clinical samples. J Microbiol Biotechnol 2009;19(10):1259–64.

29. Mingora CM, Garcia BA, Mange KC, et al. Time-to-positivity of Mycobacterium avium complex in broth culture associates with culture conversion. BMC Infect Dis 2022;22(1):246.

30. Griffith DE, Adjemian J, Brown-Elliott BA, et al. Semi-quantitative culture analysis during therapy for Mycobacterium avium complex lung disease. Am J Respir Crit Care Med 2015;192(6):754–60.

31. Forbes BA, Hall GS, Miller MB, et al. Practical guidance for clinical microbiology laboratories: mycobacteria. Clin Microbiol Rev 2018;31(2).

32. Spaulding AB, Lai YL, Zelazny AM, et al. Geographic distribution of nontuberculous mycobacterial species identified among clinical isolates in the United States, 2009-2013. Ann Am Thorac Soc 2017;14(11):1655–61.

33. Hoefsloot W, van Ingen J, Andrejak C, et al. The geographic diversity of nontuberculous mycobacteria isolated from pulmonary samples: an NTM-NET collaborative study. Eur Respir J 2013;42(6): 1604–13.

34. Caulfield AJ, Wengenack NL. Diagnosis of active tuberculosis disease: from microscopy to molecular techniques. J Clin Tuberc Other Mycobact Dis 2016; 4:33–43.

35. Hologic. Letter of Discontinuation (press release). San Diego, CA: Hologic; 2021.

36. Rodriguez-Temporal D, Rodriguez-Sanchez B, Alcaide F. Evaluation of MALDI biotyper interpretation criteria for accurate identification of nontuberculous mycobacteria. J Clin Microbiol 2020;58(10).

37. Alcaide F, Amlerova J, Bou G, et al. How to: identify non-tuberculous Mycobacterium species using MALDI-TOF mass spectrometry. Clin Microbiol Infect 2018;24(6):599–603.

38. van Eck K, Faro D, Wattenberg M, et al. Matrix-assisted laser desorption ionization-time of flight mass spectrometry fails to identify nontuberculous mycobacteria from primary cultures of respiratory samples. J Clin Microbiol 2016;54(7):1915–7.

39. Toney NC, Zhu W, Jensen B, et al. Evaluation of MALDI biotyper mycobacteria library for identification of nontuberculous mycobacteria. J Clin Microbiol 2022;60(9):e0021722.

40. Saleeb PG, Drake SK, Murray PR, et al. Identification of mycobacteria in solid-culture media by matrix-assisted laser desorption ionization-time of flight mass spectrometry. J Clin Microbiol 2011;49(5): 1790–4.

41. Luo L, Cao W, Chen W, et al. Evaluation of the VITEK MS knowledge base version 3.0 for the identification of clinically relevant Mycobacterium species. Emerg Microbes Infect 2018;7(1):114.

42. Huang WC, Yu MC, Huang YW. Identification and drug susceptibility testing for nontuberculous mycobacteria. J Formos Med Assoc 2020;119(Suppl 1): S32–41.

43. Padilla E, Gonzalez V, Manterola JM, et al. Comparative evaluation of the new version of the INNO-LiPA Mycobacteria and genotype Mycobacterium assays for identification of Mycobacterium species from MB/BacT liquid cultures artificially inoculated with Mycobacterial strains. J Clin Microbiol 2004;42(7):3083–8.

44. Decurtis E, Machado I, Durbin D, et al. MALDI-TOF mass spectrometry from nucleic acid: development of a novel platform for identification of mycobacteria to the species and subspecies level. Astract CPHM: 156 - 2943. ASM Microbe Conference Washington DC; 2022.

45. Dohal M, Porvaznik I, Solovic I, et al. Whole genome sequencing in the management of non-tuberculous mycobacterial infections. Microorganisms 2021;9(11).

46. Slany M, Pavlik I. Molecular detection of nontuberculous mycobacteria: advantages and limits of a broad-range sequencing approach. J Mol Microbiol Biotechnol 2012;22(4):268–76.

47. Kim SH, Shin JH. Identification of nontuberculous mycobacteria using multilocous sequence analysis of 16S rRNA, hsp65, and rpoB. J Clin Lab Anal 2018;32(1).

48. Turenne CY, Tschetter L, Wolfe J, et al. Necessity of quality-controlled 16S rRNA gene sequence databases: identifying nontuberculous Mycobacterium species. J Clin Microbiol 2001;39(10):3637–48.

49. Hatakeyama S, Ohama Y, Okazaki M, et al. Antimicrobial susceptibility testing of rapidly growing mycobacteria isolated in Japan. BMC Infect Dis 2017; 17(1):197.

50. Broda A, Jebbari H, Beaton K, et al. Comparative drug resistance of Mycobacterium abscessus and M. chelonae isolates from patients with and without cystic fibrosis in the United Kingdom. J Clin Microbiol 2013;51(1):217–23.

51. Nie W, Duan H, Huang H, et al. Species identification of Mycobacterium abscessus subsp. abscessus and Mycobacterium abscessus subsp. bolletii using rpoB and hsp65, and susceptibility testing to eight antibiotics. Int J Infect Dis 2014;25:170–4.

52. Perkins KM, Lawsin A, Hasan NA, et al. Notes from the field: Mycobacterium chimaera contamination of heater-cooler devices used in cardiac surgery - United States. MMWR Morb Mortal Wkly Rep 2016; 65(40):1117–8.

53. Baker AW, Lewis SS, Alexander BD, et al. Two-phase hospital-associated outbreak of Mycobacterium abscessus: investigation and mitigation. Clin Infect Dis 2017;64(7):902–11.

54. Davidson RM, Hasan NA, de Moura VC, et al. Phylogenomics of Brazilian epidemic isolates of Mycobacterium abscessus subsp. bolletii reveals relationships of global outbreak strains. Infect Genet Evol 2013;20: 292–7.

55. Wallace RJ Jr, Zhang Y, Brown-Elliott BA, et al. Repeat positive cultures in Mycobacterium intracellulare lung disease after macrolide therapy represent new infections in patients with nodular bronchiectasis. J Infect Dis 2002;186(2):266–73.

56. Griffith DE, Brown-Elliott BA, Langsjoen B, et al. Clinical and molecular analysis of macrolide resistance in Mycobacterium avium complex lung disease. Am J Respir Crit Care Med 2006;174(8):928–34.

57. Wuzinski M, Bak AK, Petkau A, et al. A multilocus sequence typing scheme for Mycobacterium abscessus complex (MAB-multilocus sequence typing) using whole-genome sequencing data. Int J Mycobacteriol 2019;8(3):273–80.

58. CLSI. Susceptibility testing of mycobacteria, Nocardia spp., and other aerobic actinomycetes, M24. 3rd edition. USA: Clinical and Laboratory Standards Institute; 2018.

59. Brown-Elliott BA, Nash KA, Wallace RJ Jr. Antimicrobial susceptibility testing, drug resistance mechanisms, and therapy of infections with nontuberculous mycobacteria. Clin Microbiol Rev 2012;25(3):545–82.

60. Brown-Elliott BA, Iakhiaeva E, Griffith DE, et al. In vitro activity of amikacin against isolates of Mycobacterium avium complex with proposed MIC breakpoints and finding of a 16S rRNA gene mutation in treated isolates. J Clin Microbiol 2013;51(10): 3389–94.

61. CLSI. Performance standards for susceptibility testing of mycobacteria, nocardia spp., and other aerobic actinomycetes, 2nd edition CLSI supplement M24S. USA: Clinical and Laboratory Standards Institute; 2023.

62. Griffith DE, Eagle G, Thomson R, et al. Amikacin liposome inhalation suspension for treatment-refractory lung disease caused by Mycobacterium avium complex. (CONVERT). A prospective, open-label, randomized study. Am J Respir Crit Care Med 2018;198(12):1559–69.

63. Brown BA, Wallace RJ Jr, Onyi GO, et al. Activities of four macrolides, including clarithromycin, against Mycobacterium fortuitum, Mycobacterium chelonae, and M. chelonae-like organisms. Antimicrob Agents Chemother 1992;36(1):180–4.

64. Wallace RJ Jr, Dunbar D, Brown BA, et al. Rifampin-resistant Mycobacterium kansasii. Clin Infect Dis 1994;18(5):736–43.

65. Prammananan T, Sander P, Brown BA, et al. A single 16S ribosomal RNA substitution is responsible for resistance to amikacin and other 2-deoxystreptamine aminoglycosides in Mycobacterium abscessus and Mycobacterium chelonae. J Infect Dis 1998;177(6):1573–81.

66. Wallace RJ Jr, Wiss K, Bushby MB, et al. In vitro activity of trimethoprim and sulfamethoxazole against the nontuberculous mycobacteria. Rev Infect Dis 1982;4(2):326–31.

67. Brown-Elliott BA, Wallace RJ Jr. In Vitro susceptibility testing of eravacycline against nontuberculous mycobacteria. Antimicrob Agents Chemother 2022; 66(9):e0068922.

68. Brown-Elliott BA, Wallace RJ Jr. In Vitro susceptibility testing of omadacycline against nontuberculous mycobacteria. Antimicrob Agents Chemother 2021; 65(3).

69. Koh WJ, Jeon K, Lee NY, et al. Clinical significance of differentiation of Mycobacterium massiliense from Mycobacterium abscessus. Am J Respir Crit Care Med 2011;183(3):405–10.

70. Davidson RM, Benoit JB, Kammlade SM, et al. Genomic characterization of sporadic isolates of the dominant clone of Mycobacterium abscessus subspecies massiliense. Sci Rep 2021;11(1):15336.

71. Nash KA, Andini N, Zhang Y, et al. Intrinsic macrolide resistance in rapidly growing mycobacteria. Antimicrob Agents Chemother 2006;50(10):3476–8.

72. Bastian S, Veziris N, Roux AL, et al. Assessment of clarithromycin susceptibility in strains belonging to the Mycobacterium abscessus group by erm(41) and rrl sequencing. Antimicrob Agents Chemother 2011;55(2):775–81.

73. Brown-Elliott BA, Vasireddy S, Vasireddy R, et al. Utility of sequencing the erm(41) gene in isolates of Mycobacterium abscessus subsp. abscessus with low and intermediate clarithromycin MICs. J Clin Microbiol 2015;53(4):1211–5.

74. Meier A, Heifets L, Wallace RJ Jr, et al. Molecular mechanisms of clarithromycin resistance in Mycobacterium avium: observation of multiple 23S rDNA mutations in a clonal population. J Infect Dis 1996; 174(2):354–60.

75. Wallace RJ Jr, Meier A, Brown BA, et al. Genetic basis for clarithromycin resistance among isolates of Mycobacterium chelonae and Mycobacterium abscessus. Antimicrob Agents Chemother 1996; 40(7):1676–81.

76. Bruker. Nontuberculous Mycobacteria. Available at: https://www.hain-lifescience.de/uploadfiles/file/produkte/mikrobiologie/mykobakterien/ntm_eng.pdf. Accessed June 30, 2023.

77. LG-Chem. AdvanSure TB/NTM real-time PCR. Package insert. LGI-TBP02-02. Korea: LG Chem Ltd.; 2020.

78. YD-Diagnostics. MolecuTech molecular diagnostic system. In: Diagnostics Y, editor. CAT.NO.YDC-044(Rev.04/2018-01-17. Republic of Korea. . YD Diagnostic Corp; 2002.

79. Nipro. Genoscholar NTM+NDRTB II. In: Instructions for Use. D-CE-AK-MDRTB2-02. Mechelen, Belgium.

80. Anyplex™ MTB/NTM Real-time Detection. https://www.seegene.com/assays/anyplex_mtb_ntm_real time_detection. Accessed 9/29/2022.

81. Kogene. PowerChek TB/NTM Real-time PCR Kit series. 2013; https://www.kogene.co.kr/eng/sub/product/clinical_dx/tuberculosis.asp. Accessed 9/29/2022.

82. GenoScreen. Deeplex Myc-TB - user manual. Deeplex® Myc-TB user manual RUO (V3 - july 2020). Lille, France: GenoScreen Innovative Genomics; 2020.

83. BioCore. TB/NTM PCR KIT - Package Insert. Rev.03 (2022.09.15) ed. Republic of Korea: invites BioCore Co, Ltd; 2022.

84. BioCore. TB/NTM PCR (one tube) KIT - Package Insert. Rev.03 (2022.09.15) ed. Republic of Korea: invites BioCore Co, Ltd; 2022.

85. BioCore. TB/NTM Real Time PCR Kit - Package Insert. Rev.03 (2022.09.15) ed. Republic of Korea: invites BioCore Co, Ltd; 2022.

86. Hologic. AccuProbe Culture Identification Tests. 2022; http://www.hologic.ca/products/clinical-diagnostics-and-blood-screening/assays-and-tests/accuprobe-culture-identification. Accessed 09/29, 2022.

87. Bruker. GenoType NTM-DR VER 1.0. https://www.hain-lifescience.de/en/products/microbiology/mycobacteria/ntm/genotype-ntm-dr.html. Accessed 9/29/2022.

88. Bruker. FluoroType® Mycobacteria VER 1.0 – powered by LiquidArray®. https://www.hain-lifescience.de/en/products/microbiology/mycobacteria/ntm/fluorotype-mycobacteria.html. Accessed 9/29/2022.

89. Ramis IB, Cnockaert M, Von Groll A, et al. Evaluation of the Speed-Oligo Mycobacteria assay for the identification of nontuberculous mycobacteria. J Med Microbiol 2015;64(Pt 3):283–7.

90. Fujirebio. INNO-LiPA® MYCOBACTERIA v2, FAQ: INNO-LiPA MYCOBACTERIA. https://www.fujirebio.com/en/products-solutions/innolipa-mycobacteria-v2, 9/29/2022.

91. bioMerieux. 510(k) SUBSTANTIAL EQUIVALENCE DETERMINATION DECISION SUMMARY. 510(k) Number: K162950. Available at: https://www.accessdata.fda.gov/cdrh_docs/reviews/K162950.pdf. Accessed June 30, 2023.

92. Bruker. Mycobacteria Identification MALDI BioTyper - Pamphlet. Bruker 06-2021, 1889142 ed. Bruker Daltonics GmbH & Co. KG; 2021.

Diagnostic Criteria and the Decision to Treat Nontuberculous Mycobacterial Pulmonary Disease

David E. Griffith, MD[a],*, Timothy R. Aksamit, MD[b]

KEYWORDS

- Nontuberculous mycobacteria (NTM) • Mycobacterium avium complex • Diagnostic criteria
- "Watchful waiting"

KEY POINTS

- Diagnostic criteria for nontuberculous mycobacterial pulmonary disease involve three elements: symptoms, radiographic appearance, and microbiologic findings.
- The microbiologic diagnostic criterion is complicated by the need to have at least two positive acid-fast bacilli cultures from sputum or one positive culture from a bronchoscopic specimen to make the diagnosis.
- Not all patients who meet diagnostic criteria require immediate therapy, but can be followed by "watchful waiting.
- There are clinical findings that predict disease progression and mitigate against "watchful waiting."
- Newer objective markers for predicting disease progression are emerging.

INTRODUCTION

Among all clinical aspects of nontuberculous mycobacterial (NTM) pulmonary disease, confidently diagnosing NTM pulmonary disease and knowing when to start antimycobacterial therapy remain stubbornly elusive. Even in a field notoriously slow to show progress, the ambiguity about disease diagnosis and uncertainty about when to initiate antimycobacterial therapy stand out as especially stagnant and frustrating.[1–3]

A singularly important priority is the need for objective ways to predict the level of risk for NTM disease progression, thereby identifying patients who will have progressive NTM pulmonary disease and require early initiation of therapy and those that can be observed safely without starting treatment. The decisions we make as clinicians currently are based on empirical observations

often hampered by subjective interpretation. Owing to an unprecedented level of NTM clinical and basic science research interest, there are many investigators globally searching for objective diagnostic "gold standard(s)" to accurately predict the risk of disease progression. Although there is progress toward that goal, we are currently left with making the best of decades old empirical clinical parameters. We emphasize the essential elements of current NTM pulmonary disease diagnosis and treatment decision analyses: (1) an understanding of relative NTM species virulence, (2) an understanding of NTM pulmonary disease pathophysiology and natural history, and (3) dedication to unrelenting longitudinal follow-up of patients either with or suspected of having NTM pulmonary disease.

Historically, a major impediment to diagnosing NTM pulmonary disease was an underestimation

a Department of Medicine, Division of Mycobacterial Disease and Pulmonary Infections, National Jewish Health, 1400 Jackson Street, Denver, CO 80206, USA; b Pulmonary Disease and Critical Care Medicine, Mayo Clinic, 200 First Street, Southwest, Rochester, MN 55905, USA
* Corresponding author.
E-mail address: griffithd@njhealth.org

Clin Chest Med 44 (2023) 757–769
https://doi.org/10.1016/j.ccm.2023.07.003
0272-5231/23/© 2023 Elsevier Inc. All rights reserved.

chestmed.theclinics.com

of NTM virulence or disease-causing potential. In the absence of frank cavitary lung disease, patients with a noncavitary form of NTM disease, especially those with nodular/bronchiectatic (NB) *Mycobacterium avium* complex (MAC) lung disease, were generally dismissed as being "colonized" with MAC.[4] The assumption was that the respiratory tract can be "colonized" with NTM without invasive disease, particularly in patients with chronic respiratory disease such as bronchiectasis and/or chronic obstructive pulmonary disease (COPD). "Colonization" without infection (ie, no tissue invasion) is an unproven condition for NTM that has never been rigorously tested. No pathologic studies have been done to demonstrate the *absence* of tissue invasion associated with isolation of NTM in respiratory specimens. Recent studies with chest computed tomography (CT) have shown that "colonized" patients often have a combination of multifocal bronchiectasis and nodular parenchymal disease believed to be due to invasive mycobacterial infection.[3] There is not enough known about the pathophysiology of NTM lung disease to be sure that "colonization" is not, in fact, transient, indolent, or slowly progressive infection. The term "colonization" by MAC or other NTM should be avoided as it implies a benign process. We prefer NTM or MAC "infection," with a modifier indicating the activity and/or severity of the infection.

Diagnostic Criteria for Nontuberculous Mycobacterial Pulmonary Disease

The NTM diagnostic guidelines have not changed significantly in approximately 25 years[1–3] (**Box 1**). The 2007 guideline included clinical, radiographic, and microbiologic criteria for diagnosing NTM pulmonary disease.[2] The 2020 guideline also recommends the use of these criteria to classify patients as having NTM pulmonary disease.[3] Based on these diagnostic criteria, the minimum evaluation of a patient suspected of NTM lung disease should include[1] chest radiograph or, in the absence of cavitation, chest high resolution computed tomography (HRCT) scan[2]; three or more sputum specimens (spontaneous or induced) for acid-fast bacilli (AFB) analysis; and[3] exclusion of other disorders such as tuberculosis (TB) and lung malignancy. In most patients, a diagnosis can be made without bronchoscopy or lung biopsy.[2,3]

Given the large number of identified NTM species (approximately 200), the wide spectrum of NTM virulence, and variable host susceptibility for NTM, it would be impossible for a single set of diagnostic criteria to be accurate or practical for all NTM species in all clinical circumstances. A

Box 1

Clinical and microbiologic criteria for diagnosing nontuberculous mycobacterial lung disease

Clinical (both required)

1. Pulmonary symptoms, nodular or cavitary opacities on chest radiograph, or a high-resolution computed tomography scan that shows multifocal bronchiectasis with multiple small nodules

    And

2. Appropriate exclusion of other diagnoses

Microbiologic

1. Positive culture results from at least two separate expectorated sputum samples (A, II). If the results from[1] are nondiagnostic, consider repeat sputum AFB smears and cultures

    Or

2. Positive culture result from at least one bronchial wash or lavage

    Or

3. Transbronchial or other lung biopsy with mycobacterial histopathologic features (granulomatous inflammation or AFB) and positive culture for NTM or biopsy showing mycobacterial histopathologic features (granulomatous inflammation or AFB) and one or more sputum or bronchial washings that are culture positive for NTM.

4. Expert consultation should be obtained when NTM are recovered that are either infrequently encountered or that usually represent environmental contamination

5. Patients who are suspected of having NTM lung disease but do not meet the diagnostic criteria should be followed until the diagnosis is firmly established or excluded

6. Making the diagnosis of NTM lung disease does not, per se, necessitate the institution of therapy, which is a decision based on potential risks and benefits of therapy for individual patients

---

limitation of the NTM diagnostic criteria developed so far is that, by necessity, they were developed based on experience with common and well-described respiratory pathogens such as MAC, *Mycobacterium kansasii,* and *Mycobacterium abscessus.* By consensus, the same diagnostic assumptions are applied to other common NTM respiratory pathogens including *Mycobacterium xenopi, Mycobacterium malmoense,* and *Mycobacterium szulgai.* For nearly every other NTM respiratory isolate, the applicability of the diagnostic criteria is not established.

Figs. 1A, B and **2**A, B are NTM pulmonary disease cases for consideration as you read the article. These cases will be revisited at the end of this article.

Clinical: Symptoms

The symptoms of NTM pulmonary disease are variable and nonspecific. However, virtually all patients have chronic or recurring cough, with or without sputum production. Other symptoms include fatigue, malaise, dyspnea, fever, hemoptysis, chest pain, and weight loss. Constitutional symptoms are sometimes predominant, especially fatigue. Evaluation is complicated by similar symptoms caused by coexisting lung diseases, such as bronchiectasis, chronic bronchitis, emphysema, cystic fibrosis (CF), and interstitial lung disease (ILD).

Other important symptomatic clues to the presence of bronchiectasis and NTM pulmonary disease include early onset and recurrent respiratory problems such as frequent episodes of bronchitis or pneumonia or frequent antibiotic use for respiratory infections. For some patients, this history is more illuminating than current symptoms.

A major delay in the diagnosis of NTM-related abnormalities, especially bronchiectasis, is a delay in radiographic evaluation for patients with chronic cough. Patients sometimes undergo a standard diagnosis/treatment algorithm for chronic cough but without early chest radiography and without follow-up once the standard diagnostic evaluation and therapeutic trials are unsuccessful.[5,6] The persistence of the cough without overall clinical decline can result in the doctor and patient accepting the cough as "normal" for that patient. The most recent American College of Chest Physicians cough guidelines suggest that a cough lasting more than 8 weeks is a "chronic cough" deserving further diagnostic evaluation including chest radiography.[5,6] In most cases, a chest radiograph is an acceptable start with a low threshold for following up with a chest CT scan.

Physical findings are not specifically addressed in the current guidelines, but it is important to recognize the typical physical characteristics associated with the NB form of NTM (especially MAC) disease. Patients are typically female, thin, relatively tall, and sometimes with scoliosis and/or pectus excavatum. For patients with chronic cough and the typical NB MAC lung disease morphotype, early radiographic evaluation, including chest CT scan, is justified.

Clinical: Radiography

Radiographic features of NTM lung disease depend on whether the disease is primarily fibrocavitary (FC), similar to TB or characterized by nodules and bronchiectasis, NB disease (**Figs. 3** and **4**). Compared with the radiographic findings in TB, patients with NTM FC radiographic changes tend to have the following characteristics: (1) thin-walled cavities with less surrounding parenchymal opacity, (2) less bronchogenic but more contiguous spread of disease, and (3) more marked involvement of pleura over the involved areas of the lungs.[3] None of these differences, however, is sufficiently specific to exclude the diagnosis of TB from the radiographic appearance. NTM may also produce dense airspace disease or a solitary pulmonary nodule without cavitation. Basal pleural disease is not often found, and pleural effusion is rare.

A plain chest radiograph may be adequate for diagnosing patients with FC disease. Chest CT is still important for identifying comorbid problems such as emphysema, pulmonary fibrosis, and primary or secondary malignancy in the lungs. The chest CT also aids in an accurate measurement of cavity dimensions to facilitate follow-up of the cavity size on therapy. Chest CT is also necessary before surgical referral.

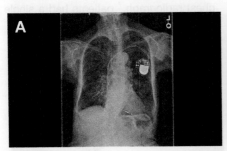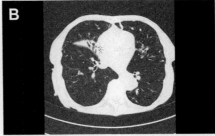

Fig. 1. (*A*) Posterior/anterior (PA) chest radiograph from an 89-year-old female patient with bronchiectasis and sputum that is AFB smear positive and culture positive for MAC. Her BMI is 18 and she is losing weight. She also has coronary artery disease and congestive heart failure. Would you start MAC therapy? (*B*) Chest CT cut from the same patient showing right middle lobe collapse and scattered tree in bud densities and bronchiectasis with mucus plugging.

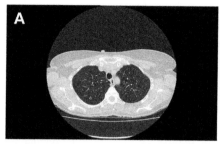
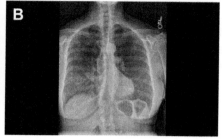

Fig. 2. (*A*) Chest CT cut from a 58-year-old woman with chronic cough and sputum AFB smear negative but culture positive for MAC. Mild chronic cough, active, weight stable. Not using airway clearance. "Watchful waiting" recommended. (*B*) PA chest radiograph 2 years after CT from (*A*). Patient's symptoms unchanged, weight stable. Sputum AFB smear negative but culture positive for MAC. Chest radiograph shows right middle lobe (RML) collapse, previously noted on prior CT scan. Would you start MAC therapy?

Chest CT is necessary to demonstrate the characteristic abnormalities of NB NTM lung disease. Routine chest radiographs are not adequate for this purpose. For patients with predominantly noncavitary disease, the abnormalities on chest radiograph are primarily found in the mid and lower lung field. Studies with chest CT show that up to 90% of patients with mid- and lower lung field noncavitary disease with MAC have associated multifocal bronchiectasis, with many patients having clusters of small (5 mm) nodules in associated areas of the lung.[3] These findings correspond histopathologically to bronchiectasis, bronchiolar and peribronchiolar inflammation, and granuloma formation.[3] Small but evolving cavitation also frequently accompanies these abnormalities. Essentially any NTM respiratory pathogen can be associated with this radiographic appearance but *M avium* and *Mycobacterium intracellulare* by far the most common NTM pathogens associated with this radiographic pattern.[2,3]

Microbiology

Presumptive diagnosis based on clinical and radiographic features is not adequate for initiation of antimycobacterial therapy. The isolation of NTM in culture is necessary for the diagnosis of NTM lung disease and to direct the appropriate therapy. The variable antibiotic susceptibility differences between NTM species make a "one size fits all" empirical therapy for presumed NTM disease impossible.

NTM is ubiquitous in the environment, including municipal (potable) water; therefore, NTM can be isolated from a respiratory specimen due to environmental contamination anywhere along the specimen processing pathway from collection of expectorated sputum to inoculation of mycobacterial cultures. In addition, some patients who have NTM isolated from their respiratory tract do not show the evidence of progressive disease. Therefore, a single positive NTM culture from expectorated sputum is not adequate to diagnose NTM lung disease.[1–3] More than one culture-positive specimen for the same NTM species or subspecies (*M abscessus*) is necessary for diagnostic purposes.

Patients should have at least three sputum specimens collected on separate days (ideally a week apart) and analyzed for AFB. In a study evaluating the association of MAC isolated from sputum and new cavitary or infiltrative lesions on chest radiograph,[7] patients had a single isolation

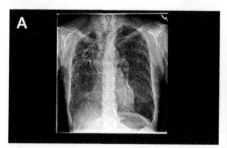
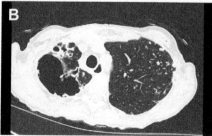

Fig. 3. (*A*) PA chest radiograph from a 66-year-old patient, ex-smoker with bilateral nodular densities and large right apical cavity. (*B*) Chest CT cut from the same patient showing the large right apical cavity with smaller satellite cavities with nodular and tree in bud densities in the left lung. Sputum is AFB smear and culture positive for MAC.

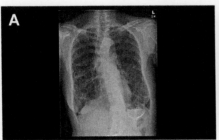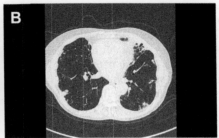

Fig. 4. (A) PA chest radiograph from a 79-year-old patient with multiple sputum AFB cultures positive for AFB. The chest radiograph shows primarily mid and lower lung densities and scoliosis. (B) Chest CT cut from the patient in (A) showing right middle lobe and lingular bronchiectasis and scattered nodules with tree-in-bud densities.

of MAC (from three specimens) and only two of these patients, both with specimens that were AFB smear positive, subsequently developed new chest radiographic abnormalities. Alternatively, 26 of 29 (90%) patients who had MAC isolated from two specimens and 39 of 40 (98%) patients with MAC isolated from three specimens had progressive radiographic abnormalities. All 116 patients who had four or more MAC isolates had progressive radiographic abnormalities. Furthermore, 181 of 185 (98%) patients who had two or more MAC isolates, generally on the initial three sputum specimens collected, also had progressive radiographic abnormalities. Clinically significant MAC pulmonary disease is unlikely in patients who have a single positive sputum culture during the initial evaluation but can be as high as 98% in those with two or more positive cultures.[7]

The exception to the requirement for two positive cultures to make a diagnosis is the patient with classic symptoms and radiographic findings for NB NTM lung disease who is unable to produce sputum for AFB analysis. For this specific type of patient, the isolation of NTM, especially MAC, from one bronchoscopic specimen is considered adequate for NTM pulmonary disease diagnosis (see **Box 1**).

Clinical studies have established bronchial washings as a valid culture source for *Mycobacterium tuberculosis*, but there are only limited data suggesting that bronchial washings and lavage may also be useful for diagnosing NTM (MAC) lung disease.[8,9] Current expert consensus is that bronchial washings are more sensitive than routine expectorated sputum testing and less likely to be affected by environmental contamination if the bronchoscopic specimens are protected from tap water contamination. Those assumptions are not validated and there are no studies demonstrating the superiority of bronchoscopically obtained specimens for NTM cultures over induced sputum for the majority of NTM pulmonary disease patients. The routine use of bronchoscopy for

NTM pulmonary disease patient follow-up is not established. We do not recommend routine follow-up bronchoscopies but rather advocate ongoing efforts to induce sputum in patients who have difficulty producing sputum.

In retrospect, the requirement for only one bronchoscopically obtained NTM culture as diagnostic was based on a practical consideration. Patients could not be expected to undergo two or more bronchoscopies to meet the two positive cultures requirement for expectorated sputum. The diagnosis of NTM lung disease with one bronchoscopy specimen requires a careful review of the patient's overall clinical circumstance and hopefully confirmation with induced or expectorated sputum.

In patients with nondiagnostic microbiologic and radiographic studies (ie, patients who do not clearly meet diagnostic criteria), or if there is concern about the presence of another disease producing radiographic abnormalities, a lung biopsy (bronchoscopic or surgical) may be required for diagnosis (see **Box 1**). If a tissue sample from a transbronchial, percutaneous, or open-lung biopsy yields an NTM organism and shows histopathologic changes typical of mycobacterial disease (ie, granulomatous inflammation with or without the presence of AFB), this by itself is sufficient to establish the diagnosis of NTM lung disease. If the lung biopsy is negative on culture (which may occur when transbronchial biopsies are performed because of the small size of the tissue sample) but demonstrates mycobacterial histopathology features (without a history of other granulomatous or mycobacterial disease), NTM lung disease is considered to be present when one or more sputum specimens or bronchial washes are culture positive for NTM.

Applying the Nontuberculous Mycobacterial Diagnostic Guidelines

There are significant limitations of applying NTM diagnostic guidelines to specific patient groups and atypical clinical circumstances in the context of a single bronchoscopically obtained NTM culture. In general, more diagnostic weight is afforded a smear positive AFB specimen from bronchoscopy than one that is a smear negative.

NTM species that are generally not pathogenic and usually isolated due to contamination when recovered from respiratory specimens include Mycobacterium gordonae, Mycobacterium terrae complex, and Mycobacterium mucogenicum. Other species known to be present in tap water that can cause pulmonary infection but may reflect contamination when recovered from a single sample include Mycobacterium simiae and Mycobacterium lentiflavum. For any of these NTM species, there should be a high bar for making a diagnosis even if diagnostic criteria are met. Expert consultation may be helpful for making this decision and consideration should be given to more invasive diagnostic evaluation such as lung biopsy.

It is increasingly common for laboratories to isolate and report new or rare NTM species from clinical specimens. The rapid expansion of NTM species identification makes it impossible for clinicians to maintain familiarity with newly identified NTM species. In many cases, the clinical experience with these organisms consists of isolated case reports that are difficult to interpret as there is no overall assessment of the disease-causing potential of the organism. Expert consultation may be helpful, although the experts are confined in their assessment to the few published reports of disease caused by the rare NTM. Reference laboratories can be helpful by summarizing how often and from what source these rare NTM are isolated. The applicability of the current diagnostic guidelines for these rarely isolated NTM species is unknown, as it is for the majority of the 200 identified NTM species. Patients who are suspected of having NTM pulmonary disease but do not meet the diagnostic criteria should be followed until the diagnosis is firmly established or excluded.

Another common problem is a single positive bronchoscopic NTM culture from patients with ILD, sarcoidosis, emphysema, lung cancer, or other chronic lung disease. These patients frequently do not have radiographic findings consistent with mycobacterial disease or symptoms that are related to their underlying chronic lung disease.

One scenario is a patient with ILD, with no prior history of mycobacterial disease, undergoing bronchoscopy (**Fig. 5**A, B). The patient has chronic, perhaps progressive symptoms and the chest radiograph/CT is invariably abnormal due to the patient's underlying ILD. In the absence of the ILD, the approach to the patient would likely be a conservative one with further collection of sputum for AFB analysis and periodic chest CT scans. However, for these patients with progressive and potentially life-threatening disease, the concern is that antimycobacterial treatment might improve symptoms and prevent radiographic progression caused by active mycobacterial disease.

Another scenario is a patient with chronic lung disease such as sarcoidosis who will receive immunosuppressive therapy, especially biologic agents, who has NTM isolated from a bronchoscopic specimen (**Fig. 6**A, B). As with the first example, it is usually difficult to unambiguously demonstrate active NTM disease symptomatically and radiographically. For these patients, the major concern is the potential for NTM dissemination due to the immunosuppressive agent.

For both patients, our approach if MAC is isolated is to initiate therapy with a macrolide and ethambutol, avoiding rifamycin-related drug–drug interactions. Clearly, if one of these patients has symptomatic and/or radiographic changes consistent with progressive mycobacterial disease, then more aggressive antimycobacterial treatment would be indicated. A more difficult scenario is the patient who has M abscessus isolated from a respiratory specimen obtained specimen where decisions are more difficult because of the need for intravenous antibiotics.

Another scenario is the patient with severe emphysema who has an NTM isolated from sputum or bronchoscopic specimen (**Fig. 7**A, B). There may not be convincing evidence of active NTM disease radiographically. Mycobacterial therapy may not improve either the patient's symptoms or prognosis which is a function of their underlying emphysema. It could be argued that the addition of macrolide and ethambutol in this circumstance would do little harm but is unlikely to produce meaningful benefit.

The significance of an NTM isolated from a patient during therapy for pulmonary TB is variable.[10,11] The co-isolation of NTM with TB can confound the evaluation of TB therapy adequacy, as sputum may be persistently AFB smear positive by NTM. Fortunately, the rapid identification of NTM associated with smear positivity can reassure clinicians that TB therapy is not failing. For patients with co-isolation of NTM and TB, more frequent radiographic analysis is important to confirm the adequacy of TB therapy and/or to alert the clinician to progressive NTM disease.

Limited data suggest that NTM cultured from patients on TB therapy do not require immediate change in the antimycobacterial regimen to cover the NTM isolate as well as the TB isolate.[10,11] The opinion among many TB experts is that the

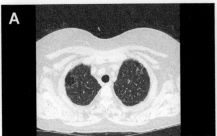 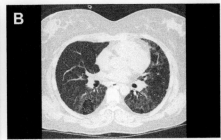

Fig. 5. (A, B) Chest CT cuts from a 48-year-old patient with recent diagnosis of ILD. A bronchoscopic specimen is AFB smear negative but culture positive for MAC. The chest CT cuts do not show the evidence of active mycobacterial disease.

approach to these patients is to adequately treat the TB and then address the significance of the NTM isolate using the guideline-based diagnostic criteria. Unfortunately, there are patients who do have progressive NTM disease while on TB therapy and require a pivot in antimycobacterial treatment for coverage of both TB and the NTM. Perhaps the most troublesome situation is a patient to have TB and progressive *M abscessus* disease where initiating intravenous medication for coverage of *M abscessus* would be necessary. Fortunately, drugs typically used to treat *M abscessus* such as amikacin and linezolid/tedizolid also have activity against TB.

The significance of two NTM species co-isolated simultaneously from a patient is also challenging. The combination of MAC and *M abscessus* isolation during MAC therapy is especially common.[12] Co-isolation of MAC and *M abscessus* typically occurs in a patient with NB disease and is infrequently reported from patients with cavitary disease. Radiographically, it is not possible to reliably determine which organism is most responsible for mycobacterial disease-related abnormalities. Similarly, there are no symptoms that distinguish the two organisms.

Some experts feel that the relative disease burden is reflected by semiquantitative analysis of AFB cultures, which can be used as a guide to which organism to approach first or whether both organisms need to be treated initially. Unfortunately, semiquantitation of sputum cultures is not widely available. Another approach is to treat the more easily treatable organism which in this case would be MAC. MAC therapy would become both a therapeutic and diagnostic intervention requiring very close patient follow-up microbiologically and radiographically. If the patient improves symptomatically and radiographically, MAC therapy could be continued to completion regardless of the sputum AFB cultures status for *M abscessus.* Conversely, if while on MAC therapy there is radiographic progression then it is more likely that the patient requires treatment for both MAC and *M abscessus*. The third option is to begin treatment for MAC and *M abscessus* immediately. There is very little guidance on criteria that would facilitate these decisions. There is also little overlap in the antimycobacterial treatment of MAC and *M abscessus,* which almost always requires intravenous antibiotics, so the decision to treat both organisms is not simple or easily accomplished.

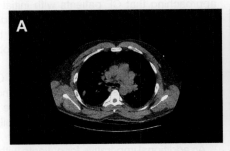 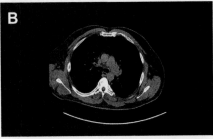

Fig. 6. (A) Chest CT mediastinal window for 52-year-old patient found to have bulky mediastinal adenopathy. Endobronchial ultrasound-guided, transbronchial needle aspiration (EBUS) biopsy consistent with sarcoid. (B) Chest CT mediastinal window showing spontaneous improvement in mediastinal adenopathy. Bronchoscopically obtained specimen AFB smear negative but culture positive for MAC. The lung windows also showed improvement and no evidence of active mycobacterial disease. No radiographic abnormalities consistent with progressive MAC lung disease. Patient found to have cardiac sarcoid involvement and placed on immunosuppressive agent.

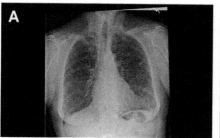 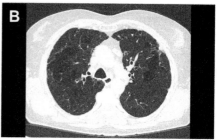

Fig. 7. (*A*) PA chest radiograph from a 61-year-old patient, ex-smoker with emphysema and one positive broncho-scopic AFB culture for MAC. (*B*) CT cut from the same patient showing diffuse emphysematous changes and nonspecific interstitial densities without abnormalities consistent with progressive MAC disease.

One situation that deserves special attention is the co-isolation of MAC with a macrolide susceptible *M abscessus* isolate. *M abscessus* subspecies *massiliense* does not have an active *erm* gene and is therefore macrolide susceptible. It is also important to emphasize that approximately 20% of *M abscessus* subspecies *abscessus* have a mutation in the *erm* gene that inactivates it.[13] If the patient has a macrolide susceptible *M abscessus* isolate and is given standard MAC therapy with azithromycin, ethambutol, and rifampin that patient would be receiving macrolide monotherapy for the *M abscessus* which would place the patient at high risk for developing acquired mutational macrolide resistant *M abscessus*. It is important to remember that treatment success for *M abscessus* is approximately 80% with a macrolide susceptible isolate and approximately 30% with a macrolide resistant isolate.[3] If a clinician chooses to treat MAC without therapy for *M abscessus* then the *erm* gene status of the *M abscessus* isolate must be known so that a patient's macrolide susceptible *M abscessus* isolate is not inadvertently exposed to macrolide monotherapy.

The interpretation of NTM in the sputum of HIV-infected patients presents a particular problem. In general, for patients with abnormal chest radiographs, the diagnostic criteria recommended for immunocompetent hosts are still applicable, with an emphasis on the exclusion of other possible pulmonary pathogens. With or without radiographic evidence of pulmonary disease, respiratory isolates of NTM, especially MAC, in HIV-seropositive persons with severely impaired immune function may be due to disseminated NTM disease or can be a harbinger of disseminated disease.[14] In addition, some NTM species that are generally considered nonpathogenic have been associated with pulmonary disease in the HIV-infected host. Given these considerations, the diagnosis of lung disease caused by NTM is usually not difficult in patients with preserved immune function if the usual combination of clinical,

radiographic, and bacteriologic criteria is used. The better the host immune system the more likely the current diagnostic criteria would be applicable but with poor immune function any NTM respiratory isolate is cause for concern.

In general, the diagnostic criteria for NTM lung disease in recent guidelines are applicable for patients with CF as well.[15,16] However, diagnosing NTM disease can be quite difficult due to overlapping symptoms and radiographic changes attributable to the underlying CF and other respiratory pathogens. All aspects of CF care should be reviewed and optimized to determine the clinical significance of NTM in the sputum. Specifically, consider a trial of NTM-sparing intravenous antibiotics that target conventional bacteria and assess for CF-related diabetes, uncontrolled gastrointestinal reflux disease, and clinical and immunologic features of allergic bronchopulmonary aspergillosis (ABPA). Likewise, adequate treatment of sinus disease, nutritional support, and effective airway clearance strategies should be implemented.[16] If after treating all identified reversible factors there is still evidence of ongoing lung infection, then antimycobacterial therapy is initiated. The current management of non-CF bronchiectasis patients with NTM isolated in the sputum is approaching that CF patients with initial aggressive airway clearance and treatment and/or suppression of bronchiectasis-related bacterial pathogens before starting antimycobacterial therapy.

Although most of the patients with CF from whom NTM are recovered will likely not meet microbiologic criteria for disease at the time of an initial positive culture, the close surveillance of these patients is warranted.

An additional imperative for patients with CF and other chronic lung diseases (ILD, COPD) is the potential consequences of the low-dose and long-term azithromycin therapy and the risk of developing macrolide-resistant NTM. A careful evaluation for possible pulmonary NTM infection, including multiple sputum cultures for NTM, should precede any initiation of macrolide monotherapy, and cultures for NTM should be obtained periodically thereafter.

Decision to Treat Nontuberculous Mycobacterial Pulmonary Disease

The first population/patient/problem, intervention, comparison, outcome (PICO) question in the 2020 NTM Treatment guidelines is, "Should patients with NTM pulmonary disease be treated with antimicrobial therapy or followed for evidence of progression (watchful waiting)?"[3]

The provided answer is, "In patients who meet the diagnostic criteria for NTM pulmonary disease, *we suggest initiation of treatment rather than watchful waiting*, especially in the context of positive AFB sputum smears and/or cavitary lung disease." The caveat for AFB smear positivity is unambiguous; a specimen is or is not AFB smear positive. The presence of cavitation is not so simple. What is the definition of a cavity?

Juhn and colleagues studied patients with newly diagnosed treatment-naïve NTM-PD and analyzed risk factors for mortality.[17] Increased mortality was significantly associated with the radiological form of NTM pulmonary disease for the cavitary NB form and the FC form compared with the non-cavitary NB form. Cavities in the cavitary NB form were not defined by size but rather by radiographic location. The FC form was characterized by cavitary lesions typically located in the upper lobes, and the NB form was characterized by bilateral bronchiectasis with nodular infiltrates involving the middle lung zones.

Chae and colleagues compared treatment outcomes between the FC and C-NB types treated with guideline-based therapy (GBT) composed of daily three-drug oral antibiotics with or without injectable aminoglycoside.[18] The culture conversion rates of patients with the cavitary NB type were higher than that of patients with the FC type. The conversion rates of those who received oral medications alone and those treated with oral medications and an injectable aminoglycoside were similar. They concluded the culture conversion rates of the patients with cavitary NB type treated with GBT were significantly higher than those of patients with the FC type and that the cavitary NB type could be treated with oral medications alone. As with the Jhun study, cavities were not defined by size but rather by location.

Defining a cavity is not a moot exercise. Rather, it has significant prognostic and therapeutic implications. For study protocol purposes, some experts define cavities, regardless of location as

greater than 2 cm in diameter. It is apparent, however, that apical cavities with FC disease differ pathophysiologically from mid and lower lung cavities with NB disease. There is little disagreement about the use of parenteral antibiotic for cavities associated with FC disease. The two cited studies offer different perspectives on cavitary NB disease. Our recommendation is that any cavity greater than 2 cm qualifies as cavitary disease requiring parenteral antibiotic in addition to daily oral antibiotic. Smaller cavities associated with NB disease may be treated with oral antibiotic but require very close follow-up to monitor treatment response with a low threshold for adding parenteral antibiotic especially in the context of enlarging cavities.

Elsewhere in the document it is stated: "Importantly, just because a patient meets diagnostic criteria for NTM pulmonary disease does not necessarily mean antibiotic treatment is required." Some patients with MAC have stable, indolent, or slowly progressive disease. In some instances, "watchful waiting" may be the preferred course of action." Although this statement seems to contradict the guidance from the PICO question, there is a rationale for both approaches.

In a study of 305 patients who met guideline-based diagnostic criteria, progression was more likely to occur in patients who were AFB smear positive, had FC disease or more extensive radiographic disease.[19] Among 115 patients who met diagnostic criteria for MAC pulmonary disease and in whom treatment was not initiated, 51.6% (20% of the original cohort) underwent spontaneous sputum conversion during a median follow-up of 5.6 years.[19] The predictors of spontaneous sputum culture conversion included younger age, higher body mass index, and negative sputum AFB smears at initial diagnosis.

Conversely, factors that predict progressive MAC disease include demographic factors— gender, older age, presence of comorbidities, low body mass index; laboratory factors— elevated inflammatory indices (erythrocyte sedimentation rate [ESR], C-reactive protein [CRP]), anemia, hypoalbuminemia; radiographic factors—FC disease, extent of disease and bacteriologic; and microbiologic factors—bacterial load (as reflected by sputum AFB smear status or semi-quantitative AFB culture analysis) and pathogenicity of NTM species.[19–22]

Major symptoms such as severe fatigue with marked decrease in quality of life can also be important factors influencing therapy initiation. Conversely, mild signs and symptoms of disease, higher potential for medication intolerance/toxicity, and organisms less responsive to treatment (eg, *M abscessus*) would move the balance toward watchful waiting. Any treatment decision should include a discussion with the patient that outlines the potential adverse effects of antimicrobial therapy, the uncertainties surrounding the benefits of antimicrobial therapy, and the potential for recurrence including reinfection (particularly in the setting of NB disease).

Finally, watchful waiting should not be a passive process. NB MAC lung disease is in general a very indolent (glacial) process. There is usually time for appropriate data collection and a deliberate risk/benefit assessment about treatment. Patients should be started on airway clearance for bronchiectasis which can be transformative symptomatically. Airway clearance is likely a necessary element for any successful antibiotic therapy of NB NTM/MAC lung disease. Patients seek engagement with a physician who will manage bronchiectasis and evaluate status of NTM/MAC indefinitely. If the diagnosis remains in question, the patient should remain under observation and expert consultation sought. Most diagnostic uncertainty can be overcome with this approach.

Objective Indicators for Determining Risk of Nontuberculous Mycobacterial Disease Progression

In addition to clinical NTM disease progression indicators, several new objective laboratory-based indicators are being assessed.

Time to positive sputum culture detection (TTP) offers potential prognostic and monitoring value for NTM pulmonary disease. Standard liquid culture techniques detect the growth of mycobacteria according to oxygen consumption in the tube of growth medium. It is theorized that a heavier mycobacterial burden in the specimen will lead to earlier detection in the indicator tube.[23] Edwards and colleagues evaluated 125 patients, 65% of whom fulfilled NTM disease criteria.[23] TTP and AFB smear grades were negatively correlated. TTP was associated with NTM disease, AFB smear positivity, and treatment initiation by 3 and 6 months. A threshold TTP of 10 days or less was associated with MAC PD, AFB smear positivity, treatment by 3 and 6 months. After 3 and 6 months of treatment, the median change in TTP decreased significantly. Overall, TTP is associated with bacterial burden and infection severity and increases in response to treatment. TTP before and on treatment is also associated with microbiological treatment response in patients with MAC-PD.[24,25] TTP is an easily obtained biomarker that should be routinely reported and combined with other markers to predict NTM disease progression. It also should be routinely incorporated as a study objective in NTM treatment trials.

Anti-Glycopeptidolipid-Core Immunoglobulin-A Antibody

Glycopeptidolipid (GPL) core is a common major cell wall component of the *M avium* and *M intracellulare*.[26] Other mycobacterial species do not have this core component except for rapidly growing mycobacteria including *M abscessus*. Structurally, GPLs consist of a lipopeptide core and a variable oligosaccharide.[26]

Hernandez and colleagues studied serum samples from 25 MAC patients starting treatment at enrollment and 18 control subjects with or without bronchiectasis.[27] Mean levels of anti-GPL-core immunoglobulin A (IgA) antibodies were tested between 0 and 3, 6, or 12 months after treatment. At baseline, IgA antibody concentrations in MAC patients were significantly higher than in controls without bronchiectasis. Sensitivity and specificity for MAC-PD in this population was 48% and 89%, respectively. Among MAC patients starting antimicrobial therapy, mean IgA levels decreased at month 3, month 6, and at 1 year. The Quality of Life-Bronchiectasis Respiratory Symptom Scale improvement correlated with decreasing IgA titers after 12 months of treatment in MAC patients. The authors concluded that anti-GPL-core IgA antibody levels are relatively specific for MAC-PD and decrease with treatment. Measurable levels of MAC-specific IgA in controls might

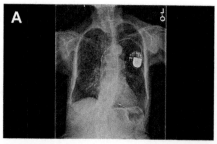 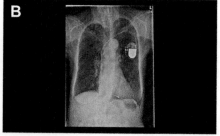

Fig. 8. (*A, B*) An 89-year-old patient from **Fig. 1**. (*A*) The initial chest film, and (*B*) the film after being in assisted living for 9 months. Her sputum is still AFB culture positive for MAC.

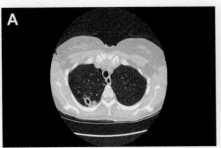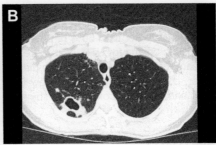

Fig. 9. (A) Follow-up chest CT from patient in **Fig. 2** shows new RUL cavities. In retrospect, early cavitation appears visible on the PA chest radiograph in **Fig. 2**B. (B) Chest CT cut done 10 months after the CT in (A) showing an enlarging RUL cavity. Patient started on multidrug MAC therapy including intravenous amikacin.

be indicative of subclinical or prior MAC infection and reflective of the diagnostic sensitivity of serologic methods.

Another recent study suggests that the anti-GPL-core IgA antibody level could be used as a "second positive sputum culture" for diagnosing MAC lung disease in patients with only one positive culture. The IgA antibody level would be a surrogate for a confirmatory culture thereby satisfying NTM disease microbiologic diagnostic criteria.[28]

Studies in various countries have also reported satisfactory diagnostic efficacies of the anti-GPL-core IgA antibody enzyme immunoassay.[26] A meta-analysis of 16 studies by Shibata and colleagues[24] reported summary estimates of sensitivity and specificity of 0.70 and 0.91 using the 0.7 U/mL cutoff.[26] A US study reported a sensitivity of 51.7% and specificity 93.9% with the 0.7 U/mL cutoff, and it determined a best combination of sensitivity and specificity with the cutoff point 0.3 U/mL (70.1% and 93.9%, respectively).[29] Studies have evaluated longitudinal IgA level change with respect to MAC therapy in association with culture positivity and other unfavorable treatment responses, showing that changes in the antibody levels may reflect disease activity.[26]

The anti-GPL-core IgA antibody is also found in M abscessus making it useful for M abscessus disease as well as MAC. It also may make interpretation of anti-GPL-core IgA antibody levels difficult to interpret in patients co-isolated with MAC and M abscessus.

The role of cavitary NB and soluble programmed death protein-1 (sPD-1), an immune-related biomarker, in the disease course of NB NTM-LD, has also been evaluated.[30] Patients with NB NTM-LD and low sPD-1, low BMI, high smear grade, and cavitary NB were at high risk for disease progression. sPD-1 was low in patients with cavitary NB phenotype and dose-responsively associated with disease progression.

We return to the patients in **Figs. 1** and **2**. The patient in **Fig 1** appeared to be a good candidate for antimycobacterial therapy, as well as airway clearance, but declined both. She was living alone and during her evaluation, she moved into an assisted living situation with regular meals and supervised activity. She subsequently had remarkable clinical and radiographic improvement with persistently positive sputum AFB cultures (**Fig. 8**A, B).

The patient in **Fig 2** was not started on MAC therapy by mutual agreement with her physician. They chose a "watchful waiting" strategy. Her chest radiograph 2 years after this decision shows a developing cavity in the right upper lobe (RUL) which was confirmed 1 year later on chest CT scan. After discussion with her physician, no antimycobacterial therapy was started. The most recent chest CT shows enlargement of the RUL cavity (**Fig. 9**A, B). The patient now consents to antimycobacterial therapy.

These cases illustrate the unpredictability of MAC lung disease and the limitations of our current diagnostic efforts to predict disease progression and the limitations of the "watchful waiting" approach.

SUMMARY

Outside of cavitary NTM pulmonary disease, the current NTM diagnosis criteria are not easily applied. They require knowledge about individual NTM species pathogenicity and host susceptibility as well as other subjective clinical assessments. Overly rigorous criteria might delay or prevent the diagnosis, with the subsequent risk for progressive disease. Conversely, criteria that are too lenient could result in unnecessary exposure of patients to potentially toxic and expensive therapy. Because NTM pulmonary disease is generally slowly progressive, there is usually sufficient time to collect adequate clinical material, specifically multiple respiratory specimens, and serial radiographic analysis, necessary for confidently making a diagnosis. Overall, greater than 50% of patients who meet diagnostic criteria for NTM-LD progress within 3 to 5 years. For patients in whom the diagnosis is unclear, continued longitudinal follow-up is mandatory and expert consultation highly recommended.

CLINICS CARE POINTS

- It is incumbant upon the clinician to know the relative virulence of NTM isolated from respiratory specimens to determine which NTM species are contaminants, which NTM species rarely cause progressive disease and which are likely to cause progressive disease.
- Know the clinical and laboratory factors that predict disease progression for each patient.
- For patients without risk factors for disease progression an period of "watchful waiting" may be appropriate if accompanied by clinical, microbiologic and radiographic monitoring on an indefinite basis.
- Expert consultation is strongly encouraged when the diagnosis is in doubt due to isolation of an unusual NTM species or difficult risk/benefit decision about starting therapy.

DISCLOSURE

Potential COI for Dr D.E. Griffith Insmed Inc: Consultant, Speaker, Grant recipient AN2 Therapeutics: Consultant Paratek Pharmaceuticals: Consultant; Potential COI for Dr T.R. Aksamit: None.

REFERENCES

1. Wallace RJ Jr, Cook JL, Glassroth J, et al. American Thoracic Society statement: diagnosis and treatment of disease caused by nontuberculous mycobacteria. Am J Respir Crit Care Med 1997;156:S1–25.
2. Griffith DE, Aksamit T, Brown-Elliott BA, et al. ATS Mycobacterial Diseases Subcommittee; American Thoracic Society; Infectious Disease Society of America. An official ATS/IDSA statement: diagnosis, treatment, and prevention of nontuberculous mycobacterial diseases. Am J Respir Crit Care Med 2007;175(4):367–416. Erratum in: Am J Respir Crit Care Med. 2007 Apr 1;175(7):744-5. Dosage error in article text. PMID: 17277290.
3. Daley CL, Iaccarino JM, Lange C, et al. Treatment of nontuberculous mycobacterial pulmonary disease: an official ATS/ERS/ESCMID/IDSA clinical practice guideline. Clin Infect Dis 2020;71(4):e1–36. Erratum in: Clin Infect Dis. 2020 Dec 31;71(11):3023.4.
4. Wolinsky E. Nontuberculous mycobacteria and associated diseases. Am Rev Respir Dis 1979; 119(1):107–59.
5. Irwin RS, French CL, Chang AB, et al, CHEST Expert Cough Panel. Classification of cough as a symptom in adults and management algorithms: CHEST guideline and expert panel report. Chest 2018; 153(1):196–209.
6. Gibson P, Wang G, McGarvey L, et al. CHEST Expert Cough Panel. Treatment of unexplained chronic cough: CHEST Guideline and expert panel report. Chest 2016;149(1):27–44.
7. Tsukamura M. Diagnosis of disease caused by Mycobacterium avium complex. Chest 1991;99(3): 667–9.
8. Anderson C, Inhaber N, Menzies D. Comparison of sputum induction with fiber-optic bronchoscopy in the diagnosis of tuberculosis. Am J Respir Crit Care Med 1995;152:1570–4.
9. Sugihara E, Hirota N, Niizeki T, et al. Usefulness of bronchial lavage for the diagnosis of pulmonary disease caused by Mycobacterium avium-intracellulare complex (MC) infection. J Infect Chemother 2003;9: 328–32.
10. Jun HJ, Jeon K, Um SW, et al. Nontuberculous mycobacteria isolated during the treatment of pulmonary tuberculosis. Respir Med 2009;103(12):1936–40.
11. Hwang SM, Lim MS, Hong YJ, et al. Simultaneous detection of Mycobacterium tuberculosis complex and nontuberculous mycobacteria in respiratory specimens. Tuberculosis 2013;93(6):642–6.
12. Griffith DE, Philley JV, Brown-Elliott BA, et al. The significance of Mycobacterium abscessus subspecies abscessus isolation during Mycobacterium avium complex lung disease therapy. Chest 2015;147(5): 1369–75.
13. Brown-Elliott BA, Vasireddy S, Vasireddy R, et al. Utility of sequencing the erm(41) gene in isolates of Mycobacterium abscessus subsp. abscessus with low and intermediate clarithromycin MICs. J Clin Microbiol 2015;53(4):1211–5.
14. Chin DP, Hopewell P, Stone EN, et al. Mycobacterium avium complex in the respiratory or gastrointestinal tract and the risk of Mycobacterium avium complex bacteremia in patients with human immunodeficiency virus infection. J Infect Dis 1994;169:289–95.
15. Richards CJ, Olivier KN. Nontuberculous mycobacteria in cystic fibrosis. Semin Respir Crit Care Med 2019;40(6):737–50.
16. Floto RA, Olivier KN, Saiman L, et al. US cystic fibrosis foundation and European cystic fibrosis society. US cystic fibrosis foundation and European cystic fibrosis society consensus recommendations for the management of non-tuberculous

mycobacteria in individuals with cystic fibrosis. Thorax 2016;71(Suppl 1):i1–22.

17. Jhun BW, Moon SM, Jeon K, et al. Prognostic factors associated with long-term mortality in 1445 patients with nontuberculous mycobacterial pulmonary disease: a 15-year follow-up study. Eur Respir J 2020; 55(1):1900798.

18. Chae G, Park YE, Chong YP, et al. Treatment outcomes of cavitary nodular bronchiectatic-type *Mycobacterium avium* complex pulmonary disease. Antimicrob Agents Chemother 2022;66(9):e0226121.

19. Hwang JA, Kim S, Jo KW, et al. Natural history of *Mycobacterium avium* complex lung disease in untreated patients with stable course. Eur Respir J 2017;49(3):1600537.

20. Kwon BS, Lee JH, Koh Y, et al. The natural history of non- cavitary nodular bronchiectatic *Mycobacterium avium* complex lung disease. Respir Med 2019;150: 45–50.

21. Moon SM, Jhun BW, Baek SY, et al. Long-term natural history of non-cavitary nodular bronchiectatic nontuberculous mycobacterial pulmonary disease. Respir Med 2019;151:1–7.

22. Ito Y, Hirai T, Maekawa K, et al. Predictors of 5-year mortality in pulmonary *Mycobacterium avium-intracellulare* complex disease. Int J Tuberc Lung Dis 2012;16(3):408–14.

23. Edwards BD, Brode SK, Mehrabi M, et al. Time to positive culture detection predicts *Mycobacterium avium* pulmonary disease severity and treatment initiation. Ann Am Thorac Soc 2022 Jun;19(6):925–32.

24. Mingora CM, Garcia BA, Mange KC, et al. Time-to-positivity of *Mycobacterium avium* complex in broth culture associates with culture conversion. BMC Infect Dis 2022;22(1):246.

25. Danho R, Schildkraut JA, Zweijpfenning SMH, et al. Mycobacterium growth indicator tube time-to-positivity can serve as an early biomarker of treatment response in *Mycobacterium avium* complex pulmonary disease. Chest 2022;161(2):370–2.

26. Shibata Y, Horita N, Yamamoto M, et al. Diagnostic test accuracy of anti-glycopeptidolipid-core IgA antibodies for *Mycobacterium avium* complex pulmonary disease: systematic review and meta-analysis. Sci Rep 2016;6:29325.

27. Hernandez AG, Brunton AE, Ato M, et al. Use of anti-glycopeptidolipid-core antibodies serology for diagnosis and monitoring of *Mycobacterium avium* complex pulmonary disease in the United States. Open Forum Infect Dis 2022;9(11):ofac528.

28. Kawasaki T, Kitada S, Fukushima K, et al. The diagnosis of nontuberculous mycobacterial pulmonary disease by single bacterial isolation plus anti-GPL-core IgA antibody. Microbiol Spectr 2022;10(1): e0140621.

29. Kitada S, Levin A, Hiserote M, et al. Serodiagnosis of *Mycobacterium avium* complex pulmonary disease in the USA. Eur Respir J 2013;42:454–60.

30. Pan SW, Su WJ, Chan YJ, et al. Disease progression in patients with nontuberculous mycobacterial lung disease of nodular bronchiectatic (NB) Pattern: the Roles of cavitary NB and soluble programmed death Protein-1. Clin Infect Dis 2022;75(2):239–47.

Treatment of *Mycobacterium avium* Complex Pulmonary Disease: When Should I Treat and What Therapy Should I Start?

Minh-Vu H. Nguyen, MD, MSc, Charles L. Daley, MD*

KEYWORDS

- *Mycobacterium avium* complex • Nontuberculous mycobacteria • Azithromycin • Amikacin
- Macrolide-resistance

KEY POINTS

- A three-drug, macrolide-based regimen is recommended over a two-drug or non-macrolide-based regimen.
- Treatment should continue for at least 12 months after culture conversion.
- Amikacin liposome inhalation suspension should be added to guideline-based therapy for treatment refractory disease.
- Novel and repurposed therapies under investigation hold promise.

INTRODUCTION

Nontuberculous mycobacteria (NTM) can produce both pulmonary and, less commonly, various extrapulmonary diseases in humans. *Mycobacterium avium* complex (MAC) is the principal cause of NTM pulmonary disease in most parts of the world[1] with considerable geographic diversity of MAC species and subspecies.[2] The most common species are *Mycobacterium avium* and *Mycobacterium intracellulare*, which are responsible for most human MAC pulmonary disease, although less common species can also produce pulmonary disease (**Table 1**).[3–9] The importance of accurate species identification of MAC is illustrated by species-related variation of propensity to cause lung disease, severity of disease and prognosis.[10,11]

This article focuses on the treatment of MAC pulmonary disease, which is a chronic, burdensome disease associated with significant morbidity and mortality. Its treatment is fraught with frequent adverse drug effects and disheartening outcomes. The 2020 NTM guideline by the American Thoracic Society (ATS), European Respiratory Society, European Society of Clinical Microbiology and Infectious Disease, and Infectious Diseases Society of America) has provided evidence-based recommendations for treatment of MAC pulmonary disease.[1] However, the reality is that MAC pulmonary disease can be difficult to manage with limited therapeutic options and evidence-base to inform management, and thus, clinicians are implored to have a nuanced understanding of its current treatment to better serve their patients.

WHAT THERAPY SHOULD I START?

The ATS-led international NTM guideline recommends three macrolide-based regimens based on the phenotype of the patient and whether the patient is treatment-naïve or treatment-refractory (**Table 2**).[1] Drug susceptibility testing should be

Division of Mycobacterial and Respiratory Infections, National Jewish Health, Denver, CO 80206, USA
* Corresponding author.
E-mail address: daleyc@njhealth.org

Clin Chest Med 44 (2023) 771–783
https://doi.org/10.1016/j.ccm.2023.06.009
0272-5231/23/© 2023 Elsevier Inc. All rights reserved.

Table 1
Species and subspecies of *Mycobacterium avium* complex

Species and Subspecies	Subspecies	Comments
M avium	avium	Primarily in birds
	hominissuis	Most common to cause disease in humans
	paratuberculosis	Rarely causes human disease Cause of Johne's disease in cattle
	silvaticum	Rarely causes human disease
M intracellulare	intracellulare	Most common subsp of *M intracellulare* to cause human pulmonary disease
	chimaera	Second most common subsp of *M intracellulare* to cause human disease; Cause of disseminated disease associated with heater cooler units
	yongonense	Third most common subsp of *M intracellulare* to cause of pulmonary disease
M arosiense	–	Uncommon cause of human disease
M bouchedurhonense	–	Uncommon cause of human disease
M colombiense	–	Uncommon cause of human disease
M lepraemurium	–	Cause of murine and feline leprosy
M marseillense	–	Uncommon cause of human disease
M paraintracellulare	–	Uncommon cause of human disease
M timonense	–	Uncommon cause of human disease
M vulneris	–	Uncommon cause of human disease

van Ingen J, et al. International Journal of Systemic and Evolutionary Microbiology,2018;69.; Tortoli E, et al. Infect, Genetics, Evol 2019;75.

Table 2
Medical treatment regimens for macrolide-susceptible *Mycobacterium avium* complex pulmonary disease

Type of Disease	No. of Drugs	Preferred Regimen	Dose	Dosing Frequency
Nodular-bronchiectatic	3	Azithromycin (clarithromycin) Rifampicin (rifabutin) Ethambutol	500 mg/d (1000 mg/d) 600 mg/d (300 mg/d) 25 mg/kg/d	3 times weekly
Cavitary	≥ 3	Azithromycin (clarithromycin) Rifampicin (rifabutin) Ethambutol Amikacin IV (streptomycin)[a]	250–500 mg/d (1000 mg/d) 600 mg/d (300 mg/d) 15 mg/kg/d 10–25 mg/d	Daily 3 times weekly
Refractory	≥ 4	Azithromycin (clarithromycin) Rifampicin (rifabutin) Ethambutol Amikacin liposome inhalation suspension Amikacin IV (streptomycin)[a]	250–500 mg/d (1000 mg/d) 600 mg/d (300 mg/d) 15 mg/kg/d 590 mg/d 10–25 mg/d	Daily 3 times weekly

IV, administered intravenously.
[a] Consider for cavitary disease, extensive nodular bronchiectatic disease, or macrolide resistant MAC.
Adapted from Daley CL, et al. Euro Respir J 2020;56:2000535.

performed to at least clarithromycin and amikacin because the cut points for resistance have been correlated with microbiologic response to therapy.[1,12,13] The composition of the regimen, administration, and duration of therapy is reviewed below. Because the treatment of MAC pulmonary disease involves prolonged administration of multiple antibiotics with the potential for significant adverse effects (AEs), the decision to treat should be informed by the patient's symptoms, radiographic progression, comorbidities, and their preferences.

COMPOSITION OF THE REGIMEN

A three-drug, macrolide-based, azithromycin preferred regimen is recommended and should be administered for at least 12 months beyond culture conversion (see **Table 2**).[1] Macrolide susceptibility has long been associated with treatment success, and the loss of the macrolide is associated with culture conversion rates as low as 5% to 36%.[1] Systematic reviews have reported that improved treatment success is seen in patients taking macrolide-based compared with macrolide-free regimens.[14–17]

The efficacy of macrolides was demonstrated by a small, open-label, non-comparative trial designed to evaluate short-term outcomes of clarithromycin monotherapy.[18] Sputum cultures converted to negative in 58% of patients with clarithromycin-susceptible isolates after 4 months of therapy. Subsequent studies supported the superiority of regimens that contained clarithromycin to those that did not.[19–21] Lower culture conversion rates were associated with clarithromycin-resistant isolates and prior mycobacterial treatment.[21]

Azithromycin is the preferred macrolide because of better tolerability, less drug interactions, lower pill burden with single daily dosing, and similar microbiologic outcomes to clarithromycin.[1] The recommended daily dose of azithromycin is 250 mg because higher doses have been associated with frequent gastrointestinal AEs and ototoxicity.[22] Unlike clarithromycin, azithromycin does not inhibit CYP3A4.[23] However, clarithromycin is a reasonable alternative if azithromycin is not available or not tolerated.

Macrolide resistance occurred in 16% of patients with MAC pulmonary disease who were treated for 4 months with macrolide monotherapy.[18] Among human immunodeficiency virus (HIV)-infected patients with disseminated MAC, 46% developed macrolide resistance after a median of 16 weeks.[24,25] Ethambutol is the preferred companion agent because it protects against the development of macrolide resistance better than

rifampin or fluoroquinolones.[1] Optic neuropathy is the principal AE and may present with reduced visual acuity or impaired red/green color discrimination. The benefit of rifamycins in the treatment regimen is unclear but they are included in the regimen because of the historical success of three-drug regimens in the treatment of pulmonary disease and evidence that rifabutin may reduce the risk of macrolide resistance in HIV-infected patients with disseminated MAC.[25]

Most providers prefer to use rifampin over rifabutin because rifabutin is poorly tolerated in elderly patients without HIV infection.[1,26] Common AEs include gastrointestinal symptoms, arthralgia, leukopenia, and uveitis. Rifampin is a potent inducer of CYP450 enzyme systems that can result in multiple drug interactions. For example, rifampin reduces serum levels of macrolides, especially clarithromycin, although the clinical significance of this remains unclear.[27] Compared with rifampin, rifabutin is a less potent inducer of CYP450 enzymes and thus, reduces serum macrolide levels less. However, because rifabutin is a CYP3A4 substrate, its levels are increased when given with clarithromycin leading to higher risk of AEs like uveitis.

Aminoglycoside Use

Aminoglycosides were used in many of the studies that established the efficacy of three-drug therapy for MAC pulmonary disease. A double-blind randomized controlled trial from Japan reported that the addition of intramuscular streptomycin to the first 3 months of a 24-month three-drug regimen was associated with a higher frequency of sputum culture conversion but mortality, microbiologic recurrence, clinical course, and radiographic findings were not significantly affected.[28] The usual starting dose is 15 to 25 mg/kg and subsequent doses are adjusted according to serum drug concentration monitoring.[1] Parenteral aminoglycosides may be administered thrice weekly for the initial 2 to 3 months of therapy.[1] Ototoxicity has been reported in over a third of patients and is frequently irreversible so surveillance for toxicity should include serial audiograms as well as serum creatinine measurements to assess for nephrotoxicity.[29]

Alternative Antibiotics

Unfortunately, there are few alternative antibiotics for treatment of MAC pulmonary disease, and for some, access can be difficult. Clofazimine is a fat-soluble riminophenazine that is approved for treatment of leprosy and commonly used to treat drug-resistant tuberculosis.[30] Clofazimine has good antimicrobial activity against MAC isolates and may be an alternative to the rifamycins for treatment of MAC pulmonary disease.[31–33] A retrospective study of patients with predominantly nodular bronchiectatic NTM disease in Canada suggested that clofazimine- and rifampin-containing three-drug regimens produce similar microbiologic outcomes and relapse rates.[34] In addition, several retrospective studies have reported good long-term safety and tolerability of clofazimine in patients with NTM pulmonary disease.[31,32,34] AEs include skin pigmentation, dry skin, gastrointestinal complaints, and prolongation of the QTc interval.

Moxifloxacin has potent activity against *Mycobacterium tuberculosis* and its use has been associated with significantly improved treat outcomes in people with multidrug-resistant tuberculosis.[35] However, moxifloxacin's role in the management of MAC pulmonary disease is limited. Moxifloxacin should not be used to substitute for ethambutol because the combination of a macrolide and fluoroquinolone has been associated with an increased risk of macrolide resistance.[36] A retrospective study demonstrated treatment success in approximately one-third of cases of macrolide-susceptible MAC, but there was no benefit in cases of macrolide-resistant MAC.[37] AEs include tendonitis, tendon rupture, and prolongation of the QTc interval.

Bedaquiline, a diarylquinoline antibiotic used for the treatment of drug-resistant tuberculosis, has excellent in vitro activity against MAC.[38,39] However, data supporting its use in treatment of MAC pulmonary disease are extremely limited. A small case series reported that bedaquiline may be efficacious for treatment-refractory MAC pulmonary disease.[40] Because rifamycins increase the clearance of bedaquiline, concomitant administration of these agents should be avoided.[41]

The utility of oxazolidinone antibiotics for MAC pulmonary disease is uncertain. The minimal inhibitory concentration (MIC) of linezolid is high and withdrawal from therapy is common due to AEs such as bone marrow suppression and peripheral neuropathy.[42,43] Tedizolid may have superior efficacy and tolerability by virtue of its favorable pharmacokinetic profile and lower MICs.[44]

Two Versus Three Drugs

Three drugs are currently suggested for the treatment of MAC pulmonary disease.[1] For some patients, such as those who are intolerant of a three-drug regimen, a two-drug regimen may be appropriate. A preliminary open-label randomized controlled trial involving HIV-negative patients with treatment-naïve pulmonary disease in Japan reported that a two-drug regimen including clarithromycin and ethambutol was non-inferior to a three-drug regimen that included rifampin and was associated with superior treatment tolerability.[45] The study was limited by its small sample size, large drop out, nonstandard drug doses, and the fact that rifampin significantly reduces the serum concentration of clarithromycin. Regarding the latter, a study from Japan, reported that the median area under the curve of clarithromycin decreased by 92.1% from 0 to 12 hour after concomitant administration of rifampin compared with clarithromycin monotherapy.[46] If a two-drug regimen is used, the preferred combination is currently azithromycin and ethambutol.

ADMINISTRATION OF THE REGIMEN

The treatment regimen can be administered either intermittently (3 days per week) or daily depending on the severity of disease as assessed on imaging studies. Thrice weekly therapy is recommended for patients with macrolide-susceptible, non-cavitary, nodular bronchiectatic disease and those who are unable to tolerate daily therapy.[1] Several prospective and retrospective studies, predominantly involving patients with nodular bronchiectasis, support the notion that intermittent therapy is of similar efficacy and superior tolerability to daily therapy.[26,47–49] A study from South Korea reported that in patients whose cultures remained positive despite 12 months of intermittent therapy, switching to daily therapy achieved treatment success in 30% of cases.[50]

Daily administration is recommended for persons with cavitary disease or severe bronchiectatic disease as well as those with treatment refractory disease. A prospective, non-comparative trial suggested that the efficacy of intermittent therapy is reduced in those with cavitary disease, previous treatment for MAC pulmonary disease, chronic obstructive pulmonary disease, or bronchiectasis.[51]

SURGERY

For some patients, adjunctive surgical therapy should be considered for treatment of MAC pulmonary disease. The indications for surgery include: (1) focal disease refractory to medical therapy; (2) intractable or life-threatening symptoms; and (3) parenchymal disease amenable to "debulking" to slow progression.[52] Antimicrobial therapy is recommended to be administered for 8 to 12 weeks before surgery. A systematic review identified 15 studies, three of which compared outcomes in those who underwent surgery plus antimicrobial therapy versus antimicrobial therapy alone. There were no differences in cure rate, recurrences, or death, although culture conversion was more likely. Complications occurred in 7% to 35% of patients, there was no operative mortality and postoperative mortality occurred in 0% to 9%. Open thoracotomy is associated with higher rates of mortality and major morbidity than thoracoscopic surgery. Surgeons should be experienced in the surgical management of mycobacterial lung disease. In an institution with a high degree of expertise, there was a low likelihood of conversion to an open procedure (3%), low morbidity (7%), no mortality, and a short length of stay (mean 3.3 days).[53]

OUTCOMES OF TREATMENT OF *MYCOBACTERIUM AVIUM* COMPLEX PULMONARY DISEASE

A systematic review that included 42 studies and 2748 patients reported treatment success in 52.8% of patients with MAC pulmonary disease.[14] Success increased to 61.4% in those who received an ATS recommended regimen and 65.7% if the regimen was taken for at least 1 year. However, two more recent studies reported treatment success in almost 80% of patients.[48,54] Factors that have been associated with poor treatment outcomes have included lack of adherence, cavitary disease, weak regimens, macrolide resistance, and possibly the species of MAC.[55–58] The most important factor associated with treatment success is clarithromycin susceptibility. A prospective study from Japan demonstrated culture conversion in 83.9% of patients with clarithromycin-susceptible MAC compared with only 25% of patients whose isolates exhibited intermediate susceptibility or resistance.[21] Unfortunately, microbiologic recurrences occur in 25% to 48% of patients after completion of therapy[48,58–60] and most of the recurrences are due to reinfection.[48,59,60]

Five-year all-cause mortality varies from 13% to 40% depending on the population studied.[61–63] Female sex, non-cavitary disease, and few comorbidities are associated with lower mortality rates. The mortality rate of macrolide-resistant MAC pulmonary disease has been reported to be as high as 47% at 5 years.[64,65]

MANAGING TREATMENT REFRACTORY DISEASE

Treatment success is not achieved in all patients—approximately 20% to 30% of patients with MAC pulmonary disease fail therapy.[47,48] Although there is no standard definition of treatment failure, a consensus definition of treatment failure described the reemergence of multiple positive cultures or persistence of positive cultures with the causative species from respiratory samples after ≥ 12 months of antimycobacterial treatment, whereas the patient is on treatment.[66] However, studies suggest that the microbiologic status of the patient within the first 6 months of therapy is predictive of the outcomes at 12 months. One such study reported that 83% of patients with MAC pulmonary disease had their first negative culture within 6 months of starting therapy and semiquantitative culture scores as early as 2 to 3 months were predictive of culture status at 12 months.[67] A study from South Korea reported that among 470 treatment-naïve patients with MAC pulmonary disease, 76% achieved culture conversion by 12 months of therapy with 24% failing to do so.[68] Of the 357 that achieved culture conversion, 96% had done so by 6 months. Of the 113 patients who did not achieve culture conversion, 93% had also failed to do so by 6 months. Factors associated with poor treatment outcomes include the presence of cavitary disease, lack of adherence, inappropriate regimen such as macrolides paired with only rifampin or a fluoroquinolone, lack of ethambutol, and macrolide resistance.

The lack of ethambutol in the treatment regimen has been associated with treatment failure. In a study from South Korea, 60 of 508 patients with MAC pulmonary disease stopped ethambutol due to adverse reactions.[57] Treatment failure occurred in 29% of those who discontinued ethambutol versus 18.3% in those who continued ethambutol and for those who had fluoroquinolones substituted for ethambutol, treatment failure occurred in 39.1%.[57] The odds of microbiological cure were higher with maintenance of macrolide, ethambutol, and rifampin (odds ratio: 5.74) and macrolide and ethambutol (odds ratio: 5.12) but not macrolide and rifampin.[56] In another study from South Korea, substitution of a fluoroquinolone (levofloxacin or moxifloxacin) for ethambutol was associated with inferior patient outcomes.[69]

The ATS-led multi-society NTM guidelines define treatment refractory as patients who fail to convert cultures to negative after at least 6 months of guideline-based therapy.[1] For treatment refractory patients, reasons for failure include nonadherence to the regimen, often due to adverse reactions to the drugs, acquired drug resistance, and poor absorption of the medication. Determination of serum drug concentrations may be helpful particularly in persons at risk for malabsorption of the medications like people with cystic fibrosis, diabetes mellitus, or HIV infection.[1]

Two randomized controlled trials of amikacin liposome inhalation suspension (ALIS) demonstrated that in patients who continued guideline-based therapy without addition of ALIS to the multidrug regimen, culture conversion was achieved in less than 10% so continuing the same regimen without alteration is not recommended.[1] The two randomized trials of ALIS demonstrated significantly better conversion at 84 days in a Phase 2 randomized, placebo-controlled study and by 6 months in a Phase 3 randomized controlled trial.[70,71] ALIS was well tolerated, the principal AEs being respiratory symptoms; dysphonia occurred in 50% of subjects and cough in about one-third. Based on these studies, the revised NTM guidelines recommend addition of ALIS to guideline-based therapy in those patients who have not converted cultures to negative by 6 months of therapy.[1] As noted previously, for those individuals who are on intermittent therapy, switching to daily administration was associated with culture conversion in 30% of patients.[50] Addition of other drugs, such as clofazimine or bedaquiline, has also been associated with improved conversion in retrospective observational studies.[32,40]

MACROLIDE-RESISTANT DISEASE

Macrolide resistance is usually caused by a point mutation at position 2058 or 2059 in the 23S ribosomal ribonucleic acid (rRNA) gene.[72] The likelihood of macrolide resistance emerging during treatment with a recommended three-drug regimen has varied from 0% to 33% among treatment naïve patients with nodular bronchiectatic disease.[47,48] Prescribing patterns that predispose to macrolide resistance have differed between retrospective studies but tend to include macrolide monotherapy, two-drug therapy with a macrolide and either a fluoroquinolone or rifampin, and omission of ethambutol.[36,64,65]

A systematic review that included nine studies reported that culture conversion was achieved in 21% of patients with macrolide-resistant MAC pulmonary disease and that mortality was 10%.[73] Outcomes may be significantly improved with the combination of aminoglycoside therapy for at least 6 months and surgical resection.[36] This approach may increase the proportion of patients achieving culture conversion from 5% to 79%.

For treatment of macrolide-resistant MAC pulmonary disease, a multiple-drug regimen should be formulated and guided by drug susceptibility testing and expert consultation (**Table 3**). The British Thoracic Society NTM guidelines suggest using a rifamycin, ethambutol, isoniazid, or a fluoroquinolone with consideration of an injectable aminoglycoside.[74] However, neither isoniazid nor fluoroquinolones have much in vitro activity against MAC. Factors associated with improved outcomes include surgical resection in conjunction with prolonged administration of parenteral aminoglycosides and a C-reactive protein less than 1.0 mg/dl.[75] Three studies had reported improved treatment outcomes in patients who undergo surgical resection and received parenteral aminoglycosides[36,64,65] with the most significant impact coming from surgery.[64] There is no difference in outcomes when a macrolide is continued or a fluoroquinolone is added.[37,64] In addition, worse outcomes are expected when stopping ethambutol or in cavitary disease.[76] Other more active candidate oral agents include clofazimine, bedaquiline, and linezolid. If patients are intolerant to parenteral aminoglycosides, ALIS should be considered given that the CONVERT trial showed that the addition of ALIS, compared with guideline-based therapy alone, had better culture conversion rates among those with clarithromycin-resistant isolates.[71]

MONITORING FOR TREATMENT RESPONSE

Clinical, radiographic, and microbiologic data are used to determine if the patient is responding to treatment. It is important to monitor for improvement in symptoms, radiographic findings, and culture conversion. A retrospective study from South Korea reported that over 75% to 82% of 217 patients with treatment naïve MAC pulmonary disease experienced symptomatic improvement, 68% to 73% had radiographic improvement and 67% to 76% converted sputum cultures to negative in a mean of 34 days.[47] A study that used semiquantitative cultures reported that the most common symptoms of cough and fatigue improved on therapy and correlated with culture conversion.[67] Because the time of culture conversion determines the length of therapy, sputum cultures should be obtained every 1 to 2 months.[1] Sputum should be induced if it cannot be collected spontaneously, and bronchoscopy should be rarely required to document conversion.

MONITORING FOR ADVERSE EFFECTS

Drug-related AEs are common during therapy: the most commonly reported AEs are listed in **Table 4**. The development of an AE can adversely affect treatment outcomes by leading to treatment interruptions, morbidity, and premature discontinuation of therapy. Up to 70% of treated patients have reported a treatment-related AE and 30%–70% of patients receiving daily antimicrobial treatment permanently discontinue at least one drug in

Table 3
Building a treatment regimen for macrolide-resistant *Mycobacterium avium* complex pulmonary disease

Action	Why?
Stop the macrolide	Does not improve outcome
Continue ethambutol	Improves outcome
Change rifampin to rifabutin	Slightly more in vitro activity with rifabutin
Add amikacin (IV), transition to inhaled	Improves outcome when combined with surgery
Add another drug(s)	Have varying degrees of in vitro activity and tolerance
Do not add isoniazid	Minimal in vitro activity—more risk than benefit
Do not add a fluoroquinolone	Minimal in vitro activity and associated with worse outcomes
Consider surgical resection	Improves outcomes but not for everyone
Consult an expert	Provides invaluable knowledge and experience

Abbreviation: IV, intravenous.

Table 4
Common drug-related adverse effects and monitoring recommendations

Drug or Class	Reactions	Monitoring Modality
Macrolides	Gastrointestinal, tinnitus, hearing loss, hepatotoxicity, prolonged QTc	Clinical visit, audiogram, liver function tests, electrocardiogram
Ethambutol	Ocular toxicity, neuropathy	Clinical visit, vision examination, color discrimination test
Rifamycins	Orange discoloration of bodily fluids, hepatotoxicity, cytopenias, hypersensitivity, uveitis (rifabutin)	Clinical visit, liver function tests, complete blood count, vision examination (rifabutin)
Aminoglycosides	Vestibular toxicity, ototoxicity, nephrotoxicity, electrolyte abnormalities	Clinical visit, audiogram, metabolic panel
Clofazimine	Skin darkening, xerosis, hepatotoxicity, prolonged QTc	Clinical visit, liver function tests, electrocardiogram
Moxifloxacin	Prolonged QTc, hepatotoxicity, tendinopathy	Clinical visit, liver function tests, electrocardiogram
Bedaquiline	Gastrointestinal, hepatotoxicity, prolonged QTc	Clinical visit, liver function tests, electrocardiogram
Oxazolidinones	Cytopenias, peripheral neuropathy, optic neuritis	Clinical visit, vision examination, color discrimination test, complete blood count
Amikacin liposome inhalation suspension	Dysphonia, cough, dyspnea, vestibular toxicity, ototoxicity, nephrotoxicity	Clinical visit, audiogram, metabolic panel

Adapted from Daley CL, et al. Euro Respir J 2020;56:2000535.

their initial regimen because of AEs.[47,48,77] As no studies have addressed the optimal approach to monitoring for AEs, the multi-society NTM guideline recommends that the approach is individualized based on the drugs used in the regimen, concurrent drugs and overlapping drug toxicities, age, comorbidities, and resources available.[1] A survey of expert clinicians in the management of NTM disease demonstrated consistent opinions on the management of hepatotoxicity, ototoxicity, tinnitus, and gastrointestinal upset.[78] Patients should be educated about potential side effects and provided with verbal and written instructions. In addition, they should be assured that they will be closely monitored for AEs so that they can be detected early and managed appropriately. When AEs occur, they should be addressed immediately. A common approach to managing less severe AEs is to temporarily hold the medication and rechallenge later. This approach has worked well with dysphonia related to ALIS.[79]

DRUGS IN DEVELOPMENT

There are several compounds in preclinical and clinical development including Phase 1 and Phase 2 clinical trials. Epetraborole is a novel boron-containing, orally available, small molecule inhibitor of bacterial leucyl-transfer ribonucleic acid (tRNA) synthetase.[80] The antimicrobial has broad antimycobacterial activity against both slowly and rapidly growing NTM including excellent in vitro activity against Mycobacterium abscessus.[80] Unpublished data show an MIC range of 0.25 to 8 mg/L with an MIC_{50} of 2 mg/L on cation adjusted Mueller–Hinton Broth against MAC.[81] In a chronic mouse MAC infection model, epetraborole demonstrated potent in vivo efficacy and significantly improved efficacy when combined with standard of care.[82] Another unpublished study using the MAC hollow fiber model reported that epetraborole was bactericidal and when combined with a standard-of-care regimen, the drug demonstrated resistance suppression.[83] Epetraborole was well tolerated at the expected dose of 500 mg a day in a phase 1b 28 day dose ranging study.[84] The most common AE was nausea (23%). A pivotal phase 2/3 randomized, placebo-controlled trial of treatment refractory MAC is currently enrolling in the United States, Australia, Japan, and South Korea (NCT05327803).

Omadacycline is a third-generation member of the tetracycline family, specifically an aminomethylcycline.[85] In vitro, omadacycline has similar activity to that of tigecycline against NTM but is better tolerated and comes in both intravenous and oral formulations. Against MAC, its MIC_{50} has been reported as high as greater than 16 mg/L,[86] but such values may be falsely elevated because omadacycline's concentration rapidly declines in testing solutions and therefore, looks less effective against slowly growing mycobacteria with long doubling time.[87] A hollow fiber model suggested that omadacycline actually has the most potent activity against MAC compared with other first- and second-line MAC drugs.[87] Small cases series have demonstrated clinical improvement when part of a multidrug regimen and reasonable tolerance in the setting of M abscessus infections.[88–90]

SPR720 is an aminobenzimidazole, gyrase B inhibitor that is converted to SPR719 which is the active moiety. In vitro, mouse and hollow fiber models have demonstrated activity against slowly growing NTM like MAC and Mycobacterium kansasii. The MIC_{90} for MAC is 2.0 mg/L with an MIC range of 0.06 to 4 mg/L.[91] A randomized, double-blind, placebo-controlled trial demonstrated that the drug was well tolerated up to doses of 1000 mg per day with mild to moderate AEs and no serious adverse events.[92] The drug is currently being evaluated in a Phase 2 trial of patients with treatment-naïve MAC pulmonary disease (NCT04553406).

Apramycin is a veterinary aminoglycoside with excellent in vitro activity against NTM and is being evaluated for therapy in humans. In vitro studies against M abscessus report that M abscessus was 100% susceptible to apramycin.[93] Further, apramycin showed potent bactericidal activity against the organism, as opposed to amikacin, which was only bacteriostatic.[93] In vitro studies against MAC are currently underway. A phase 1 clinical trial in humans had been completed, but its data are pending publication (NCT04105205).

Bacteriophages are viruses that infect bacteria and have been used to treat highly drug-resistant bacteria and mycobacteria. In the largest case series of bacteriophage therapy for NTM disease to date, the investigators describe how isolates from 200 patients with NTM infection were screened for phage susceptibility and one or more lytic phages were identified for 55 isolates.[94] Twenty patients—seventeen with M abscessus, one Mycobacterium chelonae, one disseminated BCG infection, and one M avium—received their phage therapy either intravenously, through inhalation, or both.[94] Favorable clinical or microbiologic responses were seen in 11 patients, including the patient with M avium, and no AEs were reported.[94] Of note, neutralizing antibodies were identified in eight patients which may have contributed to the lack of treatment response.[94] An FDA compassionate use protocol is now open in the United States.

Gallium, in complexes like gallium nitrate or gallium porphyrin, is a novel antimycobacterial therapeutic that interferes with the mycobacteria's iron–heme metabolism to inhibit growth.[95] In vitro studies show that various gallium complexes and their combinations, such as gallium nitrate with gallium protoporphyrin, potently inhibited both *M abscessus* and MAC growth.[95–97] Intravenous gallium is currently under investigation for adult patients with cystic fibrosis (CF) and NTM disease as a phase 1 clinical trial (NCT04294043).

Inhaled nitric oxide (NO) has been recently evaluated as therapy for NTM lung disease. NO has been shown to facilitate host immunity against pathogens in the lungs[98] and exert direct antimycobacterial activity.[99,100] A 2020 pilot prospective study of nine CF patients shows that inhaled NO was well tolerated and reduced *M abscessus* bacterial load.[101] A 2023 open-label proof of concept trial of 10 patients with refractory NTM pulmonary disease, three of whom had MAC, reports that 4 of the 10 patients culture-converted on a 3-week regimen of inhaled NO, including all three patients with MAC.[102] An open-label, multicenter trial to evaluate high-dose intermittent inhaled NO to treat both CF and non-CF patients with NTM pulmonary disease was completed in October 2022, pending publication (NCT04685720).

CLINICS CARE POINTS

- A three-drug, macrolide-based regimen is recommended over a two-drug or non-macrolide-based regimen and should be administered for at least 12 months after culture conversion.

- Non-cavitary nodular-bronchiectatic *Mycobacterium avium* complex (MAC) pulmonary disease can be treated 3 days a week but cavitary disease should receive daily therapy.

- Amikacin liposome inhalation suspension should be added to guideline-based therapy for treatment refractory disease.

- Despite lengthy combination medical therapy and sometimes surgical lung resection, recurrence is common and often due to reinfection.

- The treatment of macrolide-resistant disease is particularly challenging and expert consultation should be sought.

- New and repurposed drugs show promising activity against MAC, and ongoing clinical trials will hopefully provide new options for treatment in the near future.

DISCLOSURE

M.-V.H. Nguyen: nothing to declare. Charles L. Daley: Research contracts/grants: AN2, Bugworks, Beyond Air, Insmed, United States, Juvabis, Paratek. Advisory Board/Consultation: AN2, Aztrazeneca, Genentech, Hyfe, Insmed, MannKind, Matinas, Nob Hill, Paratek, Pfizer, Spero, Zambon. Data Monitoring Committee: Gates Foundation, Lilly, Otsuka.

ACKNOWLEDGMENT

The authors would like to thank the Lowerre Foundation for support of this work.

REFERENCES

1. Daley CL, Iaccarino JM, Lange C, et al. Treatment of nontuberculous mycobacterial pulmonary disease: an official ATS/ERS/ESCMID/IDSA clinical practice guideline. Eur Respir J 2020;56(1).

2. Hoefsloot W, van Ingen J, Andrejak C, et al. The geographic diversity of nontuberculous mycobacteria isolated from pulmonary samples: an NTM-NET collaborative study. Eur Respir J 2013;42(6): 1604–13.

3. Murcia MI, Tortoli E, Menendez MC, et al. *Mycobacterium colombiense* sp. nov., a novel member of the *Mycobacterium avium* complex and description of MAC-X as a new ITS genetic variant. Int J Syst Evol Microbiol 2006;56(Pt 9):2049–54.

4. Bang D, Herlin T, Stegger M, et al. *Mycobacterium arosiense* sp. nov., a slowly growing, scotochromogenic species causing osteomyelitis in an immunocompromised child. Int J Syst Evol Microbiol 2008; 58(Pt 10):2398–402.

5. Ben Salah I, Cayrou C, Raoult D, et al. *Mycobacterium marseillense* sp. nov., *Mycobacterium timonense* sp. nov. and *Mycobacterium bouchedurhonense* sp. nov., members of the *Mycobacterium avium* complex. Int J Syst Evol Microbiol 2009;59(Pt 11):2803–8.

6. van Ingen J, Boeree MJ, Kosters K, et al. Proposal to elevate *Mycobacterium avium* complex ITS sequevar MAC-Q to *Mycobacterium vulneris* sp. nov. Int J Syst Evol Microbiol 2009;59(Pt 9):2277–82.

7. Kim BJ, Math RK, Jeon CO, et al. *Mycobacterium yongonense* sp. nov., a slow-growing non-chromogenic species closely related to *Mycobacterium intracellulare*. Int J Syst Evol Microbiol 2013;63(Pt 1): 192–9.

8. Lee SY, Kim BJ, Kim H, et al. *Mycobacterium paraintracellulare* sp. nov., for the genotype INT-1 of *Mycobacterium intracellulare*. Int J Syst Evol Microbiol 2016;66(8):3132–41.

9. van Ingen J, Turenne CY, Tortoli E, et al. A definition of the *Mycobacterium avium* complex for

taxonomical and clinical purposes, a review. Int J Syst Evol Microbiol 2018;68(11):3666–77.

10. Koh WJ, Jeong BH, Jeon K, et al. Clinical significance of the differentiation between *Mycobacterium avium* and *Mycobacterium intracellulare* in *M. avium* complex lung disease. Chest 2012; 142(6):1482–8.

11. Kim SY, Shin SH, Moon SM, et al. Distribution and clinical significance of *Mycobacterium avium* complex species isolated from respiratory specimens. Diagn Microbiol Infect Dis 2017;88(2):125–37.

12. CLSI. Susceptibility Testing of Mycobacteria, Nocardia spp., and Other Aerobic Actinomycetes, vol. M24. Wayne, PA: Clinical and Laboratory Standards Institute; 2018.

13. CLSI. Performance standards for susceptibility testing of mycobacteria, nocardia spp, and other aerobic actinomycetes, vol. M62. Wayne, PA: Clinical and Laboratory Standards Institute; 2018.

14. Diel R, Nienhaus A, Ringshausen FC, et al. Microbiologic outcome of interventions against *Mycobacterium avium* complex pulmonary disease: a systematic review. Chest 2018;153(4):888–921.

15. Nasiri MJ, Ebrahimi G, Arefzadeh S, et al. Antibiotic therapy success rate in pulmonary *Mycobacterium avium* complex: a systematic review and meta-analysis. Expert Rev Anti Infect Ther 2020;18(3): 263–73.

16. Pasipanodya JG, Ogbonna D, Deshpande D, et al. Meta-analyses and the evidence base for microbial outcomes in the treatment of pulmonary *Mycobacterium avium-intracellulare* complex disease. J Antimicrob Chemother 2017;72(suppl_2):i3–19.

17. Kwak N, Park J, Kim E, et al. Treatment outcomes of *Mycobacterium avium* complex lung disease: a systematic review and meta-analysis. Clin Infect Dis 2017;65(7):1077–84.

18. Wallace RJ Jr, Brown BA, Griffith DE, et al. Initial clarithromycin monotherapy for *Mycobacterium avium-intracellulare* complex lung disease. Am J Respir Crit Care Med 1994;149(5):1335–41.

19. Dautzenberg B, Piperno D, Diot P, et al. Clarithromycin in the treatment of *Mycobacterium avium* lung infections in patients without AIDS. Clarithromycin Study Group of France. Chest 1995;107(4): 1035–40.

20. Wallace RJ Jr, Brown BA, Griffith DE, et al. Clarithromycin regimens for pulmonary *Mycobacterium avium* complex. The first 50 patients. Am J Respir Crit Care Med 1996;153(6 Pt 1):1766–72.

21. Tanaka E, Kimoto T, Tsuyuguchi K, et al. Effect of clarithromycin regimen for *Mycobacterium avium* complex pulmonary disease. Am J Respir Crit Care Med 1999;160(3):866–72.

22. Griffith DE, Brown BA, Girard WM, et al. Azithromycin activity against *Mycobacterium avium* complex lung disease in patients who were not infected with human immunodeficiency virus. Clin Infect Dis 1996;23(5):983–9.

23. Zuckerman JM, Qamar F, Bono BR. Review of macrolides (azithromycin, clarithromycin), ketolids (telithromycin) and glycylcyclines (tigecycline). Med Clin 2011;95(4):761–91, viii.

24. Chaisson RE, Benson CA, Dube MP, et al. Clarithromycin therapy for bacteremic *Mycobacterium avium* complex disease. A randomized, double-blind, dose-ranging study in patients with AIDS. AIDS Clinical Trials Group Protocol 157 Study Team. Ann Intern Med 1994;121(12):905–11.

25. Gordin FM, Sullam PM, Shafran SD, et al. A randomized, placebo-controlled study of rifabutin added to a regimen of clarithromycin and ethambutol for treatment of disseminated infection with *Mycobacterium avium* complex. Clin Infect Dis 1999;28(5):1080–5.

26. Griffith DE, Brown BA, Girard WM, et al. Azithromycin-containing regimens for treatment of *Mycobacterium avium* complex lung disease. Clin Infect Dis 2001;32(11):1547–53.

27. Koh WJ, Jeong BH, Jeon K, et al. Therapeutic drug monitoring in the treatment of *Mycobacterium avium* complex lung disease. Am J Respir Crit Care Med 2012;186(8):797–802.

28. Kobashi Y, Matsushima T, Oka M. A double-blind randomized study of aminoglycoside infusion with combined therapy for pulmonary *Mycobacterium avium* complex disease. Respir Med 2007;101(1): 130–8.

29. Peloquin CA, Berning SE, Nitta AT, et al. Aminoglycoside toxicity: daily versus thrice-weekly dosing for treatment of mycobacterial diseases. Clin Infect Dis 2004;38(11):1538–44.

30. Hwang TJ, Dotsenko S, Jafarov A, et al. Safety and availability of clofazimine in the treatment of multidrug and extensively drug-resistant tuberculosis: analysis of published guidance and meta-analysis of cohort studies. BMJ Open 2014;4(1):e004143.

31. Yang B, Jhun BW, Moon SM, et al. Clofazimine-containing regimen for the treatment of *Mycobacterium abscessus* lung disease. Antimicrob Agents Chemother 2017;61(6).

32. Martiniano SL, Wagner BD, Levin A, et al. Safety and effectiveness of clofazimine for primary and refractory nontuberculous mycobacterial infection. Chest 2017;152(4):800–9.

33. van Ingen J, Totten SE, Helstrom NK, et al. In vitro synergy between clofazimine and amikacin in treatment of nontuberculous mycobacterial disease. Antimicrob Agents Chemother 2012;56(12):6324–7.

34. Jarand J, Davis JP, Cowie RL, et al. Long-term follow-up of *Mycobacterium avium* complex lung disease in patients treated with regimens Including clofazimine and/or rifampin. Chest 2016;149(5): 1285–93.

35. Falzon D, Schunemann HJ, Harausz E, et al. World Health Organization treatment guidelines for drug-resistant tuberculosis, 2016 update. Eur Respir J 2017;49(3).

36. Griffith DE, Brown-Elliott BA, Langsjoen B, et al. Clinical and molecular analysis of macrolide resistance in Mycobacterium avium complex lung disease. Am J Respir Crit Care Med 2006;174(8):928–34.

37. Koh WJ, Hong G, Kim SY, et al. Treatment of refractory Mycobacterium avium complex lung disease with a moxifloxacin-containing regimen. Antimicrob Agents Chemother 2013;57(5):2281–5.

38. Brown-Elliott BA, Philley JV, Griffith DE, et al. In vitro susceptibility testing of bedaquiline against Mycobacterium avium complex. Antimicrob Agents Chemother 2017;61(2).

39. Kim DH, Jhun BW, Moon SM, et al. In vitro activity of bedaquiline and delamanid against nontuberculous mycobacteria, including macrolide-resistant clinical isolates. Antimicrob Agents Chemother 2019;63(8).

40. Philley JV, Wallace RJ Jr, Benwill JL, et al. Preliminary results of bedaquiline as salvage therapy for patients with nontuberculous mycobacterial lung disease. Chest 2015;148(2):499–506.

41. Svensson EM, Murray S, Karlsson MO, et al. Rifampicin and rifapentine significantly reduce concentrations of bedaquiline, a new anti-TB drug. J Antimicrob Chemother 2015;70(4):1106–14.

42. Brown-Elliott BA, Crist CJ, Mann LB, et al. In vitro activity of linezolid against slowly growing nontuberculous Mycobacteria. Antimicrob Agents Chemother 2003;47(5):1736–8.

43. Winthrop KL, Ku JH, Marras TK, et al. The tolerability of linezolid in the treatment of nontuberculous mycobacterial disease. Eur Respir J 2015;45(4):1177–9.

44. Brown-Elliott BA, Wallace RJ Jr. In vitro susceptibility testing of tedizolid against nontuberculous mycobacteria. J Clin Microbiol 2017;55(6):1747–54.

45. Miwa S, Shirai M, Toyoshima M, et al. Efficacy of clarithromycin and ethambutol for Mycobacterium avium complex pulmonary disease. A preliminary study. Ann Am Thorac Soc 2014;11(1):23–9.

46. Iketani O, Komeya A, Enoki Y, et al. Impact of rifampicin on the pharmacokinetics of clarithromycin and 14-hydroxy clarithromycin in patients with multidrug combination therapy for pulmonary Mycobacterium avium complex infection. J Infect Chemother 2022;28(1):61–6.

47. Jeong BH, Jeon K, Park HY, et al. Intermittent antibiotic therapy for nodular bronchiectatic Mycobacterium avium complex lung disease. Am J Respir Crit Care Med 2015;191(1):96–103.

48. Wallace RJ Jr, Brown-Elliott BA, McNulty S, et al. Macrolide/azalide therapy for nodular/bronchiectatic Mycobacterium avium complex lung disease. Chest 2014;146(2):276–82.

49. Griffith DE, Brown BA, Murphy DT, et al. Initial (6-month) results of three-times-weekly azithromycin in treatment regimens for Mycobacterium avium complex lung disease in human immunodeficiency virus-negative patients. J Infect Dis 1998;178(1):121–6.

50. Koh WJ, Jeong BH, Jeon K, et al. Response to switch from intermittent therapy to daily therapy for refractory nodular bronchiectatic Mycobacterium avium complex lung disease. Antimicrob Agents Chemother 2015;59(8):4994–6.

51. Lam PK, Griffith DE, Aksamit TR, et al. Factors related to response to intermittent treatment of Mycobacterium avium complex lung disease. Am J Respir Crit Care Med 2006;173(11):1283–9.

52. Mitchell JD. Surgical treatment of pulmonary nontuberculous mycobacterial infections. Thorac Surg Clin 2019;29(1):77–83.

53. Yu JA, Pomerantz M, Bishop A, et al. Lady Windermere revisited: treatment with thoracoscopic lobectomy/segmentectomy for right middle lobe and lingular bronchiectasis associated with nontuberculous mycobacterial disease. Eur J Cardio Thorac Surg 2011;40(3):671–5.

54. Jhun BW, Moon SM, Kim SY, et al. Intermittent antibiotic therapy for recurrent nodular bronchiectatic Mycobacterium avium complex lung disease. Antimicrob Agents Chemother 2018;62(2).

55. Asakura T, Nakagawa T, Suzuki S, et al. Efficacy and safety of intermittent maintenance therapy after successful treatment of Mycobacterium avium complex lung disease. J Infect Chemother 2019;25(3):218–21.

56. Kim HJ, Lee JS, Kwak N, et al. Role of ethambutol and rifampicin in the treatment of Mycobacterium avium complex pulmonary disease. BMC Pulm Med 2019;19(1):212.

57. Kwon YS, Kwon BS, Kim OH, et al. Treatment outcomes after discontinuation of ethambutol due to adverse events in Mycobacterium avium complex lung disease. J Kor Med Sci 2020;35(9):e59.

58. Boyle DP, Zembower TR, Reddy S, et al. Comparison of clinical features, virulence, and relapse among Mycobacterium avium complex species. Am J Respir Crit Care Med 2015;191(11):1310–7.

59. Koh WJ, Moon SM, Kim SY, et al. Outcomes of Mycobacterium avium complex lung disease based on clinical phenotype. Eur Respir J 2017;50(3).

60. Boyle DP, Zembower TR, Qi C. Relapse versus reinfection of Mycobacterium avium complex pulmonary disease. Patient characteristics and macrolide susceptibility. Ann Am Thorac Soc 2016;13(11):1956–61.

61. Andrejak C, Thomsen VO, Johansen IS, et al. Nontuberculous pulmonary mycobacteriosis in Denmark:

incidence and prognostic factors. Am J Respir Crit Care Med 2010;181(5):514–21.

62. Gochi M, Takayanagi N, Kanauchi T, et al. Retrospective study of the predictors of mortality and radiographic deterioration in 782 patients with nodular/bronchiectatic *Mycobacterium avium* complex lung disease. BMJ Open 2015;5(8):e008058.

63. Fleshner M, Olivier KN, Shaw PA, et al. Mortality among patients with pulmonary non-tuberculous mycobacteria disease. Int J Tubercul Lung Dis 2016;20(5):582–7.

64. Morimoto K, Namkoong H, Hasegawa N, et al. Macrolide-resistant *Mycobacterium avium* complex lung disease: analysis of 102 consecutive cases. Ann Am Thorac Soc 2016;13(11):1904–11.

65. Moon SM, Park HY, Kim SY, et al. Clinical characteristics, treatment outcomes, and resistance mutations associated with macrolide-resistant *Mycobacterium avium* complex lung disease. Antimicrob Agents Chemother 2016;60(11):6758–65.

66. van Ingen J, Aksamit T, Andrejak C, et al. Treatment outcome definitions in nontuberculous mycobacterial pulmonary disease: an NTM-NET consensus statement. Eur Respir J 2018;51(3).

67. Griffith DE, Adjemian J, Brown-Elliott BA, et al. Semiquantitative culture analysis during therapy for *Mycobacterium avium* complex lung disease. Am J Respir Crit Care Med 2015;192(6):754–60.

68. Moon SM, Jhun BW, Daley CL, et al. Unresolved issues in treatment outcome definitions for nontuberculous mycobacterial pulmonary disease. Eur Respir J 2019;53(5).

69. Lee JH, Park YE, Chong YP, et al. Efficacy of fluoroquinolones as substitutes for ethambutol or rifampin in the treatment of *Mycobacterium avium* complex pulmonary disease according to radiologic types. Antimicrob Agents Chemother 2022; 66(2):e0152221.

70. Olivier KN, Griffith DE, Eagle G, et al. Randomized trial of liposomal amikacin for inhalation in nontuberculous mycobacterial lung disease. Am J Respir Crit Care Med 2017;195(6):814–23.

71. Griffith DE, Eagle G, Thomson R, et al. Amikacin liposome inhalation suspension for treatment-refractory lung disease caused by *Mycobacterium avium* complex (CONVERT). A prospective, open-label, randomized study. Am J Respir Crit Care Med 2018;198(12):1559–69.

72. Nash KA, Zhang Y, Brown-Elliott BA, et al. Molecular basis of intrinsic macrolide resistance in clinical isolates of *Mycobacterium fortuitum*. J Antimicrob Chemother 2005;55(2):170–7.

73. Park Y, Lee EH, Jung I, et al. Clinical characteristics and treatment outcomes of patients with macrolide-resistant *Mycobacterium avium* complex pulmonary disease: a systematic review and meta-analysis. Respir Res 2019;20(1):286.

74. Haworth CS, Banks J, Capstick T, et al. British Thoracic Society guidelines for the management of non-tuberculous mycobacterial pulmonary disease (NTM-PD). Thorax 2017;72(Suppl 2):ii1–64.

75. Kadota T, Matsui H, Hirose T, et al. Analysis of drug treatment outcome in clarithromycin-resistant *Mycobacterium avium* complex lung *disease*. BMC Infect Dis 2016;16:31.

76. Adachi Y, Tsuyuguchi K, Kobayashi T, et al. Effective treatment for clarithromycin-resistant *Mycobacterium avium* complex lung disease. J Infect Chemother 2020;26(7):676–80.

77. Zweijpfenning S, Kops S, Magis-Escurra C, et al. Treatment and outcome of non-tuberculous mycobacterial pulmonary disease in a predominantly fibro-cavitary disease cohort. Respir Med 2017; 131:220–4.

78. van Ingen J, Aliberti S, Andrejak C, et al. Management of drug toxicity in *Mycobacterium avium* complex pulmonary disease: an expert panel survey. Clin Infect Dis 2021;73(1):e256–9.

79. Swenson C, Lapinel NC, Ali J. Clinical management of respiratory adverse events associated with amikacin liposome inhalation suspension: results from a patient survey. Open Forum Infect Dis 2020;7(4):ofaa079.

80. Ganapathy US, Gengenbacher M, Dick T. Epetraborole is active against *Mycobacterium abscessus*. Antimicrob Agents Chemother 2021;65(10): e0115621.

81. De Stefano MSSC, Alley MRK, Cynamon MH. *In vitro* activities of epetraborole, a novel bacterial leucyl-tRNA synthetase inhibitor, against *Mycobacterium avium* complex isolates. Open Forum Infect Dis 2022;9:S659–60.

82. De KDM, Shoen CA, Cynamon MH, et al. Epetraborole, a novel bacterial leucyl-tRNA synthetase inhibitor, demonstrates potent efficacy and improves efficacy of a standard of care regimen against *Mycobacterium avium* complex in a chronic mouse lung infection model. Open Forum Infect Dis 2022;9:S655–6.

83. Chapagain M, Howe D, Alley MRK, et al. Dose-response studies of the novel bacterial leucyl-tRNA synthetase inhibitor, epetraborole, in the intracellular hollow fiber system model of *Mycobacterium avium* complex lung disease. Open Forum Infect Dis 2022;9:S652–3.

84. Eckburg PBCD, Long J, Chanda S, et al. Tolerability and pharmacokinetics of oral epetraborole at the predicted therapeutic dosage for *Mycobacterium avium* complex (MAC) lung disease: a phase 1b dose-ranging and food effect study. Open Forum Infect Dis 2022;9:S664–5.

85. Tanaka SK, Steenbergen J, Villano S. Discovery, pharmacology, and clinical profile of omadacycline, a novel aminomethylcycline antibiotic. Bioorg Med Chem 2016;24(24):6409–19.

86. Brown-Elliott BA, Wallace RJ Jr. In Vitro susceptibility testing of omadacycline against nontuberculous mycobacteria. Antimicrob Agents Chemother 2021;65(3).

87. Chapagain M, Pasipanodya JG, Athale S, et al. Omadacycline efficacy in the hollow fibre system model of pulmonary *Mycobacterium avium* complex and potency at clinically attainable doses. J Antimicrob Chemother 2022;77(6):1694–705.

88. Duah M, Beshay M. Omadacycline in first-line combination therapy for pulmonary *Mycobacterium abscessus* infection: a case series. Int J Infect Dis 2022;122:953–6.

89. Morrisette T, Alosaimy S, Philley JV, et al. Preliminary, real-world, multicenter experience with omadacycline for *Mycobacterium abscessus* infections. Open Forum Infect Dis 2021;8(2):ofab002.

90. Siddiqa A, Khan S, Rodriguez GD, et al. Omadacycline for the treatment of *Mycobacterium abscessus* infections: case series and review of the *literature*. IDCases 2023;31:e01703.

91. Pennings LJ, Ruth MM, Wertheim HFL, et al. The benzimidazole SPR719 shows promising concentration-dependent activity and synergy against nontuberculous mycobacteria. Antimicrob Agents Chemother 2021;65(4).

92. Talley AK, Thurston A, Moore G, et al. First-in-human evaluation of the safety, tolerability, and pharmacokinetics of SPR720, a novel oral bacterial DNA gyrase (GyrB) inhibitor for mycobacterial infections. Antimicrob Agents Chemother 2021; 65(11):e0120821.

93. Moore JE, Koulianos G, Hardy M, et al. Antimycobacterial activity of veterinary antibiotics (Apramycin and Framycetin) against *Mycobacterium abscessus*: implication for patients with cystic fibrosis. Int J Mycobacteriol 2018;7(3):265–7.

94. Dedrick RM, Smith BE, Cristinziano M, et al. Phage therapy of *Mycobacterium* infections: compassionate use of phages in 20 patients with drug-resistant mycobacterial disease. Clin Infect Dis 2023;76(1): 103–12.

95. Choi SR, Switzer B, Britigan BE, et al. Gallium porphyrin and gallium nitrate synergistically inhibit Mycobacterial species by targeting different aspects of iron/heme metabolism. ACS Infect Dis 2020;6(10):2582–91.

96. Choi SR, Talmon GA, Britigan BE, et al. Nanoparticulate beta-cyclodextrin with gallium tetraphenylporphyrin demonstrates in vitro and in vivo antimicrobial efficacy against *Mycobacteroides abscessus* and *Mycobacterium avium*. ACS Infect Dis 2021;7(8):2299–309.

97. Choi SR, Britigan BE, Narayanasamy P. Synthesis and in vitro analysis of novel gallium tetrakis(4-methoxyphenyl)porphyrin and its long-acting nanoparticle as a potent antimycobacterial agent. Bioorg Med Chem Lett 2022;62:128645.

98. Ricciardolo FL, Sterk PJ, Gaston B, et al. Nitric oxide in health and disease of the respiratory system. Physiol Rev 2004;84(3):731–65.

99. Miller CC, Rawat M, Johnson T, et al. Innate protection of *Mycobacterium smegmatis* against the antimicrobial activity of nitric oxide is provided by mycothiol. Antimicrob Agents Chemother 2007; 51(9):3364–6.

100. Yaacoby-Bianu K, Gur M, Toukan Y, et al. Compassionate nitric oxide adjuvant treatment of persistent *Mycobacterium* infection in cystic fibrosis patients. Pediatr Infect Dis J 2018;37(4):336–8.

101. Bentur L, Gur M, Ashkenazi M, et al. Pilot study to test inhaled nitric oxide in cystic fibrosis patients with refractory *Mycobacterium abscessus* lung infection. J Cyst Fibros 2020;19(2):225–31.

102. Flume PA, Garcia BA, Wilson D, et al. Inhaled nitric oxide for adults with pulmonary non-tuberculous mycobacterial infection. Respir Med 2023;206: 107069.

Treatment Approaches to *Mycobacterium abscessus* Pulmonary Disease

Michael R. Holt, BSc, MBBS, FRACP[a,b],*,
Timothy Baird, BSc, MBBS, DTM&H, FRACP[c,d,e]

KEYWORDS

• *M abscessus* • Nontuberculous mycobacteria • Pulmonary disease • Treatment

KEY POINTS

- *Mycobacterium abscessus* complex comprises three subspecies. Subspecies *abscessus* and *bolletii* usually exhibit inducible macrolide resistance, whereas subspecies *massiliense* usually does not. Macrolide susceptibility is determined by phenotypic testing after 14 days of incubation.
- Macrolide susceptibility is the key determinant of treatment outcome for *M abscessus* pulmonary disease (MAB-PD) and must be protected by adequate companion drugs in treatment regimens.
- The optimal approach to treatment of MAB-PD is undefined. Current treatment strategies result in poor outcomes, especially for macrolide-resistant isolates, and considerable drug toxicity.
- Multiple novel or repurposed therapeutic candidates are emerging.

INTRODUCTION

Mycobacterium abscessus complex is the most common cause of rapid-grower nontuberculous mycobacterial pulmonary disease (NTM-PD) and a significant contributor to the burden of NTM-PD worldwide.[1] It is distinguished from other NTM by evidence of worldwide dominant circulating clones and possible person-to-person transmission.[2] The complex comprises three taxa, the classification of which has been controversial and subject to multiple revisions.[3] In keeping with recent clinical literature, the current review refers to these taxa as subspecies: subspecies *abscessus*, subspecies *massiliense*, and subspecies *bolletii*.[4] The isolation frequency of these subspecies varies geographically, although subspecies *abscessus* is usually most common ($\approx$45–70%), followed by subspecies *massiliense* ($\approx$20–55%), and subspecies

bolletii ($\approx$1–15%).[5] Treatment outcomes for the subspecies illustrate the importance of macrolide susceptibility. Subspecies *abscessus* and *bolletii* possess a functional *erm*(41) gene, which confers inducible macrolide resistance.[6] In subspecies *massiliense*, the *erm*(41) gene is nonfunctional due to a deletion mutation.[6] A systematic review and meta-analysis reported sustained sputum culture conversion with initial macrolide-containing multidrug regimens in 35% (95% CI: 24%–46%) of patients with subspecies *abscessus* and 79% (95% CI: 52%–97%) of patients with subspecies *massiliense*.[7] In 15% to 20% of subspecies *abscessus* isolates, there is a loss-of-function T28C substitution in the *erm*(41) gene and treatment outcomes for these C28 sequevars are similar to those for subspecies *massiliense*.[8–10] Conversely, treatment outcomes for *M abscessus* complex with mutational macrolide resistance are abysmal.[11]

 a Gallipoli Medical Research Foundation, The University of Queensland, Brisbane, Queensland, Australia; b Department of Thoracic Medicine, Royal Brisbane & Women's Hospital, Butterfield Street, Herston, Brisbane, Queensland, Australia; c Sunshine Coast Health Institute, Sunshine Coast, Queensland, Australia; d University of the Sunshine Coast, Sunshine Coast, Queensland, Australia; e Department of Respiratory Medicine, Sunshine Coast University Hospital, 6 Doherty St, Birtinya, Sunshine Coast, Queensland 4575, Australia
* Corresponding author. Department of Thoracic Medicine, Royal Brisbane & Women's Hospital, Butterfield Street, Herston, Brisbane, Queensland 4029, Australia.
E-mail address: michaelrholt@outlook.com

Clin Chest Med 44 (2023) 785–798
https://doi.org/10.1016/j.ccm.2023.06.010

CLINICAL SIGNIFICANCE OF *M ABSCESSUS* AND DECISION TO TREAT

M abscessus may be a contaminant or "coloniser" of the respiratory tract, thus its isolation from respiratory samples does not necessarily indicate disease.[12] As for other NTM, the diagnosis of *M abscessus* pulmonary disease (MAB-PD) requires synthesis of serial microbiological and clinico-radiological data.[13] Decisions to initiate pharmacotherapy for MAB-PD should be patient-focused and individualized. Risk factors for NTM-PD progression and mortality, such as fibrocavitary disease, smear positivity, and immune suppression, favor therapy.[14,15] On the other hand, watchful waiting may be prudent in a low-risk, pauci-symptomatic patient, for whom treatment is anticipated to be unsuccessful or poorly tolerated. In a Korean study of 126 subjects with MAB-PD and persistently positive sputum cultures for ≥6 months without treatment, 33 subjects required treatment within 2 years of diagnosis.[16] However, spontaneous culture conversion was observed in 24 subjects and maintained in 13/18 of those with at least 6 months of follow-up (mean follow-up: 2.7 ± 1.5 years). Irrespective of the initial decision regarding pharmacotherapy, non-pharmacologic strategies are essential (**Box 1**).[17,18]

ANTIBIOTIC SUSCEPTIBILITY AND RESISTANCE MECHANISMS

M abscessus exhibits broad antibiotic resistance due to a thick, lipid-laden cell envelope, in vivo biofilm formation, and multiple internal systems.[19,20] The internal "intrinsic resistome" includes target-modifying enzymes [eg, *erm*(41)], antibiotic-modifying/inactivating enzymes (eg, beta-lactamase and rifampicin adenosine diphosphate [ADP]-ribosyltransferase) and efflux pumps.[19] As a consequence, *M abscessus*

Box 1
Non-pharmacologic measures for nontuberculous mycobacterial pulmonary disease
Smoking cessation
Airway clearance
Nutritional support
Management of gastroesophageal reflux and aspiration
Pulmonary rehabilitation
Psychosocial support
Management of predisposing conditions and risk factors

---

demonstrates limited susceptibility to beta-lactam antibiotics and possesses intrinsic resistance to ethambutol and rifampicin. Mutational resistance to macrolides and amikacin may also occur due to 23S rRNA and 16S rRNA gene mutations, respectively.[21,22]

Clinically, it is most important to determine susceptibility to macrolide antibiotics. Phenotypic antibiotic susceptibility testing (AST) demonstrates mutational macrolide resistance after 3 to 5 days of incubation. For isolates that are susceptible at day 3 to 5, the presence of inducible macrolide resistance is determined by an extended incubation period of 14 days.[23] Molecular methods may also be used to predict *erm*(41) functionality, although discrepancies between phenotypic and genotypic susceptibility may occur.[24]

Table 1 reflects the antibiotic susceptibility profile of *M abscessus* according to breakpoints defined by the Clinical and Laboratory Standards Institute (CLSI).[25–28] Susceptibility breakpoints are yet to be defined for tigecycline and clofazimine.[23] Furthermore, standardized AST procedures and interpretive strategies are lacking for clofazimine.[23] Using broth microdilution methods, minimum inhibitory concentrations (MICs) for these agents seem low. For example, a study of 218 *M abscessus* isolates from Singapore reported a MIC90 of 0.25 μg/mL for clofazimine and 1 μg/mL for tigecycline.[26]

CURRENT PRINCIPLES OF PHARMACOTHERAPY

Optimal therapeutic strategies for MAB-PD, including drug selection, administration techniques, and treatment duration, are unknown.[4] Guidelines suggest a biphasic approach (**Table 2**).[4,29,30] An initial intensive phase, which includes parenteral agents, is followed by a continuation phase that comprises oral agents, usually in combination with inhaled amikacin. The duration of treatment is 12 months beyond culture conversion. Although this approach is often successful for macrolide-susceptible isolates, enduring culture conversion is rarely achieved in macrolide-resistant disease.[7,31]

The macrolides are the only agents for which there is robust correlation between AST results and clinical outcomes. Amikacin is associated with improved microbiological outcomes, although outcomes remain poor in the setting of macrolide resistance.[32] Companion drugs are necessary to protect against emergent mutational resistance to the macrolides and amikacin. Experts recommend that at least three active drugs are used, noting that macrolides are not "counted"

Table 1
M abscessus antibiotic susceptibility according to Clinical and Laboratory Standards Institute breakpoints

Drug	Susceptible		Intermediate		Resistant	
	MIC (μg/mL)	%	MIC (μg/mL)	%	MIC (μg/mL)	%
Clarithromycin D3	≤ 2		4		≥ 8	
subspecies *abscessus*		74–83.8		0–11		12.3–17.9
subspecies *massiliense*		91.1–93		0–1.1		6–8.9
Clarithromycin D14	≤ 2		4		≥ 8	
subspecies *abscessus*		11–15.2		0.7–3		83.6–86
subspecies *massiliense*		86.7–92.6		1.1–2.2		6.3–11.1
Amikacin	≤ 16	76–94.7	32	1.8–18.7	≥ 64	0.9–5.3
Imipenem	≤ 4	0–25	8–16	1.8–71.4	≥ 32	16–98.3
Cefoxitin	≤ 16	3.7–23.8	32–64	65.9–88.1	≥ 128	8–16.7
Linezolid	≤ 8	27.5–67.6	16	19–34.2	≥ 32	8.7–48
Ciprofloxacin	≤ 1	0.5–5.3	2	0.9–6.2	≥ 4	92.1–95.4
Moxifloxacin	≤ 1	0–5	2	1.4–10.1	≥ 4	86.8–98.6
Doxycycline	≤ 1	0.5–1.8	2–4	0–1.1	≥ 8	98–99.1
Minocycline	≤ 1	0.5–6	2–4	5.5–8	≥ 8	86–94
TMP-SMX	≤ 2/38	2.6–21.7	N/A	N/A	≥ 4/76	78.3–97.4

Abbreviations: MIC, minimum inhibitory concentration; D3, incubation day 3 to 5; D14, incubation day 14; TMP-SMX, trimethoprim–sulfamethoxazole.
   Adapted from ref.[25–28]

for resistant isolates but may be used for their immunomodulatory properties.[18] Although guidelines recommend that other drugs are selected based on AST, a paucity of data precludes predicting in vivo susceptibility and treatment outcomes from in vitro results. *M abscessus* is often resistant to many of the oral agents recommended by older guidelines (see **Table 1**), creating an urgent need for new therapeutic options.[29,30] Antibiotic dosing and side effects are outlined in **Table 3**. Monitoring for adverse effects is further detailed elsewhere in this issue.

The duration of the intensive phase is undefined. Some guidelines suggest a minimum of 4 weeks.[29] Longer durations are often recommended, especially in macrolide-resistant disease, according to clinical response and tolerance of therapy.[29] A retrospective Korean study suggested that subspecies *massiliense* can be effectively treated with shorter durations of intensive phase and overall therapy than subspecies *abscessus*, although the mean duration of the briefer intensive phase was 4.7 months.[33] Given the paucity of effective non-parenteral treatment options, experts caution against arbitrarily deescalating therapy.[18] The decision to switch from intensive to continuation phase therapy should be based on microbiological and clinico-radiological response. In the absence of culture conversion, the appropriate course of action is unclear. A recent retrospective Korean study demonstrated diminishing conditional probability of microbiological cure, defined by enduring culture conversion, with extended parenteral amikacin therapy.[34] After 12 weeks of therapy, the conditional probability of cure was 8.8%. In this scenario, more appropriate treatment outcome measures are clinical and radiological improvement. The treatment approach may need to be adapted accordingly, such as a transition to episodic parenteral therapy, perhaps with chronic suppressive therapy with oral or inhaled agents.[13]

MACROLIDES

Macrolide susceptibility is the key determinant of treatment outcome.[7,31] Thus, azithromycin or clarithromycin should be included in treatment regimens for *M abscessus* isolates without inducible or mutational macrolide resistance.[4] Regarding isolates with inducible or mutational resistance, the current multi-society guidelines suggest inclusion of a macrolide if this agent is being used for its immunomodulatory properties, whilst emphasizing that the macrolide is not considered an active drug in this context.[4] This approach is subtly different from the British Thoracic Society guidelines, which recommend inclusion of a macrolide (where tolerated) in treatment regimens for isolates with inducible, but not mutational, macrolide resistance.[29]

Table 2
Recent guidelines for treatment of *M abscessus* pulmonary disease

	ATS/ERS/ESCMID/IDSA 2020[4]	BTS 2017[29]	CFF/ECFS 2016[30]
Intensive phase	*Macrolide-susceptible:* 1–2 IV agents, plus 2 PO agents (macrolide prioritized) *Inducible or mutational macrolide resistance:* 2–3 IV agents, plus 2–3 PO agents (macrolide not counted)	*Macrolide-susceptible or inducible macrolide resistance‡:* IV amikacin, plus IV tigecycline, plus IV imipenem (if tolerated), plus PO azithromycin, or clarithromycin (if tolerated) *Mutational macrolide resistance‡:* IV amikacin, plus IV tigecycline, plus IV imipenem (if tolerated)	2 IV drugs, plus ≥1 PO drug Typically: IV amikacin, plus IV imipenem, plus IV tigecycline, plus PO azithromycin
Continuation phase	*Macrolide-susceptible:* 2–3 PO/NEB agents (macrolide prioritized) *Inducible or mutational macrolide resistance:* 2–3 PO/NEB agents (macrolide not counted)	*Macrolide-susceptible or inducible macrolide resistance:* NEB amikacin, plus PO clarithromycin or azithromycin, plus 1–3 PO agents§ guided by AST and tolerance *Mutational macrolide resistance:* NEB amikacin, plus 2–4 PO agents§ guided by AST and tolerance	≥ 2 PO drugs, plus azithromycin or clarithromycin, ± NEB amikacin Typically: PO azithromycin, plus PO clofazimine, plus PO minocycline, plus PO moxifloxacin, plus NEB amikacin
Notes	IV agents: amikacin, imipenem (or cefoxitin), tigecycline PO agents: azithromycin (or clarithromycin), clofazimine, linezolid NEB agents: amikacin	§PO agents: clofazimine (start during intensive phase if tolerated), linezolid, minocycline, moxifloxacin, TMP-SMX ‡An intensive phase of ≥ 4 wk is recommended, with extension to 3–6 mo if tolerated for inducible or mutational macrolide resistance.	

Abbreviations: IV, intravenous; PO, by mouth; NEB, nebulized; AST, antibiotic susceptibility testing; TMP-SMX, trimethoprim–sulfamethoxazole.
  ‡, §, They denote the corresponding explanatory text in the Notes row.

AMIKACIN (PARENTERAL AND INHALED)

Amikacin exhibits concentration-dependent bactericidal activity against NTM. Efficacy is predicted by the ratio of peak serum concentration (Cmax) to MIC. Recommended intravenous doses of amikacin are 15 mg/kg (ideal body weight) daily or 25 mg/kg thrice weekly. Calculated Cmax is 35 to 45 μg/mL for the former and 65 to 80 μg/mL for the latter.[35] Given the MIC distribution of *M abscessus* and unpredictable penetrance of amikacin into lung tissue and macrophages, these levels may not achieve optimal Cmax/MIC at the point of infection, especially with daily dosing.[36,37] In gram-negative bacterial infections and tuberculosis, optimal Cmax/MIC values of 8 to 12 have been suggested.[37,38] A hollow fiber model of *M abscessus* infection suggested a lower optimal (EC80) Cmax/MIC of 3.2.[38] The administration of high doses is limited by significant renal and eighth cranial nerve toxicities. In a prospective, randomized trial, there was no significant

Table 3
Antibiotic dosing, side effects, and monitoring

	Antibiotic	Dose	Side Effects	Monitoring[a]
Intravenous	Amikacin [R]	15 mg/kg daily, or 25 mg/kg thrice weekly[b]	Ototoxicity Nephrotoxicity Electrolyte disorders	Audiogram Electrolytes, renal function
	Tigecycline [H]	25–50 mg, 1–2 times per day[c]	Nausea/vomiting Hepatitis Acute pancreatitis	Clinical monitoring LFTs Amylase/lipase
	Imipenem [R]	500–1000 mg, 2–3 times per day	Rash Nausea/vomiting Cytopenia Nephrotoxicity	Clinical monitoring Full blood count Electrolytes, renal function
	Cefoxitin [R]	2–4 g, 2–3 times per day	Cytopenia Hepatotoxicity Nephrotoxicity (rare)	Full blood count LFTs Electrolytes, renal function
Oral	Azithromycin Clarithromycin [R]	250–500 mg daily 500 mg twice per day	Gastrointestinal Ototoxicity Hepatotoxicity QTc prolongation	Clinical monitoring Audiogram LFTs ECG (QTc)
	Clofazimine [H]	100–200 mg daily	Skin dryness/irritation Enteropathy (rare) QTc prolongation Hepatotoxicity	Clinical monitoring ECG (QTc) LFTs
	Linezolid	600 mg, 1–2 times per day[d]	Cytopenia Peripheral neuropathy Optic neuritis	Full blood count Clinical monitoring Visual acuity and color discrimination
	Minocycline	100 mg twice per day	Photosensitivity Gastrointestinal	Clinical monitoring
	Moxifloxacin	400 mg daily	QTc prolongation Hepatotoxicity Tendinopathy	ECG (QTc) LFTs Clinical monitoring
	TMP-SMX [H, R]	800/160 mg twice per day	Gastrointestinal Photosensitivity Cytopenia	Clinical monitoring Full blood count
Inhaled	Amikacin (ALIS) Amikacin (PF)	590 mg daily 250–500 mg per day	Dysphonia Cough Dyspnoea Ototoxicity Nephrotoxicity	Clinical monitoring Audiogram Electrolytes, renal function

[R]: dose adjustment recommended in renal impairment.

[H]: caution or dose adjustment recommended in hepatic impairment.

Abbreviations: TMP-SMX, trimethoprim–sulfamethoxazole; ALIS, amikacin liposome inhalation solution; PF, parenteral formulation.

[a] Intermittent testing of full blood count, electrolytes, renal function, and liver function tests should be performed throughout antibiotic treatment for NTM-PD.

[b] Therapeutic drug monitoring is recommended, with dose titration to achieve peak concentrations of 35 to 45 μg/mL (daily dosing) or 65 to 80 μg/mL (thrice weekly dosing).

[c] A lower initial dose is suggested (eg, 25 mg once or twice daily) and titration to the maximally tolerated dose with antiemetic premedication.

[d] Many patients will be unable to tolerate 600 mg twice daily. Toxicity may be minimized with therapeutic drug monitoring.

Adapted from refs.[4,29]

difference in toxicity profile between daily and thrice-weekly dosing regimens.[39] Ototoxicity was associated with cumulative amikacin exposure.

Our approach is to dose amikacin thrice-weekly, targeting the higher Cmax of 65 to 80 μg/mL with therapeutic drug monitoring (TDM). We consider targeting a lower range for isolates with low MIC. Given the in vitro synergy of clofazimine with amikacin, we routinely combine these two agents when building a regimen.[40]

The potential for nebulized parenteral amikacin to improve microbiological and clinical outcomes in MAB-PD was suggested by a small retrospective study of patients with NTM-PD, predominantly caused by M abscessus.[41] Nebulization of the parenteral formulation was most commonly tolerated at doses of 250 mg daily or twice daily. Owing to systemic and pulmonary side effects, 35% of patients ceased therapy. Amikacin liposome inhalation suspension (ALIS, 590 mg daily) has since been formulated to achieve superior uptake by pulmonary macrophages and its role in refractory Mycobacterium avium complex pulmonary disease (MAC-PD) was established by phase 2 and 3 randomized controlled trials.[42,43] Of note, ALIS was efficacious for MAC isolates with amikacin MICs up to 64 μg/mL, and the CLSI breakpoint for ALIS resistance in MAC is defined by a higher MIC than for intravenously administered amikacin.[23,43] ALIS has predominantly been used in MAB-PD as a component of continuation phase treatment.[44] Discontinuation due to adverse effects occurs in approximately 15% of cases. Retrospective studies have reported possible efficacy and the results of an open-label clinical trial are pending (ClinicalTrials.gov ID: NCT03038178).[45,46]

TIGECYCLINE

Tigecycline produced an exceptional 1-log kill in a hollow-fiber system model of pulmonary M abscessus infection.[47] However, the derived optimal clinical dose of 200 mg is not attainable in practice due to adverse effects. Retrospective studies have associated tigecycline with clinico-radiological improvement and significantly more frequent short-term culture conversion.[48–51] Nausea and vomiting are the main barriers to therapy. In our experience, these can be mitigated by premedication with an antiemetic and gradual dose escalation.

IMIPENEM-CILASTATIN AND CEFOXITIN

Imipenem–cilastatin (hereinafter referred to as "imipenem") and cefoxitin are beta-lactam antibiotics with some activity against M abscessus. Imipenem, but not cefoxitin, was independently associated

with treatment success in a meta-analysis of individual patient data.[32] Imipenem is also preferred due to superior tolerability. In a retrospective study of Korean patients with MAB-PD, cefoxitin was discontinued in 60% of cases due to leukopenia, thrombocytopenia, or hepatotoxicity.[52]

Cefoxitin and especially, imipenem, exhibit in vitro instability.[53] As a result, MICs are influenced by incubation time, and the typical intermediate-range results may underrepresent the efficacy of these agents. The instability of imipenem also presents a challenge to outpatient administration. Cefoxitin is better suited to situations that require continuous infusion.

CLOFAZIMINE

Clofazimine is safe and efficacious in MAB-PD.[54,55] A recent study of Korean subjects with MAC-PD or MAB-PD suggested superior culture conversion for isolates with a clofazimine MIC ≤ 0.25 μg/mL.[56] In vitro, clofazimine synergises with amikacin and clarithromycin against M abscessus and prevents the regrowth that is observed with either agent alone.[57] The half-life of clofazimine is 36 days and time to reach steady-state conditions is 144 days.[58] The therapeutic and adverse effects of clofazimine relate to gradual accumulation of the drug in tissue. Side effects include skin-tanning and electrocardiographic QT prolongation. The former may be associated with skin irritation or stigma in certain cultures. A recent study of the pharmacokinetics of clofazimine in NTM-PD reported progressive QT prolongation with cumulative exposure, even in steady-state settings, and the investigators suggested monitoring of the QT interval throughout therapy.[58] Rarely, severe clofazimine-related enteropathy may occur.[59]

We routinely use clofazimine in the treatment of M abscessus. Owing to its long half-life and synergy with amikacin, we introduce clofazimine during the intensive phase and consider it reasonable to reduce the dose if skin changes become problematic for the patient.

OTHER ORAL AGENTS

Guidelines recommend that other oral agents are selected according to AST results. Options may include linezolid, minocycline, moxifloxacin, and trimethoprim–sulfamethoxazole. M abscessus is more frequently susceptible to linezolid than these other oral agents (see **Table 1**), although MICs for linezolid are often high.[60] A recent retrospective Chinese study of patients with MAB-PD reported superior microbiological outcomes with an ntensified regimen that included linezolid and high-dose cefoxitin, despite the latter being withdrawn in 37.5% of cases.[61] Nonetheless, long-term administration of linezolid at recommended doses is often limited by cytopenias and neurotoxicity. A retrospective cohort study of patients with NTM disease in the United States reported toxicity-related cessation or interruption in 87% of cases.[62] TDM is likely instrumental in optimal administration of this agent.[63] Regarding other oral agents, our experience concords with international reports that M abscessus is usually resistant to minocycline, moxifloxacin, and trimethoprim–sulfamethoxazole (see **Table 1**).

EMERGING THERAPIES

The outcomes and toxicity of guidelines-based therapy for MAB-PD remain suboptimal.[4,29,30,64] Fortunately, there is growing momentum to meet the need for better treatment strategies. There are multiple promising new and/or "repurposed" emerging therapies, including oral, intravenous and nebulized antibiotics (**Table 4**), and nonantibiotic antimicrobial agents.[64,65] Many are presently being assessed in clinical studies (**Table 5**). Some experts currently recommend omadacycline, tedizolid, and bedaquiline for treatment of MAB-PD, and certain dual beta-lactams for salvage therapy.[18]

RIFABUTIN

Rifamycins have traditionally not been used in MAB-PD due to resistance of M abscessus to rifampicin. However, recent in vitro data indicate that rifabutin may have bactericidal activity against all 3 M abscessus subspecies.[66,67] Several in vitro studies have demonstrated synergistic activity against M abscessus with clarithromycin, tigecycline, imipenem, linezolid, and tedizolid.[68–71] Furthermore, rifabutin potentially suppresses inducible macrolide resistance by preventing induction of whiB7 and erm(41) gene expression.[72] The clinical implications of these in vitro findings remain unknown, although rifabutin is included in the FORMaT trial (see **Table 5**). We consider rifabutin an attractive additional oral agent when building a regimen against M abscessus, particularly if inducible macrolide resistance is present.

BEDAQUILINE

Bedaquiline is an oral diarylquinolone that was formulated and approved for the treatment of multidrug-resistant tuberculosis.[73,74] It decreases mycobacterial ATP production through inhibition of ATP synthase and has demonstrated in vitro bacteriostatic activity against M abscessus,

extremely low MICs and possible synergy with clofazimine.[65,73–77] Although no randomized trials have assessed the efficacy of bedaquiline in MAB-PD, Philley and colleagues explored its use as salvage therapy in 10 patients with treatment-refractory NTM-PD (four with MAB-PD).[78] Treatment was well-tolerated overall, with some improvements noted in symptoms, radiology, and bacterial load. However, culture conversion was not sustained for 6 months in any patient.[78] Concerningly, more recent in vitro studies suggested that bedaquiline may decrease the activity of cefoxitin and imipenem by suppressing the beta-lactam-induced ATP burst, although the clinical implications of this finding remain unclear.[79]

NOVEL TETRACYCLINE ANALOGUES

Omadacycline, a first-in-class aminomethylcycline, is available in both oral and intravenous formulations. It received FDA approval in 2019 for the treatment of bacterial community-acquired pneumonia and acute bacterial skin and skin structure infections (ABSSSI) and has demonstrated potent in vitro activity against M abscessus with similar MICs to tigecycline.[80–82] Several small case reports and series have demonstrated promising clinical efficacy against MAB-PD with minimal toxicity; however, larger trials are required before recommendations for routine use can be made.[83–85] Eravacycline is a novel fluorocycline that is currently approved by the FDA for complicated intra-abdominal infections.[65] It has shown superior in vitro activity against M abscessus with MICs twofold lower than both tigecycline and omadacycline; however, in vivo efficacy in MAB-PD is unknown.[86]

TEDIZOLID

Tedizolid, the second-in-class oral oxazolidinone, has FDA approval for the treatment of ABSSSI in adults and may also provide an alternative to linezolid for treating MAB-PD. It has demonstrated superior in vitro activity against M abscessus to linezolid and possible synergy with imipenem.[71,87–89] A retrospective cohort study compared tedizolid and linezolid in 24 solid-organ transplant patients with NTM infection (predominantly M abscessus).[90] Drug tolerance and safety outcomes were similar between the two agents and treatment success in the tedizolid group was 58%.

DUAL BETA-LACTAMS

Dual beta-lactam agents have interestingly demonstrated potential for the treatment of MAB-PD. Recent in vitro studies suggest

Table 4
Emerging novel and "repurposed" antibiotics for *M abscessus* pulmonary disease

Antibiotic (Class)	Suggested Adult Dose[a] (Route)	Evidence	References
Rifabutin (rifamycin)	300 mg daily (PO)	• In vitro bactericidal activity against *M abscessus* • Synergistic activity with clarithromycin, tigecycline, imipenem, and tedizolid	Refs[66–70,72]
Bedaquiline (diarylquinoline)	400 mg daily for 2 weeks (PO); followed by 200 mg thrice weekly (PO)	• In vitro bacteriostatic activity against MAC and *M abscessus* • Synergy with clofazimine • May decrease the activity of cefoxitin and imipenem	Refs[73–77]
Omadacycline (tetracycline)	300 mg daily (PO); or 100 mg daily (IV)	• In vitro activity against *M abscessus* with similar MIC to tigecycline • Case reports and series demonstrating efficacy with minimal toxicity	Refs[80–85]
Eravacycline (tetracycline)	1 mg/kg twice per day (IV)	Superior in vitro activity against *M abscessus* with MICs lower than tigecycline and omadacycline	Ref[86]
Tedizolid (oxazolidinone)	200 mg daily (PO or IV)	• Superior in vitro activity against *M abscessus* compared with linezolid • Possible synergy against NTM when combined with imipenem and ethambutol	Refs[71,87–89]
Dual Beta-lactams (possible options)		• In vitro synergy between amoxicillin and imipenem + cilastatin + relebactam • In vitro synergy between imipenem + cilastatin and ceftaroline	Refs[71,91–95]
Amoxicillin	1 g, 3 times per day (PO)		
Cefoxitin	2–4 g, 2–3 times per day (IV)		
Ceftaroline	600 mg twice per day (IV)		
Ceftazidime + avibactam	2.5 g, 3 times per day (IV)		
Imipenem + cilastatin	0.5–1 g, 2–3 times per day (IV)		
Imipenem + cilastatin + relebactam	1.25 g, 4 times per day (IV)		
Inhaled antibiotics			Refs[4,96–98]
ALIS	590 mg/8.4 mL daily (INH)	Recommended for continuation phase of treatment[b] Reduction in pulmonary bacterial load in a GM-CSF knockout model	
Tigecycline	Unknown	Improved bacterial elimination from the lungs in NTM-infected mouse models (MAC and *M abscessus*)	
Clofazimine	Unknown		
Imipenem + cilastatin	250 mg twice per day (INH)	Well-tolerated in two pediatric CF patients with *M abscessus* with stabilization of lung function over 9 mo	

Abbreviations: ALIS, amikacin liposome inhalation suspension; GM-CSF, granulocyte-macrophage colony-stimulating factor; INH, inhaled; IV, intravenous; MAC, *Mycobacterium avium* complex; MIC, minimum inhibitory concentration; NTM, nontuberculous mycobacteria; PO, oral.

[a] Suggested doses extrapolated from case reports, case series, and literature concerning for infections.

[b] 2020 ATS/ERS/ESCMID/IDSA Guidelines recommend inhaled amikacin in the continuation phase of treatment with no specification for ALIS versus the standard nebulized intravenous formulation.

Table 5
Interventional studies for *M abscessus* pulmonary disease

ClinicalTrials.gov Identifier	Description	Region	Updated Date	Accessed Date
NCT04310930	Platform, phase 2 and 3, interventional RCT to assess the optimal drug regimen for MAB-PD ("FORMaT")	Multinational	15th September 2022	23rd November 2022
NCT04922554	Phase 2 RCT of omadacycline vs placebo in MAB-PD	USA	21st November 2022	23rd November 2022
NCT04163601	Retrospective, observational study of ALIS in MAB-PD	France	12th February 2020	23rd November 2022
NCT04685720	Pilot study to assess the safety of high-dose intermittent inhaled NO for MAC-PD or MAB-PD	Australia	28th December 2020	23rd November 2022
NCT04294043	Phase 1b interventional study of IV gallium for MAC or Mabs pulmonary infection in patients with cystic fibrosis ("ABATE")	USA	2nd November 2022	23rd November 2022

Abbreviations: ALIS, amikacin liposome inhalation suspension; Mabs, *M abscessus*; MAC, *M avium* complex; NO, nitric oxide; PD, pulmonary disease; RCT, randomized controlled trial.

synergistic activity between a number of beta-lactam agents and reduced MICs with the addition of the new-age beta-lactamase inhibitors, avibactam, and relebactam.[71,91] Although there are currently no published in vivo data using this approach, possible therapeutic combinations that warrant further exploration based on in vitro data include ceftazidime with ceftaroline, ceftazidime with imipenem, ceftazidime + avibactam with imipenem, imipenem + relebactam with amoxicillin, and ceftaroline with impenem.[92–95]

INHALED ANTIBIOTICS

Inhaled antibiotics may play an increasing role in MAB-PD due to their potential to achieve higher drug concentrations in target tissue with reduced systemic toxicity. Inhaled amikacin, discussed above, is currently recommended for the continuation phase of MAB-PD treatment. Interest in other "re-purposed" inhaled antibiotics against NTM is growing. Inhaled imipenem was well-tolerated in two pediatric cystic fibrosis (CF) patients with MAB-PD, with stabilization of lung function over 9 months.[96] Inhaled tigecycline demonstrated a reduction in pulmonary bacterial load in granulocyte-macrophage colony-stimulating factor (GM-CSF) knockout mice with *M abscessus* infection.[97] Inhaled clofazimine was shown to be well-tolerated in mouse models of NTM-PD and associated with significantly lesser bacterial

recovery from lung tissue than the oral formulation.[98] A phase 2/3 clinical trial of clofazimine inhalation suspension is in development.[99] Further in vitro and in vivo studies are warranted to better investigate the delivery, safety, and efficacy of these antibiotics as inhaled therapies for MAB-PD.

NONANTIBIOTIC AGENTS

Multiple nonantibiotic antimicrobial agents have demonstrated promising therapeutic potential for MAB-PD and are discussed elsewhere in this issue. Case reports, small case series, and ongoing trials using inhaled nitric oxide, inhaled GM-CSF, and engineered bacteriophage therapy have all demonstrated therapeutic potential.[100–102] Gallium potently inhibits growth of *M abscessus* in vitro, and a clinical trial of intravenous gallium is underway (ClinicalTrials.gov ID: NCT04294043).[103]

SURGERY

Surgical resection for NTM-PD is detailed elsewhere in this issue. Few studies have specifically reported outcomes in MAB-PD (**Table 6**). One retrospective, observational study reported a significantly greater rate of culture enduring conversion in patients treated with adjunctive surgery, rather than medical therapy alone (57% vs 28%, $P = .022$).[104] Owing to the poor outcomes and significant toxicity of medical therapy for MAB-PD, we suggest consideration

Table 6
Surgical outcomes in *M abscessus* pulmonary disease

Indications for Surgery	Culture Conversion Rate	Study Design	Reference
Failure of sputum conversion or relapse, other complications (eg, haemoptysis)	7/8 (88%)	Retrospective observational study	Jeon et al,[52] 2009
Focal bronchiectasis, cavitation, haemoptysis	15/23 (65%)	Retrospective observational study	Jarand et al,[104] 2011
Failure of medical therapy, focal bronchiectasis, cavitation, haemoptysis	16/23 (70%)	Retrospective observational study	Kang et al,[105] 2015

of surgery for select individuals with relatively localized bronchiectasis or cavitary disease, failure of medical therapy, and adequate fitness for surgery. Important prerequisites for surgery include multidisciplinary discussion with experts in the management of NTM-PD, preoperative and postoperative antibiotic treatment, and local expertise in surgical and medical management of NTM-PD.[4,29]

The controversies regarding lung transplantation in patients with cystic fibrosis and *M abscessus* infection are discussed elsewhere in this issue. In short, transplantation is not necessarily contraindicated, if sequential negative cultures are achieved with medical therapy.[29,30]

SUMMARY

MAB-PD presents a significant therapeutic challenge due to the poor treatment outcomes and toxicity of current guidelines-based therapy. Macrolide susceptibility is a key prognostic factor and should be protected by adequate companion drugs during intensive and continuation phases. Optimal drug combinations, duration of therapy, and management of refractory disease are unknown. Fortunately, there are multiple emerging therapeutic candidates to address the unmet need for efficacious and tolerable treatment options.

CLINICS CARE POINTS

- Isolation of *M abscessus* from respiratory samples does not necessarily define disease.
- Determination of macrolide susceptibility is critical to prognostication and treatment planning.
- Expert opinion remains paramount in guiding treatment decisions.
- Therapeutic regimens must include adequate numbers of active agents.

- The decision to de-escalate from intensive phase therapy should be informed by clinical, radiological, and/or microbiological progress.
- Owing to intensive investigation of novel and "repurposed" agents, treatment approaches are likely to evolve in the coming years.

DISCLOSURE

Dr M.R. Holt has received a speaker's stipend from Sandoz, outside of the scope of this article. Dr T. Baird has received a grant from MSD for work outside the scope of this article.

REFERENCES

1. Prevots DR, Marras TK. Epidemiology of human pulmonary infection with nontuberculous mycobacteria: a review. Clin Chest Med 2015;36(1): 13–34.
2. Ruis C, Bryant JM, Bell SC, et al. Dissemination of *Mycobacterium abscessus* via global transmission networks. Nat Microbiol 2021;6(10):1279–88.
3. Tortoli E, Kohl TA, Brown-Elliott BA, et al. *Mycobacterium abscessus*, a taxonomic puzzle. Int J Syst Evol Microbiol 2018;68(1):467–9.
4. Daley CL, Iaccarino JM, Lange C, et al. Treatment of nontuberculous mycobacterial pulmonary disease: an official ATS/ERS/ESCMID/IDSA clinical practice guideline. Eur Respir J 2020;56(1).
5. Koh WJ, Stout JE, Yew WW. Advances in the management of pulmonary disease due to *Mycobacterium abscessus* complex. Int J Tubercul Lung Dis 2014;18(10):1141–8.
6. Nash KA, Brown-Elliott BA, Wallace RJ Jr. A novel gene, *erm*(41), confers inducible macrolide resistance to clinical isolates of *Mycobacterium abscessus* but is absent from *Mycobacterium chelonae*. Antimicrob Agents Chemother 2009; 53(4):1367–76.
7. Pasipanodya JG, Ogbonna D, Ferro BE, et al. Systematic review and meta-analyses of the effect of

chemotherapy on pulmonary *Mycobacterium abscessus* outcomes and disease recurrence. Antimicrob Agents Chemother 2017;61(11). https://doi.org/10.1128/AAC.01206-17.

8. Brown-Elliott BA, Vasireddy S, Vasireddy R, et al. Utility of sequencing the *erm*(41) gene in isolates of *Mycobacterium abscessus* subsp. *abscessus* with low and intermediate clarithromycin MICs. J Clin Microbiol 2015;53(4):1211–5.

9. Choi H, Jhun BW, Kim SY, et al. Treatment outcomes of macrolide-susceptible *Mycobacterium abscessus* lung disease. Diagn Microbiol Infect Dis 2018;90(4):293–5.

10. Mougari F, Amarsy R, Veziris N, et al. Standardized interpretation of antibiotic susceptibility testing and resistance genotyping for *Mycobacterium abscessus* with regard to subspecies and erm41 sequevar. J Antimicrob Chemother 2016; 71(8):2208–12.

11. Choi H, Kim SY, Kim DH, et al. Clinical characteristics and treatment outcomes of patients with acquired macrolide-resistant *Mycobacterium abscessus* lung disease. Antimicrob Agents Chemother 2017; 61(10). https://doi.org/10.1128/AAC.01146-17.

12. van Ingen J, Boeree MJ, van Soolingen D, et al. Are phylogenetic position, virulence, drug susceptibility and in vivo response to treatment in mycobacteria interrelated? Infect Genet Evol 2012;12(4): 832–7.

13. Griffith DE, Aksamit T, Brown-Elliott BA, et al. An official ATS/IDSA statement: diagnosis, treatment, and prevention of nontuberculous mycobacterial diseases. Am J Respir Crit Care Med 2007; 175(4):367–416.

14. Hwang JA, Kim S, Jo KW, et al. Natural history of *Mycobacterium avium* complex lung disease in untreated patients with stable course. Eur Respir J 2017;49(3). https://doi.org/10.1183/13993003.00537-2016.

15. Marras TK, Vinnard C, Zhang Q, et al. Relative risk of all-cause mortality in patients with nontuberculous mycobacterial lung disease in a US managed care population. Respir Med 2018;145:80–8.

16. Jo KW, Park YE, Chong YP, et al. Spontaneous sputum conversion and reversion in *Mycobacterium abscessus* complex lung disease. PLoS One 2020;15(4):e0232161.

17. Ali J. A multidisciplinary approach to the management of nontuberculous mycobacterial lung disease: a clinical perspective. Expet Rev Respir Med 2021;15(5):663–73.

18. Griffith DE, Daley CL. Treatment of *Mycobacterium abscessus* pulmonary disease. Chest 2022;161(1): 64–75.

19. Nessar R, Cambau E, Reyrat JM, et al. *Mycobacterium abscessus*: a new antibiotic nightmare. J Antimicrob Chemother 2012;67(4):810–8.

20. Fennelly KP, Ojano-Dirain C, Yang Q, et al. Biofilm formation by *Mycobacterium abscessus* in a lung cavity. Am J Respir Crit Care Med 2016;193(6):692–3.

21. Wallace RJ Jr, Meier A, Brown BA, et al. Genetic basis for clarithromycin resistance among isolates of *Mycobacterium chelonae* and *Mycobacterium abscessus*. Antimicrob Agents Chemother 1996; 40(7):1676–81.

22. Prammananan T, Sander P, Brown BA, et al. A single 16S ribosomal RNA substitution is responsible for resistance to amikacin and other 2-deoxystreptamine aminoglycosides in *Mycobacterium abscessus* and *Mycobacterium chelonae*. J Infect Dis 1998;177(6):1573–81.

23. Brown-Elliott BA, Woods GL. Antimycobacterial susceptibility testing of nontuberculous mycobacteria. J Clin Microbiol 2019;57(10). https://doi.org/10.1128/JCM.00834-19.

24. Yoshida S, Tsuyuguchi K, Kobayashi T, et al. Discrepancies between the genotypes and phenotypes of clarithromycin-resistant *Mycobacterium abscessus* complex. Int J Tubercul Lung Dis 2018;22(4):413–8.

25. Cho EH, Huh HJ, Song DJ, et al. Drug susceptibility patterns of *Mycobacterium abscessus* and *Mycobacterium massiliense* isolated from respiratory specimens. Diagn Microbiol Infect Dis 2019;93(2): 107–11.

26. Chew KL, Octavia S, Go J, et al. In vitro susceptibility of *Mycobacterium abscessus* complex and feasibility of standardizing treatment regimens. J Antimicrob Chemother 2021;76(4):973–8.

27. Kamada K, Yoshida A, Iguchi S, et al. Nationwide surveillance of antimicrobial susceptibility of 509 rapidly growing mycobacteria strains isolated from clinical specimens in Japan. Sci Rep 2021; 11(1):12208.

28. Liu CF, Song YM, He WC, et al. Nontuberculous mycobacteria in China: incidence and antimicrobial resistance spectrum from a nationwide survey. Infect Dis Poverty 2021;10(1):59.

29. Haworth CS, Banks J, Capstick T, et al. British Thoracic Society Guideline for the management of non-tuberculous mycobacterial pulmonary disease (NTM-PD). BMJ Open Respir Res 2017;4(1): e000242.

30. Floto RA, Olivier KN, Saiman L, et al. US Cystic Fibrosis Foundation and European Cystic Fibrosis Society consensus recommendations for the management of non-tuberculous mycobacteria in individuals with cystic fibrosis. Thorax 2016;71(Suppl 1):i1–22.

31. Diel R, Ringshausen F, Richter E, et al. Microbiological and clinical outcomes of treating non-*Mycobacterium avium* complex nontuberculous mycobacterial pulmonary disease: a systematic review and meta-analysis. Chest 2017;152(1):120–42.

32. Kwak N, Dalcolmo MP, Daley CL, et al. *Mycobacterium abscessus* pulmonary disease: individual patient data meta-analysis. Eur Respir J 2019;54(1).

33. Lyu J, Kim BJ, Kim BJ, et al. A shorter treatment duration may be sufficient for patients with *Mycobacterium massiliense* lung disease than with *Mycobacterium abscessus* lung disease. Respir Med 2014;108(11):1706–12.

34. Park YE, Park SY, Jhun BW, et al. Treatment outcome of continuation of intravenous amikacin for *Mycobacterium abscessus* pulmonary disease with a persistent culture positivity after the treatment initiation. J Infect Chemother 2022;28(8):1098–104.

35. Egelund EF, Fennelly KP, Peloquin CA. Medications and monitoring in nontuberculous mycobacteria infections. Clin Chest Med 2015;36(1):55–66.

36. Raaijmakers J, Schildkraut JA, Hoefsloot W, et al. The role of amikacin in the treatment of nontuberculous mycobacterial disease. Expert Opin Pharmacother 2021;22(15):1961–74.

37. Sturkenboom MGG, Simbar N, Akkerman OW, et al. Amikacin dosing for MDR tuberculosis: a systematic review to establish or revise the current recommended dose for tuberculosis treatment. Clin Infect Dis 2018;67(suppl_3):S303–7.

38. Ferro BE, Srivastava S, Deshpande D, et al. Amikacin pharmacokinetics/pharmacodynamics in a novel hollow-fiber *Mycobacterium abscessus* disease model. Antimicrob Agents Chemother 2015;60(3):1242–8.

39. Peloquin CA, Berning SE, Nitta AT, et al. Aminoglycoside toxicity: daily versus thrice-weekly dosing for treatment of mycobacterial diseases. Clin Infect Dis 2004;38(11):1538–44.

40. van Ingen J, Totten SE, Helstrom NK, et al. In vitro synergy between clofazimine and amikacin in treatment of nontuberculous mycobacterial disease. Antimicrob Agents Chemother 2012;56(12):6324–7.

41. Olivier KN, Shaw PA, Glaser TS, et al. Inhaled amikacin for treatment of refractory pulmonary nontuberculous mycobacterial disease. Ann Am Thorac Soc 2014;11(1):30–5.

42. Olivier KN, Griffith DE, Eagle G, et al. Randomized trial of liposomal amikacin for inhalation in nontuberculous mycobacterial lung disease. Am J Respir Crit Care Med 2017;195(6):814–23.

43. Griffith DE, Eagle G, Thomson R, et al. Amikacin liposome inhalation suspension for treatment-refractory lung disease caused by *Mycobacterium avium* complex (CONVERT). A prospective, open-label, randomized study. Am J Respir Crit Care Med 2018;198(12):1559–69.

44. Henriette Zweijpfenning SM, Chiron R, Essink S, et al. Safety and outcomes of amikacin liposome inhalation suspension for *Mycobacterium abscessus* pulmonary disease: a NTM-NET study. Chest 2022;162(1):76–81.

45. Kang N, Jeon K, Kim H, et al. Outcomes of inhaled amikacin-containing multidrug regimens for *Mycobacterium abscessus* pulmonary disease. Chest 2021;160(2):436–45.

46. Chiron R, Hoefsloot W, Van Ingen J, et al. Amikacin liposomal inhalation suspension in the treatment of *Mycobacterium abscessus* lung infection: a French observational experience. Open Forum Infect Dis 2022;9(10):ofac465.

47. Ferro BE, Srivastava S, Deshpande D, et al. Tigecycline is highly efficacious against *Mycobacterium abscessus* pulmonary disease. Antimicrob Agents Chemother 2016;60(5):2895–900.

48. Wallace RJ Jr, Dukart G, Brown-Elliott BA, et al. Clinical experience in 52 patients with tigecycline-containing regimens for salvage treatment of *Mycobacterium abscessus* and *Mycobacterium chelonae* infections. J Antimicrob Chemother 2014;69(7):1945–53.

49. Yang JH, Wang PH, Pan SW, et al. Treatment outcome in patients with *Mycobacterium abscessus* complex lung disease: the impact of tigecycline and amikacin. Antibiotics (Basel) 2022; 11(5). https://doi.org/10.3390/antibiotics11050571.

50. Kwon YS, Levin A, Kasperbauer SH, et al. Efficacy and safety of tigecycline for *Mycobacterium abscessus* disease. Respir Med 2019;158:89–91.

51. Kim SR, Jang M, Kim SY, et al. Outcomes of short-term tigecycline-containing regimens for *Mycobacterium abscessus* pulmonary disease. Antimicrob Agents Chemother 2022;66(10):e0077422.

52. Jeon K, Kwon OJ, Lee NY, et al. Antibiotic treatment of *Mycobacterium abscessus* lung disease: a retrospective analysis of 65 patients. Am J Respir Crit Care Med 2009;180(9):896–902.

53. Rominski A, Schulthess B, Muller DM, et al. Effect of beta-lactamase production and beta-lactam instability on MIC testing results for *Mycobacterium abscessus*. J Antimicrob Chemother 2017;72(11):3070–8.

54. Martiniano SL, Wagner BD, Levin A, et al. Safety and effectiveness of clofazimine for primary and refractory nontuberculous mycobacterial infection. Chest 2017;152(4):800–9.

55. Yang B, Jhun BW, Moon SM, et al. Clofazimine-containing regimen for the treatment of *Mycobacterium abscessus* lung disease. Antimicrob Agents Chemother 2017;61(6). https://doi.org/10.1128/AAC.02052-16.

56. Kwak N, Whang J, Yang JS, et al. Minimal inhibitory concentration of clofazimine among clinical isolates of nontuberculous mycobacteria and its impact on treatment outcome. Chest 2021;159(2):517–23.

57. Ferro BE, Meletiadis J, Wattenberg M, et al. Clofazimine prevents the regrowth of *Mycobacterium abscessus* and *Mycobacterium avium* type strains exposed to amikacin and clarithromycin. Antimicrob Agents Chemother 2016;60(2):1097–105.

58. Watanabe F, Furuuchi K, Hanada K, et al. Pharmacokinetics and adverse effects of clofazimine in the treatment of pulmonary non-tuberculous mycobacterial infection. Antimicrob Agents Chemother 2022;66(8):e0044122.

59. Szeto W, Garcia-Buitrago MT, Abbo L, et al. Clofazimine enteropathy: a rare and underrecognized complication of mycobacterial therapy. Open Forum Infect Dis 2016;3(3). https://doi.org/10.1093/ofid/ofw004.

60. Wallace RJ Jr, Brown-Elliott BA, Ward SC, et al. Activities of linezolid against rapidly growing mycobacteria. Antimicrob Agents Chemother 2001;45(3):764–7.

61. Li H, Tong L, Wang J, et al. An intensified regimen containing linezolid could improve treatment response in Mycobacterium abscessus lung disease. BioMed Res Int 2019;2019:8631563.

62. Winthrop KL, Ku JH, Marras TK, et al. The tolerability of linezolid in the treatment of nontuberculous mycobacterial disease. Eur Respir J 2015;45(4):1177–9.

63. Komatsu T, Nakamura M, Uchiyama K, et al. Initial trough concentration may be beneficial in preventing linezolid-induced thrombocytopenia. J Chemother 2022;34(6):375–80.

64. Kumar K, Daley CL, Griffith DE, et al. Management of Mycobacterium avium complex and Mycobacterium abscessus pulmonary disease: therapeutic advances and emerging treatments. Eur Respir Rev 2022;(163):31. https://doi.org/10.1183/16000617.0212-2021.

65. Laudone TW, Garner L, Kam CW, et al. Novel therapies for treatment of resistant and refractory nontuberculous mycobacterial infections in patients with cystic fibrosis. Pediatr Pulmonol 2021;56(Suppl 1):S55–68.

66. Aziz DB, Low JL, Wu ML, et al. Rifabutin Is active against Mycobacterium abscessus complex. Antimicrob Agents Chemother 2017;61(6). https://doi.org/10.1128/AAC.00155-17.

67. Ganapathy US, Dartois V, Dick T. Repositioning rifamycins for Mycobacterium abscessus lung disease. Expert Opin Drug Discov 2019;14(9):867–78.

68. Pryjma M, Burian J, Thompson CJ. Rifabutin acts in synergy and is bactericidal with frontline Mycobacterium abscessus antibiotics clarithromycin and tigecycline, suggesting a potent treatment combination. Antimicrob Agents Chemother 2018;62(8). https://doi.org/10.1128/AAC.00283-18.

69. Cheng A, Tsai YT, Chang SY, et al. In vitro synergism of rifabutin with clarithromycin, imipenem, and tigecycline against the Mycobacterium abscessus complex. Antimicrob Agents Chemother 2019;63(4). https://doi.org/10.1128/AAC.02234-18.

70. Chen J, Zhang H, Guo Q, et al. In vitro activity of rifabutin against Mycobacterium abscessus, clinical isolates. Clin Exp Pharmacol Physiol 2022;49(7):767–75.

71. Le Run E, Arthur M, Mainardi JL. In vitro and intracellular activity of imipenem combined with tedizolid, rifabutin, and avibactam against Mycobacterium abscessus. Antimicrob Agents Chemother 2019;63(4). https://doi.org/10.1128/AAC.01915-18.

72. Aziz DB, Go ML, Dick T. Rifabutin suppresses inducible clarithromycin resistance in Mycobacterium abscessus by blocking induction of whiB7 and erm41. Antibiotics (Basel) 2020;9(2). https://doi.org/10.3390/antibiotics9020072.

73. Andries K, Verhasselt P, Guillemont J, et al. A diarylquinoline drug active on the ATP synthase of. Mycobacterium tuberculosis. Science. 2005;307(5707):223–7.

74. Borisov SE, Dheda K, Enwerem M, et al. Effectiveness and safety of bedaquiline-containing regimens in the treatment of MDR- and XDR-TB: a multicentre study. Eur Respir J 2017;49(5). https://doi.org/10.1183/13993003.00387-2017.

75. Vesenbeckh S, Schonfeld N, Roth A, et al. Bedaquiline as a potential agent in the treatment of Mycobacterium abscessus infections. Eur Respir J 2017;49(5). https://doi.org/10.1183/13993003.00083-2017.

76. Ruth MM, JJN Sangen, Remmers K, et al. A bedaquiline/clofazimine combination regimen might add activity to the treatment of clinically relevant non-tuberculous mycobacteria. J Antimicrob Chemother 2019;74(4):935–43. https://doi.org/10.1093/jac/dky526.

77. Brown-Elliott BA, Wallace RJ Jr. In vitro susceptibility testing of bedaquiline against Mycobacterium abscessus complex. Antimicrob Agents Chemother 2019;63(2). https://doi.org/10.1128/AAC.01919-18.

78. Philley JV, Wallace RJ Jr, Benwill JL, et al. Preliminary results of bedaquiline as salvage therapy for patients with nontuberculous mycobacterial lung disease. Chest 2015;148(2):499–506. https://doi.org/10.1378/chest.14-2764.

79. Lindman M, Dick T. Bedaquiline eliminates bactericidal activity of beta-lactams against Mycobacterium abscessus. Antimicrob Agents Chemother 2019;63(8). https://doi.org/10.1128/AAC.00827-19.

80. Bax HI, de Vogel CP, Mouton JW, et al. Omadacycline as a promising new agent for the treatment of infections with Mycobacterium abscessus. J Antimicrob Chemother 2019;74(10):2930–3. https://doi.org/10.1093/jac/dkz267.

81. Brown-Elliott BA, Wallace RJ Jr. In vitro susceptibility testing of omadacycline against nontuberculous mycobacteria. Antimicrob Agents Chemother 2021;(3):65. https://doi.org/10.1128/AAC.01947-20.

82. Shoen C, Benaroch D, Sklaney M, et al. In vitro activities of omadacycline against rapidly growing mycobacteria. Antimicrob Agents Chemother 2019;63(5). https://doi.org/10.1128/AAC.02522-18.

83. Minhas R, Sharma S, Kundu S. Utilizing the promise of omadacycline in a resistant, non-tubercular mycobacterial pulmonary infection. Cureus 2019; 11(7):e5112. https://doi.org/10.7759/cureus.5112.

84. Pearson JC, Dionne B, Richterman A, et al. Omadacycline for the treatment of Mycobacterium abscessus disease: a case series. Open Forum Infect Dis 2020;7(10):ofaa415. https://doi.org/10.1093/ofid/ofaa415.

85. Morrisette T, Alosaimy S, Philley JV, et al. Preliminary, real-world, multicenter experience with omadacycline for Mycobacterium abscessus infections. Open Forum Infect Dis 2021;8(2): ofab002. https://doi.org/10.1093/ofid/ofab002.

86. Kaushik A, Ammerman NC, Martins O, et al. In vitro activity of new tetracycline analogs omadacycline and eravacycline against drug-resistant clinical isolates of Mycobacterium abscessus. Antimicrob Agents Chemother 2019;63(6). https://doi.org/10.1128/AAC.00470-19.

87. Wen S, Gao X, Zhao W, et al. Comparison of the in vitro activity of linezolid, tedizolid, sutezolid, and delpazolid against rapidly growing mycobacteria isolated in Beijing, China. Int J Infect Dis 2021;109: 253–60. https://doi.org/10.1016/j.ijid.2021.06.055.

88. Compain F, Soroka D, Heym B, et al. In vitro activity of tedizolid against the Mycobacterium abscessus complex. Diagn Microbiol Infect Dis 2018;90(3):186–9. https://doi.org/10.1016/j.diagmicrobio.2017.11.001.

89. Ruth MM, Koeken V, Pennings LJ, et al. Is there a role for tedizolid in the treatment of nontuberculous mycobacterial disease? J Antimicrob Chemother 2020;75(3):609–17. https://doi.org/10.1093/jac/dkz511.

90. Poon YK, La Hoz RM, Hynan LS, et al. Tedizolid vs linezolid for the treatment of nontuberculous mycobacteria infections in solid organ transplant recipients. Open Forum Infect Dis 2021;8(4):ofab093. https://doi.org/10.1093/ofid/ofab093.

91. Dubee V, Bernut A, Cortes M, et al. beta-Lactamase inhibition by avibactam in Mycobacterium abscessus. J Antimicrob Chemother 2015;70(4): 1051–8. https://doi.org/10.1093/jac/dku510.

92. Pandey R, Chen L, Manca C, et al. Dual beta-lactam combinations highly active against Mycobacterium abscessus complex in vitro. mBio 2019;10(1). https://doi.org/10.1128/mBio.02895-18.

93. Lopeman RC, Harrison J, Rathbone DL, et al. Effect of amoxicillin in combination with imipenem-relebactam against Mycobacterium abscessus. Sci Rep 2020;10(1):928. https://doi.org/10.1038/s41598-020-57844-8.

94. Story-Roller E, Galanis C, Lamichhane G. Beta-lactam combinations that exhibit synergy against Mycobacteroides abscessus clinical isolates. Antimicrob Agents Chemother 2021;(4):65. https://doi.org/10.1128/AAC.02545-20.

95. Dousa KM, Kurz SG, Taracila MA, et al. Insights into the l,d-transpeptidases and d,d-carboxypeptidase of Mycobacterium abscessus: ceftaroline, imipenem, and novel diazabicyclooctane inhibitors. Antimicrob Agents Chemother 2020;(8):64. https://doi.org/10.1128/AAC.00098-20.

96. Jones LA, Doucette L, Dellon EP, et al. Use of inhaled imipenem/cilastatin in pediatric patients with cystic fibrosis: a case series. J Cyst Fibros 2019;18(4): e42–4. https://doi.org/10.1016/j.jcf.2019.04.017.

97. Pearce C, Ruth MM, Pennings LJ, et al. Inhaled tigecycline is effective against Mycobacterium abscessus in vitro and in vivo. J Antimicrob Chemother 2020;75(7):1889–94. https://doi.org/10.1093/jac/dkaa110.

98. Banaschewski B, Verma D, Pennings LJ, et al. Clofazimine inhalation suspension for the aerosol treatment of pulmonary nontuberculous mycobacterial infections. J Cyst Fibros 2019;18(5):714–20. https://doi.org/10.1016/j.jcf.2019.05.013.

99. MannKind. MannKind's inhaled clofazimine will advance to an adaptive phase 2/3 study for potential treatment of rare lung disease. 2023. Available at: https://investors.mannkindcorp.com/news-releases/news-release-details/mannkinds-inhaled-clofazimine-will-advance-adaptive-phase-23. Accessed May 26, 2023.

100. Bentur L, Gur M, Ashkenazi M, et al. Pilot study to test inhaled nitric oxide in cystic fibrosis patients with refractory Mycobacterium abscessus lung infection. J Cyst Fibros 2020;19(2):225–31. https://doi.org/10.1016/j.jcf.2019.05.002.

101. Scott JP, Ji Y, Kannan M, et al. Inhaled granulocyte-macrophage colony-stimulating factor for Mycobacterium abscessus in cystic fibrosis. Eur Respir J 2018;51(4). https://doi.org/10.1183/13993003.02127-2017.

102. Dedrick RM, Guerrero-Bustamante CA, Garlena RA, et al. Engineered bacteriophages for treatment of a patient with a disseminated drug-resistant Mycobacterium abscessus. Nat Med 2019;25(5):730–3. https://doi.org/10.1038/s41591-019-0437-z.

103. Abdalla MY, Switzer BL, Goss CH, et al. Gallium compounds exhibit potential as new therapeutic agents against Mycobacterium abscessus. Antimicrob Agents Chemother 2015;59(8):4826–34. https://doi.org/10.1128/AAC.00331-15.

104. Jarand J, Levin A, Zhang L, et al. Clinical and microbiologic outcomes in patients receiving treatment for Mycobacterium abscessus pulmonary disease. Clin Infect Dis 2011;52(5):565–71. https://doi.org/10.1093/cid/ciq237.

105. Kang HK, Park HY, Kim D, et al. Treatment outcomes of adjuvant resectional surgery for nontuberculous mycobacterial lung disease. BMC Infect Dis 2015;15:76. https://doi.org/10.1186/s12879-015-0823-1.

Treatment of the Less Common Nontuberculous Mycobacterial Pulmonary Disease

Marie Yan, MD[a,b], Sarah K. Brode, MD, MPH[a,c,d],
Theodore K. Marras, MD, MSc[a,c],*

KEYWORDS

- Nontuberculous mycobacteria • *Mycobacterium kansasii* • *Mycobacterium xenopi*
- *Mycobacterium malmoense* • *Mycobacterium simiae* • *Mycobacterium szulgai*
- *Mycobacterium gordonae*

KEY POINTS

- Species-specific considerations have important implications in the diagnosis and management of nontuberculous mycobacterial pulmonary disease.
- Not every patient requires antimicrobial therapy and many patients do well with nonpharmacologic management.
- The decision to institute antimicrobial therapy should incorporate clinical, radiologic, and microbiologic considerations.
- Drug susceptibility testing is used to guide regimen selection, but the correlation between in vitro activity and clinical response is unclear for most drugs.

INTRODUCTION

In the United States, *Mycobacterium avium* complex (MAC) and *Mycobacterium abscessus* are the two predominant causes of nontuberculous mycobacterial pulmonary disease (NTM-PD).[1] Numerous other species of NTM are also capable of causing lung disease, and this review focuses on disease caused by *Mycobacterium kansasii*, *Mycobacterium xenopi*, *Mycobacterium malmoense*, *Mycobacterium simiae*, *Mycobacterium szulgai*, and *Mycobacterium gordonae*. These species are regarded as less common in the United States; however, some are frequently encountered in other regions. The ensuing sections discuss the evaluation and

management of lung disease associated with these organisms, with particular emphasis on species-specific considerations. Rapidly growing species, such as *Mycobacterium chelonae* and *Mycobacterium fortuitum*, and the slowly growing species *Mycobacterium genavense* are not covered in this article, but treatment recommendations are found in a recent international consensus paper.[2]

EVALUATION OF PATIENTS WITH SUSPECTED NONTUBERCULOUS MYCOBACTERIAL PULMONARY DISEASE

Diagnosis of NTM-PD should follow the criteria outlined in the international guidelines (endorsed

[a] Department of Medicine, University of Toronto, Toronto, Ontario, Canada; [b] Clinician Investigator Program, University of British Columbia, Suite 200 City Square East Tower South, 555 West 12th Avenue, Vancouver, British Columbia V5Z 3X7, Canada; [c] Division of Respirology, University Health Network, Toronto, Ontario, Canada; [d] Division of Respiratory Medicine, West Park Healthcare Centre, 82 Buttonwood Avenue, Toronto, Ontario M6M 2J5, Canada
* Corresponding author. Toronto Western Hospital, 7E-452, 399 Bathurst Street, Toronto, Ontario M5T 2S8, Canada.
E-mail address: ted.marras@uhn.ca

Clin Chest Med 44 (2023) 799–813
https://doi.org/10.1016/j.ccm.2023.06.011
0272-5231/23/© 2023 Elsevier Inc. All rights reserved.

Table 1
Diagnostic criteria for nontuberculous mycobacterial pulmonary disease

Clinical	Pulmonary or Systemic Symptoms
Radiologic	Chest radiograph: Nodular or cavitary opacities High-resolution computed tomography: Bronchiectasis with multiple small nodules
Microbiologic[a]	Positive culture results for NTM from at least 2 separate expectorated sputum samples (if the results are nondiagnostic, consider repeat sputum acid-fast bacilli and cultures) or positive culture results for NTM from at least 1 bronchial wash or lavage or transbronchial or other lung biopsy with mycobacterial histologic features (granulomatous inflammation or acid-fast bacilli) and positive culture for NTM or biopsy showing mycobacterial histologic features (granulomatous inflammation or acid-fast bacilli) and 1 or more expectorated sputum or bronchial washings that are culture positive for NTM
Appropriate exclusion of other diagnoses	

[a] When two positive cultures are obtained, the isolates should be the same NTM species (or subspecies in the case of *M abscessus*) to meet disease criteria.
Adapted from American Thoracic Society/European Respiratory Society/European Society of Clinical Microbiology and Infectious Diseases/Infectious Diseases Society of America guidelines[3]

by the American Thoracic Society/European Respiratory Society/European Society of Clinical Microbiology and Infectious Diseases/Infectious Diseases Society of America), which consist of three domains: (1) clinical, (2) radiologic, and (3) microbiologic (**Table 1**),[3] discussed in Chapter 6 of this issue. To meet the definition of disease, all three domains must be fulfilled, in addition to the appropriate exclusion of alternative causes. As ubiquitous environmental organisms, it is not uncommon to isolate NTM species in clinical samples, even in the absence of any pathology. Therefore, it is important to follow the multidomain evaluation outlined in the diagnostic criteria to distinguish disease versus contamination/colonization. While the same criteria are often used for all NTM species, the diagnostic threshold should be calibrated by differences in clinical relevance and pathogenicity, though variable estimates have been reported (**Fig. 1**).

To satisfy the microbiologic definition, a minimum of two positive sputum cultures of the same species are required; however, many experts believe that an exception may be made for *M kansasii*, such that a single sputum isolate may be sufficient for diagnosis in the proper context. *M kansasii* is closely related to *Mycobacterium tuberculosis* and generally regarded as the most virulent NTM species. Previous studies consistently showed a higher ratio of disease to isolation for *M kansasii* compared with *M avium* (see **Fig. 1**).[4–7] Therefore, the diagnostic threshold is sometimes lowered for *M kansasii* because of its

higher pathogenicity. However, this perception has been questioned in several recent studies, which found that patients with a single isolate of *M kansasii* do not necessarily experience a high rate of subsequent disease.[8–10]

There is also evidence to support regional differences in pathogenicity. For instance, most cases of *M malmoense* disease seem to be confined to Northern Europe, where local studies estimate that between 73% and 83% of isolates reflect true disease.[7,11] In contrast, a study from the United States reported that only 10% of isolates were clinically relevant.[11] Another example is *M szulgai*. This species is rarely encountered in clinical practice; according to a large Japanese study, it was found in only 0.1% of all patients with respiratory NTM isolates (32/26,059) over a 2-year period.[6] The same study reported that only 19% of *M szulgai* isolates met the microbiologic definition of the diagnostic criteria. In comparison, studies from South Korea and the Netherlands reported that 43% and 73% of isolates were clinically relevant.[12,13]

M xenopi and *M simiae* seem to be on the lower end of the pathogenicity spectrum. Isolation of these organisms from respiratory samples often does not indicate disease. Both species have been frequently found as contaminants and implicated in various pseudo-outbreaks. Most studies estimate that only around 20% of *M simiae* isolates meet disease criteria (although one study from Iran reported 49%).[14–16] For *M xenopi*, between 5% and 48% of isolates have been found to be clinically significant.[6,7,17,18]

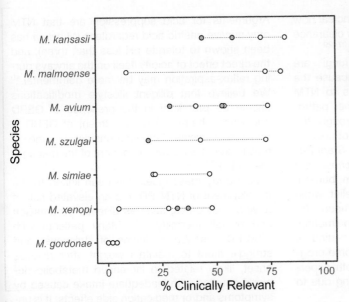

Fig. 1. Clinical relevance of less common nontuberculous mycobacteria (and *Mycobacterium avium* for reference) in respiratory isolates, as defined by the proportion of patients meeting either the full definition (*white circle*) or the microbiologic definition (*gray circle*) of the contemporaneous American Thoracic Society diagnostic criteria from a limited selection of representative studies. Each circle represents a publication describing the clinical relevance of the NTM species (Appendix 1 for sources). Note substantial variability between studies.

M gordonae is generally considered nonpathogenic. It is a common contaminant and the second most isolated NTM species worldwide.[1,19] True disease secondary to *M gordonae* is exceedingly rare. When it does occur, it is typically extrapulmonary and in the setting of impaired immunity.[20] To make a diagnosis of *M gordonae* lung disease, there must be compelling evidence of infection (eg, repeatedly positive cultures over an extended period) and every effort should be made to search for alternative diagnoses.[2] One study suggested that time to culture positivity in liquid medium may be a clue, because the median time for culture detection was 8 days in patients with definite disease compared with 24 days in cases attributed to contamination. The authors also proposed using a more stringent microbiologic definition for *M gordonae*: three or more positive cultures with one or more smear positive.[21]

Compared with MAC, patients with NTM-PD secondary to less common slowly growing NTM are more often male, typically with risk factors, such as chronic obstructive pulmonary disease (COPD) or prior tuberculosis. Presenting symptoms can be any combination of cough, sputum production, hemoptysis, weight loss, night sweats, and so forth. On imaging, patients affected by *M kansasii*, *M malmoense*, and *M szulgai* commonly have features resembling tuberculosis, such as cavitary lesions and upper lobe involvement.[4,12,13]

GENERAL TREATMENT PRINCIPLES

There are several principles of treatment that are applicable to all patients with NTM-PD, regardless of the causative species.

At the time of NTM-PD diagnosis, clinicians should evaluate for and address any predisposing conditions to minimize their clinical impact. These include structural lung diseases (eg, bronchiectasis and COPD) and immunocompromising conditions, including the use of immunosuppressive drugs. Bronchiectasis in the setting of NTM infection may be de novo or preexisting, and for many patients the timeline is unclear. In all cases, further evaluation is warranted to exclude other causes of bronchiectasis, as described in Chapter 4 of this issue. A substantial proportion of patients with MAC present with midzone-predominant bronchiectasis in the absence of overt immune impairment. This characteristic phenotype (older women with tall, lean body types, often associated with skeletal and mitral valve abnormalities) likely has a complex genetic basis and may also be seen with other NTM species (see Chapter 3 in this issue).[22–24]

Airway clearance therapy is an important component of long-term management for patients with bronchiectasis, whether de novo or preexisting (see Chapter 4 of this issue). Airway clearance routines typically include a combination of cough and breathing techniques, assistive devices (eg, oscillatory positive expiratory pressure devices), and postural drainage, with or without hypertonic saline nebulization. The exact routine should be customized to the patient's anatomy, lifestyle, and preferences.[25,26] Most of the data on airway clearance come from the general bronchiectasis population, with fewer studies that exclusively examined patients with NTM-PD. Observational studies suggest that between 30% and 52% of patients with mild disease may achieve culture conversion with airway clearance therapy alone, although it is unclear how much benefit can be attributed to airway clearance therapy given the lack of control groups.[27–29]

Coinfection with bacteria and fungi are commonly seen in NTM-PD, likely because the same factors that predispose patients to NTM also increase their susceptibility to other pathogens. This should be monitored through the routine collection of sputum cultures. Not uncommonly, bacterial pathogens, such as *Staphylococcus aureus* or *Pseudomonas aeruginosa*, are responsible for most of the symptom burden, and patients experience significant relief when these are treated, negating the need for antimycobacterial therapy. Chronic pulmonary aspergillosis can also develop in the setting of NTM-PD and this is associated with worse prognosis.[30–32] Concurrent treatment of both aspergillus and NTM is particularly challenging due to the issue of drug interactions.

NTM are widely identified in the environment, with frequent isolation from soils and natural and built water environments. Infection occurs when NTM is introduced into the respiratory tract of a susceptible host via inhalation or aspiration.[33] In patients with NTM-PD, repeated inoculation with environmental NTM is believed to contribute to recurrence and possibly refractory disease. Accordingly, reducing environmental exposure to NTM seems intuitive but there are minimal data concerning the effectiveness of such measures.[34,35] Nevertheless, it seems prudent to counsel patients regarding behavioral modifications that could mitigate exposure, to the extent that these are acceptable for their quality of life (see Chapter 1 of this issue).

Gastroesophageal reflux disease (GERD) is common among patients with NTM-PD and may not be clinically apparent. GERD is a risk factor for incident NTM-PD and studies have shown an association with increased health care utilization (all-cause and respiratory related) and possibly disease severity in patients with NTM-PD.[36–38] The explanation for this association is not clear, but it has been hypothesized that ingested NTM (often found in potable waters) may survive in the stomach and subsequently become deposited into the lungs via microaspiration. Accordingly, patients should be screened for signs/symptoms of GERD and counseled regarding lifestyle modifications to reduce reflux. Unless there are strong indications (eg, erosive esophagitis), the role of acid-suppressing medications in NTM-PD is controversial. The argument against acid suppression is that higher gastric pH could potentially lead to increased gastric survival of NTM, as suggested by an in vitro study with *M abscessus*.[39]

Arguments for acid suppression are that NTM may survive gastric acid regardless (*M avium* has been shown to tolerate pH less than three), and the direct effect of acidity itself on the airways during reflux-aspiration may be more detrimental.[40] We believe that diligent lifestyle modifications should be practiced in the presence of GERD and when pharmacologic treatment of GERD is required, clinicians should consider whether a motility agent is a safe component of the management plan.[39]

Low body mass index has been linked to the development of NTM-PD and an elevated risk of adverse outcomes, such as disease progression and overall mortality.[41–43] Many patients with NTM-PD describe a lifetime of "thinness" and struggle more to maintain weight after disease onset, likely related to increased metabolic demand coupled with inadequate intake caused by symptoms and/or medication side effects. It is unclear whether interventions designed to increase body mass index would lead to improved outcomes, but potential benefit may be inferred based on studies of nutritional supplementation in the COPD population.[44] Therefore, weight should be monitored routinely in the course of NTM-PD management, and nutritional support should be considered.

ANTIMYCOBACTERIAL THERAPY INITIATION AND DRUG SUSCEPTIBILITY TESTING

Many patients with NTM-PD do not require immediate antimycobacterial therapy and may experience stability for years without treatment. However, the clinical course of NTM-PD can be unpredictable and it is often difficult to know when mycobacterial treatment should be started. Although international guidelines generally favor early treatment, there are no widely accepted criteria or algorithms to guide the timing of antibiotic initiation. The decision to institute treatment should involve a careful consideration of the potential risks and benefits, individualized to the patient and the NTM species at hand. **Table 2** outlines some of the key factors that may inform this process (see Chapter 6 of this issue).

Drug susceptibility testing (DST) should be performed before treatment to assist with regimen selection (see Chapter 5 in this issue). For *M kansasii*, rifampin resistance (defined as minimum inhibitory concentration [MIC] ≥ 2 µg/mL) is known to correlate with clinical outcomes.[3] Clarithromycin is another key drug to test, with resistance defined as MIC greater than or equal to 32 µg/mL. The implication of DST results is less clear for other drugs and the other NTM species in this review.

Table 2
Factors to consider in evaluating the need for antimicrobial therapy

Patient	Patient preferences and values Severity and progression of symptoms Immunocompromising conditions Comorbidities/contraindications Age and frailty
Radiologic	Extent and severity of abnormalities Presence of cavities Progression over time
Microbiologic	Bacterial burden based on smear positivity and frequency of isolation Pathogenicity of species Potential for recurrence

For instance, there is currently no consensus on the appropriate definition for isoniazid resistance in *M kansasii*. Some studies have reported isoniazid resistance rates of up to 100% using an MIC breakpoint of 1 μg/mL; however, this seems to be clinically irrelevant considering that isoniazid has been successfully used for many years.[45] Therefore, further studies are needed to determine whether in vitro drug activity is predictive of in vivo response and establish clinically meaningful breakpoints for interpretation. In the meantime, DST is still recommended to help guide the construction of a multidrug regimen, but it must be emphasized that in vitro activity and specific MICs do not necessarily correlate with clinical outcomes.

Mycobacterium Kansasii

Rifamycins are the cornerstone of antimicrobial therapy for *M kansasii*. The introduction of rifampin in the 1960s led to substantial reductions in the rates of relapse and surgical intervention.[46,47] In patients with rifampin-susceptible strains, the recommended first-line regimen consists of rifampin, ethambutol, and either a macrolide or isoniazid (**Table 3**).[3] Macrolides have not been directly compared with isoniazid in a controlled setting, but previous studies have shown similar outcomes for both drugs in rifamycin-based regimens.[48–50] If thrice-weekly dosing is preferred, then only macrolides can be used as the companion drug, because there is insufficient evidence to recommend intermittent dosing for isoniazid.[3] For severe or cavitary disease, daily therapy is recommended over thrice-weekly treatment. One study did produce excellent

results with thrice-weekly treatment in cavitary disease; however, this was limited by a small sample size.[49] Rifampin-susceptible *M kansasii* generally responds well to oral regimens and parenteral therapy is usually not necessary.

Rifampin resistance rates are estimated to be low in most regions.[45] For patients with rifampin-resistant strains or intolerance to first-line treatment, a fluoroquinolone should be used along with at least two companion drugs. The combination of azithromycin, ethambutol, and a fluoroquinolone is a favored regimen, assuming there is macrolide susceptibility.[3] Other drugs that have been used include high-dose isoniazid, sulfamethoxazole/trimethoprim, streptomycin, and amikacin, and selection may be guided by DST.[51,52] Clofazimine, linezolid, and newer agents, such as bedaquiline and delamanid, have demonstrated good in vitro activity against *M kansasii*, but clinical experience is lacking.[53–55]

The recommended treatment duration is a minimum of 12 months after initiation.[3] In contrast with usual convention for NTM, the treatment duration for *M kansasii* does not need to account for time to culture conversion. This is based on data showing successful outcomes and low relapse rates after 12 months of treatment.[46,47] Treatment outcomes for *M kansasii* are quite favorable. A systematic review of treatment success for various NTM, measured by culture conversion adjusted for post-treatment relapses, observed that *M kansasii* had the highest success rate (80.2%; 95% confidence interval, 58.4%–95.2%).[56] Since sputum conversion is typically achieved within 4 months with rifamycin-based regimens, expert consultation should be obtained if cultures remain positive after 4 months.[3,46]

Mycobacterium Xenopi

The role of DST in *M xenopi* disease is unclear, and no recommendations concerning DST are provided in the international guidelines because of insufficient evidence.[3] Available data suggest that most strains are susceptible to rifamycins, clarithromycin, ciprofloxacin, clofazimine, and amikacin, with more frequent resistance to ethambutol (24%–70%) and isoniazid (43%–94%).[57–60] However, the clinical implications of in vitro MICs are uncertain.

Current data support the use of at least three drugs in the first-line treatment of *M xenopi* disease: rifampin and ethambutol combined with a macrolide and/or a fluoroquinolone (preferably moxifloxacin).[3] Macrolides and fluoroquinolones seem to be similarly efficacious in several human and animal studies, and the choice may be

Table 3
Summary of nontuberculous mycobacterial pulmonary disease diagnosis and treatment considerations by species

Species	Epidemiology and Diagnostic Considerations[a]	Antibiotic Regimen and Minimum Recommended Treatment Duration[b]	Comments
M kansasii	Common with substantial regional variation Usually considered to have high pathogenicity; diagnosis possible with a single positive culture in the appropriate clinical and radiographic context	Rifampin-susceptible: Rifampin (rifabutin) and ethambutol and either azithromycin (clarithromycin) or isoniazid 12 mo Rifampin-resistant: Moxifloxacinplus at least 2 other drugs guided by drug susceptibility testing 12 mo	Generally good outcomes with treatment, rarely is adjunctive surgery considered
M xenopi	Common in parts of Europe and North America Consider the possibility of environmental contamination or pseudo-outbreaks	Rifampin (rifabutin) and ethambutol and azithromycin (clarithromycin) and/or moxifloxacin +/− Amikacin IV for severe or cavitary disease[c] 12 mo beyond culture conversion	Highest all-cause mortality rates among NTM; adjunctive surgery may be considered in carefully selected patients
M malmoense	Common in northern Europe, less so elsewhere High proportion of isolates reported to be clinically relevant in Europe; pathogenicity may vary geographically	At least 3 of rifampin (rifabutin), ethambutol, azithromycin (clarithromycin), moxifloxacin, or clofazimine ± Amikacin IV for severe or cavitary disease[c] First 3 agents likely preferred based on extent of published data 12 mo beyond culture conversion	Adjunctive surgery may be considered in carefully selected patients
M simiae	Heterogeneous distribution; common in regions of the United States, Middle East Respiratory isolates usually not indicative of disease; maintain high diagnostic threshold and consider other potential explanations for presentation	At least 3 of: azithromycin (clarithromycin), moxifloxacin, clofazimine, or trimethoprim-sulfamethoxazole ± Amikacin IV for severe or cavitary disease[c] 12 mo beyond culture conversion	Exhibits extensive drug resistance in vitro; adjunctive surgery may be considered in carefully selected patients

M szulgai	Rarely encountered, accounts for <1% of NTM-PD	At least 3 of: rifampin (rifabutin), ethambutol, azithromycin (clarithromycin), moxifloxacin, clofazimine, or amikacin IV[c] First 3 agents likely preferred based on extent of published data 12 mo if using preferred regimen, otherwise 12 mo beyond culture conversion	Generally favorable outcomes; insufficient evidence to recommend adjunctive surgery
M gordonae	Common contaminant and essentially considered nonpathogenic; every effort should be made to look for alternative diagnoses before considering a diagnosis of NTM-PD secondary to M gordonae, and a more stringent microbiologic criterion should be applied[d], even when the diagnostic criteria is satisfied, expectant management in immunocompetent patients is usually advisable unless there are compelling indications for antibiotic treatment		

Abbreviation: IV, intravenous.

[a] American Thoracic Society/European Respiratory Society/European Society of Clinical Microbiology and Infectious Diseases/Infectious Diseases Society of America criteria should be applied in the diagnosis of nontuberculous mycobacterial pulmonary disease for all species, with additional considerations as noted.

[b] Selection of regimens for M xenopi, M malmoense, M simiae, and M szulgai should be guided by drug susceptibility testing; however, there is uncertain correlation between in vitro testing and clinical response; alternative within-class agents are in parentheses.

[c] Administer amikacin (IV) for at least several months or longer if tolerated with evidence of ongoing improvement; nebulized formulation can be used as step down therapy for remainder of treatment.

[d] One proposed criteria consist of at least three positive sputum cultures, one of which must be smear positive.

nformed by side effect profiles, comorbidities, cost, and possibly MICs. One randomized controlled trial (RCT) examined rifampin and ethambutol plus either clarithromycin or ciprofloxacin in patients with M xenopi.[61] In each group, six patients (35%) achieved a favorable outcome (alive and cured at 5 years); however, the sample size was small (17 in each group) and protocol deviations occurred in approximately half of the patients. Another RCT reported preliminary results comparing either clarithromycin or moxifloxacin in addition to rifampin and ethambutol, and found essentially identical rates of 6-month sputum culture conversion.[62]

For patients with severe or cavitary disease, the addition of intravenous (IV) amikacin is recommended. In a murine model, the addition of amikacin to either a moxifloxacin- or clarithromycin-based regimen (combined with rifampin and ethambutol) provided benefit, with a reduction in the microbiologic burden of M xenopi.[63] Nebulized amikacin requires further investigation, but may be considered as step-down therapy or in cases where IV amikacin is unfeasible or contraindicated.[64] The liposome inhalation suspension formulation has not yet been studied in M xenopi, although potential benefit might be inferred based on its successful use in MAC.[65]

M xenopi disease is associated with high all-cause mortality, with 5-year mortality estimated at 43% to 69%. In a population-based study from Canada, multivariable modeling was used to examine factors associated with mortality in NTM-PD and M xenopi was the only species that showed an increased risk of death compared with MAC as the reference (hazard ratio, 1.22 (1.13–1.31); $P < .0001$). Although it is unclear whether high mortality should be attributed to the infection itself or the large burden of comorbid conditions, considering the elevated risk associated with M xenopi, the international guidelines favor daily dosing with three or more drugs rather than thrice weekly treatment (see **Table 3**). The recommended treatment duration is a minimum of 12 months following culture conversion.[3]

Mycobacterium Malmoense

Reported DST results seem to be inconsistent between studies, possibly because of laboratory techniques or regional differences. Aside from isoniazid against which there is universal resistance, reported resistance rates are highly variable: rifampin (0%–68%), rifabutin (0%–38%), ethambutol (4%–57%), clarithromycin (0%–13%), amikacin (10%–79%), clofazimine (0%–57%), and ciprofloxacin (6%–88%).[57,58,66–69]

International consensus recommendations advise using at least three drugs, guided by DST, for a minimum of 12 months after culture conversion (see **Table 3**).[2] The preferred combination is rifampin, ethambutol, and a macrolide. Evidence to support this includes an RCT involving 167 patients who were randomized to rifampin and ethambutol combined with either clarithromycin or ciprofloxacin for 2 years.[61] At the end of 5 years, more patients in the clarithromycin group had a favorable outcome, defined as "completed treatment as allocated and were alive and cured" (38% vs 20%). However, there were more protocol deviations in the ciprofloxacin group (43% vs 24%), mostly related to unwanted side effects. A retrospective study of 30 patients, most of whom received a macrolide-based regimen, observed a favorable response in 70%.[66] Another study reported 14 patients with fibrocavitary disease who received treatment with rifampin, ethambutol, and clarithromycin for 24 months, irrespective of DST results.[69] By the end of treatment, all patients achieved culture conversion, despite an in vitro resistance rate of 23% and 8% for ethambutol and clarithromycin, respectively.

Moxifloxacin and clofazimine are suggested alternatives in the event of intolerance or resistance to macrolides, rifamycins, or ethambutol. IV amikacin is another option, especially for severe or cavitary disease.[2] Nebulized amikacin has also been proposed if IV is contraindicated or impractical.[64]

Mycobacterium Simiae

M simiae demonstrates extensive drug resistance on DST, and accordingly has a reputation as a particularly difficult infection to treat. In vitro studies of clinical and environmental isolates demonstrate near universal resistance to rifamycins, ethambutol, isoniazid, and trimethoprim-sulfamethoxazole (81%–100%). Other drugs are less predictable, and resistance rates seem to vary substantially depending on the region: clarithromycin (0%–100%), amikacin (4%–100%), moxifloxacin (8%–70%), ciprofloxacin (11%–100%), and clofazimine (0%–100%).[14–16,57,58,70–72] Considering these challenges, and the fact that most respiratory isolates are contaminants, extra scrutiny is warranted when a patient is being evaluated for antibiotic treatment for M simiae.

There is insufficient evidence to recommend a standard regimen for M simiae. Previous case series describe varying success with considerable heterogeneity among the regimens used. International consensus recommendations advise using DST to guide the selection of a suitable regimen comprising three or more drugs (see **Table 3**).[2] Potential oral options include macrolides, moxifloxacin, clofazimine, and trimethoprim-sulfamethoxazole. IV amikacin should be considered in cases of severe or cavitary disease and/or when oral options are limited. The suggested treatment duration, based on expert opinion, is a minimum of 12 months after sputum conversion.[2]

Mycobacterium Szulgai

There is little evidence in the literature to inform treatment recommendations for *M szulgai*. Based on data from case reports and case series, international consensus recommendations advise selecting three or more drugs guided by DST results (see **Table 3**).[2] *M szulgai* seems to be susceptible to most antimycobacterial agents in vitro, with resistance rates of less than 15% to all tested drugs except ciprofloxacin (26%) and isoniazid (100% using a breakpoint of 1 μg/mL).[58] The preferred regimen consists of rifampin, ethambutol, and a macrolide for 12 months (or 12 months after sputum conversion if any of the preferred drugs are omitted). Alternative options include clofazimine, moxifloxacin, and IV amikacin.[2]

Mycobacterium Gordonae

Studies have shown conflicting results with respect to DST, likely because of regional differences. One study from the Netherlands tested 278 strains and found they were highly susceptible to most antimicrobials, including rifampin, clarithromycin, ethambutol, ciprofloxacin, clofazimine, and amikacin; isoniazid was the only exception.[58] In contrast, a study from India tested 14 clinical isolates and reported universal resistance to isoniazid, rifampin, and ethambutol, in addition to a resistance rate of 71% to ciprofloxacin.[73] This discrepancy likely reflects the higher prevalence of tuberculosis and increased exposure to antituberculous agents in India.

There is limited clinical experience regarding the treatment of *M gordonae*, given the rarity of true disease attributable to this species. Even when disease definition is met, a conservative approach should generally be adopted in the management of immunocompetent patients, with antimicrobials deferred unless there are compelling indications. As noted previously, more stringent microbiologic diagnostic criteria should undoubtedly be used for *M gordonae* (eg, ≥3 positive cultures and ≥1 smear positive). Several case reports and case series have reported successful outcomes for lung disease using a combination of rifampin/rifabutin, ethambutol, and a macrolide.[20,21] The reported durations of treatment have been highly variable.

ADJUNCTIVE SURGERY

Adjunctive surgery may be considered in select patients with recalcitrant disease.[3] The goals of surgical resection include (1) improving the chance of cure, (2) alleviation of intractable symptoms or complications (eg, hemoptysis), and/or (3) slowing down disease progression through "debulking."[74,75] However, surgery is associated with significant risks, and successful surgical outcomes are contingent on careful patient selection and perioperative preparation (see Chapter 15 of this issue). Additionally, there are species-specific considerations concerning the appropriateness of surgery.

There have been two studies on the outcomes of adjuvant surgery in patient with *M xenopi* in the macrolide era. In the first study, nine patients underwent thoracic surgery with therapeutic intent, although only four patients were known to have *M xenopi* beforehand and received appropriate preoperative antibiotic treatment. The remaining five patients were diagnosed based on surgical cultures and given antibiotic treatment afterward. Postoperative complications included prolonged air leak (2/9) and pleural effusions (2/9). None of the four patients who had received preoperative therapy had positive cultures during follow-up, although their preoperative smear status was not clearly reported.[76] Another study compared outcomes of adjunctive surgery versus exclusive medical management in 27 matched cases of NTM-PD (18 MAC, 9 *M xenopi*). Surgically treated patients had a higher rate of sustained culture conversion (87.5% vs 45.8%, *P* = .002 overall; 100% vs 66.7% in *M xenopi*) after at least 1 year of follow-up. Postoperative complications occurred in six patients (20%) overall and three patients (33%) with *M xenopi*, including acute respiratory distress syndrome leading to death in two patients overall (1 MAC and 1 *M xenopi*).[77] The substantial complication rate highlights the importance of judicious patient selection.

Data concerning surgical outcomes related to *M malmoense*, *M simiae*, and *M szulgai* comprise mainly isolated case reports.[16,78–80] For *M simiae*, surgery may be advocated, at least in part, based on extensive in vitro drug resistance, which renders medical therapy particularly challenging.[2] However, the same principles regarding patient selection would still apply.

As discussed previously, *M kansasii* responds nicely to medical therapy and therefore surgery is rarely necessary.

SUMMARY

NTM-PD caused by less common NTM have distinct features depending on the species.

Diagnostic evaluation still follows the criteria established by interational guidelines, but with certain qualifications given species-specific and regional differences in pathogenicity. Many patients with NTM-PD do not require antibiotic treatment upon diagnosis; clinicians should first institute nonpharmacologic management and evaluate clinical, radiologic, and microbiologic factors in the decision regarding antimycobacterial therapy. Treatment is challenging, and evidence-based recommendations are limited for most species. DST can be used to help with regimen selection; however, this approach is imperfect given the uncertain correlation between in vitro activity and clinical response for most drugs.

CLINICS CARE POINTS

- The causative species is an important consideration in the diagnosis and management of NTM-PD, since different species have different pathogenicity and treatment regimens.

- Nonpharmacological management – including but not limited to evaluation of bronchiectasis, treatment of coinfections, airway clearance therapy, and risk factor modification – should be offered to all patients.

- Antibiotic treatment regimens are complex, typically requiring at least 3 drugs for a minimum of 12 months (the exact composition varies by species). Additionally, not every patient benefits from treatment. Therefore, the decision to initiate antibiotic therapy should be individualized, with careful consideration of various factors related to the patient, the microbiological findings, and the radiological findings.

- DST should be obtained prior to the treatment of M kansasii to determine rifampin susceptibility, which has important implications on prognosis and regimen selection.

- There is limited evidence regarding the utility of DST for other less common species of NTM. By convention, DST may be helpful to guide the construction of a suitable multidrug regimen, but clinically meaningful breakpoints have not yet been established for many drugs and it is unclear whether in vitro activity correlates with patient outcomes.

ACKNOWLEDGEMENT

MY is supported by the University of British Columbia Clinician Investigator Program.

DISCLOSURE

TKM has the following disclosures: Research grants (Insmed), consultancy (Mannkind Corporation, Partner Therapeutics, Pfizer, RedHill Biopharma, Spero Therapeutics), speaker support (AstraZeneca).

REFERENCES

1. Hoefsloot W, Ingen J van, Andrejak C, et al. The geographic diversity of nontuberculous mycobacteria isolated from pulmonary samples: an NTM-NET collaborative study. Eur Respir J 2013;42(6):1604–13.
2. Lange C, Böttger EC, Cambau E, et al. Consensus management recommendations for less common non-tuberculous mycobacterial pulmonary diseases. Lancet Infect Dis 2022;22(7):e178–90.
3. Daley CL, Iaccarino JM, Lange C, et al. Treatment of nontuberculous mycobacterial pulmonary disease: an official ATS/ERS/ESCMID/IDSA clinical practice guideline. Eur Respir J 2020;56(1):2000535.
4. Bakuła Z, Kościuch J, Safianowska A, et al. Clinical, radiological and molecular features of Mycobacterium kansasii pulmonary disease. Respir Med 2018;139:91–100.
5. Ingen J van, Bendien SA, Lange WCM de, et al. Clinical relevance of non-tuberculous mycobacteria isolated in the Nijmegen-Arnhem region, The Netherlands. Thorax 2009;64(6):502–6.
6. Morimoto K, Hasegawa N, Izumi K, et al. A laboratory-based analysis of nontuberculous mycobacterial lung disease in Japan from 2012 to 2013. Ann Am Thorac Soc 2017;14(1):49–56.
7. Vande Weygaerde Y, Cardinaels N, Bomans P, et al. Clinical relevance of pulmonary non-tuberculous mycobacterial isolates in three reference centres in Belgium: a multicentre retrospective analysis. BMC Infect Dis 2019;19(1):1061.
8. Huang HL, Cheng MH, Lu PL, et al. Predictors of developing Mycobacterium kansasii pulmonary disease within 1 year among patients with single isolation in multiple sputum samples: a retrospective, longitudinal, multicentre study. Sci Rep 2018;8:17826.
9. Koh WJ, Chang B, Ko Y, et al. Clinical significance of a single isolation of pathogenic nontuberculous mycobacteria from sputum specimens. Diagn Microbiol Infect Dis 2013;75(2):225–6.
10. Moon SM, Park HY, Jeon K, et al. Clinical Significance of Mycobacterium kansasii isolates from respiratory specimens. PLoS One 2015;10(10):e0139621.
11. Hoefsloot W, Boeree MJ, van Ingen J, et al. The rising incidence and clinical relevance of Mycobacterium malmoense: a review of the literature [review article]. Int J Tuberc Lung Dis 2008;12(9):987–93.

12. Yoo H, Jeon K, Kim SY, et al. Clinical significance of *Mycobacterium szulgai* isolates from respiratory specimens. Scand J Infect Dis 2014;46(3):169–74.

13. van Ingen J, Boeree MJ, de Lange WCM, et al. Clinical relevance of *Mycobacterium szulgai* in The Netherlands. Clin Infect Dis 2008;46(8):1200–5.

14. van Ingen J, Boeree MJ, Dekhuijzen PNR, et al. Clinical relevance of *Mycobacterium simiae* in pulmonary samples. Eur Respir J 2008;31(1):106–9.

15. Hamieh A, Tayyar R, Tabaja H, et al. Emergence of *Mycobacterium simiae*: a retrospective study from a tertiary care center in Lebanon. PLoS One 2018; 13(4):e0195390.

16. Coolen-Allou N, Touron T, Belmonte O, et al. Clinical, radiological, and microbiological characteristics of *Mycobacterium simiae* infection in 97 patients. Antimicrob Agents Chemother 2018;62(7):003955. e418.

17. Jankovic M, Sabol I, Zmak L, et al. Microbiological criteria in non-tuberculous mycobacteria pulmonary disease: a tool for diagnosis and epidemiology. Int J Tuberc Lung Dis 2016;20(7):934–40.

18. Marras TK, Mendelson D, Marchand-Austin A, et al. Pulmonary nontuberculous mycobacterial disease, Ontario, Canada, 1998-2010. Emerg Infect Dis 2013;19(11):1889–91.

19. Eckburg PB, Buadu EO, Stark P, et al. Clinical and chest radiographic findings among persons with sputum culture positive for *Mycobacterium gordonae*: a review of 19 cases. Chest 2000;117(1):96–102.

20. Chang HY, Tsai WC, Lee TF, et al. *Mycobacterium gordonae* infection in immunocompromised and immunocompetent hosts: a series of seven cases and literature review. J Formos Med Assoc 2021; 120(1, Part 2):524–32.

21. Morimoto K, Kazumi Y, Shiraishi Y, et al. Clinical and microbiological features of definite *Mycobacterium gordonae* pulmonary disease: the establishment of diagnostic criteria for low-virulence mycobacteria. Trans R Soc Trop Med Hyg 2015;109(9):589–93.

22. Kim RD, Greenberg DE, Ehrmantraut ME, et al. Pulmonary nontuberculous mycobacterial disease: prospective study of a distinct preexisting syndrome. Am J Respir Crit Care Med 2008;178(10):1066–74.

23. Namkoong H, Omae Y, Asakura T, et al. Genome-wide association study in patients with pulmonary *Mycobacterium avium* complex disease. Eur Respir J 2021;58(2):1902269.

24. Szymanski EP, Leung JM, Fowler CJ, et al. Pulmonary nontuberculous mycobacterial infection. A multisystem, multigenic disease. Am J Respir Crit Care Med 2015;192(5):618–28.

25. Polverino E, Goeminne PC, McDonnell MJ, et al. European Respiratory Society guidelines for the management of adult bronchiectasis. Eur Respir J 2017;50(3):1700629.

26. Youssefnia A, Pierre A, Hoder JM, et al. Ancillary treatment of patients with lung disease due to non-tuberculous mycobacteria: a narrative review. J Thorac Dis 2022;14(9):3575–97.

27. Huiberts A, Zweijpfenning SMH, Pennings LJ, et al. Outcomes of hypertonic saline inhalation as a treatment modality in nontuberculous mycobacterial pulmonary disease. Eur Respir J 2019;54(1):1802143.

28. Hwang JA, Kim S, Jo KW, et al. Natural history of *Mycobacterium avium* complex lung disease in untreated patients with stable course. Eur Respir J 2017;49(3):1600537.

29. Moon SM, Jhun BW, Baek SY, et al. Long-term natural history of non-cavitary nodular bronchiectatic nontuberculous mycobacterial pulmonary disease. Respir Med 2019;151:1–7.

30. Geurts K, Zweijpfenning SMH, Pennings LJ, et al. Nontuberculous mycobacterial pulmonary disease and *Aspergillus* co-infection: bonnie and Clyde? Eur Respir J 2019;54(1):1900117.

31. Lowes D, Al-Shair K, Newton PJ, et al. Predictors of mortality in chronic pulmonary aspergillosis. Eur Respir J 2017;49(2):1601062.

32. Fayos M, Silva JT, López-Medrano F, et al. Nontuberculous mycobacteria and *Aspergillus* lung co-infection: systematic review. J Clin Med 2022; 11(19):5619.

33. Falkinham JO. Environmental sources of nontuberculous mycobacteria. Clin Chest Med 2015;36(1): 35–41.

34. Gardini G, Ori M, Codecasa LR, et al, IRENE Network. Pulmonary nontuberculous mycobacterial infections and environmental factors: a review of the literature. Respir Med 2021;189:106660.

35. Morimoto K, Aono A, Murase Y, et al. Prevention of aerosol isolation of nontuberculous mycobacterium from the patient's bathroom. ERJ Open Res 2018; 4(3):00150–2017.

36. Koh WJ, Lee JH, Kwon YS, et al. Prevalence of gastroesophageal reflux disease in patients with nontuberculous mycobacterial lung disease. Chest 2007;131(6):1825–30.

37. Kim Y, Yoon JH, Ryu J, et al. Gastroesophageal reflux disease increases susceptibility to nontuberculous mycobacterial pulmonary disease. Chest 2022;163(2):270–80.

38. Kim T, Yoon JH, Yang B, et al. Healthcare utilization and medical cost of gastrointestinal reflux disease in non-tuberculous mycobacterial pulmonary disease: a population-based study, South Korea, 2009-2017. Front Med 2022;9:793453.

39. Dawrs SN, Kautz M, Chan ED, et al. *Mycobacterium abscessus* and gastroesophageal reflux: an in vitro study. Am J Respir Crit Care Med 2020;202(3): 466–9.

40. Bodmer T, Miltner E, Bermudez LE. *Mycobacterium avium* resists exposure to the acidic conditions of the stomach. FEMS (Fed Eur Microbiol Soc) Microbiol Lett 2000;182(1):45–9.

41. Song JH, Kim BS, Kwak N, et al. Impact of body mass index on development of nontuberculous mycobacterial pulmonary disease. Eur Respir J 2021;57(2):2000454.

42. Kim HJ, Kwak N, Hong H, et al. BACES Score for predicting mortality in nontuberculous mycobacterial pulmonary disease. Am J Respir Crit Care Med 2021;203(2):230–6.

43. Pan SW, Su WJ, Chan YJ, et al. Disease progression in patients with nontuberculous mycobacterial lung disease of nodular bronchiectatic (NB) pattern: the roles of cavitary NB and soluble programmed death protein-1. Clin Infect Dis 2022; 75(2):239–47.

44. Ferreira IM, Brooks D, White J, et al. Nutritional supplementation for stable chronic obstructive pulmonary disease. Cochrane Database Syst Rev 2012; 8(12):CD000998.

45. Bakuła Z, Modrzejewska M, Pennings L, et al. Drug susceptibility profiling and genetic determinants of drug resistance in *Mycobacterium kansasii*. Antimicrob Agents Chemother 2018;62(4):017888. e1817.

46. Johnston JC, Chiang L, Elwood K. Mycobacterium kansasii. Microbiol Spectr 2017;5(1). https://doi.org/10.1128/microbiolspec.TNMI7-0011-2016.

47. Santin M, Dorca J, Alcaide F, et al. Long-term relapses after 12-month treatment for *Mycobacterium kansasii* lung disease. Eur Respir J 2009;33(1): 148–52.

48. Shitrit D, Baum GL, Priess R, et al. Pulmonary *Mycobacterium kansasii* infection in Israel, 1999-2004: clinical features, drug susceptibility, and outcome. Chest 2006;129(3):771–6.

49. Griffith DE, Brown-Elliott BA, Wallace RJ. Thrice-weekly clarithromycin-containing regimen for treatment of *Mycobacterium kansasii* lung disease: results of a preliminary study. Clin Infect Dis 2003; 37(9):1178–82.

50. Moon SM, Choe J, Jhun BW, et al. Treatment with a macrolide-containing regimen for *Mycobacterium kansasii* pulmonary disease. Respir Med 2019;148: 37–42.

51. Wallace RJ, Dunbar D, Brown BA, et al. Rifampin-resistant. Mycobacterium kansasii. Clin Infect Dis 1994;18(5):736–43.

52. Ahn CH, Wallace RJJ, Steele LC, et al. Sulfonamide-containing regimens for disease caused by rifampin-resistant. Mycobacterium kansasii. Am Rev Respir Dis 1987;135(1):10–6.

53. Guna R, Muñoz C, Domínguez V, et al. In vitro activity of linezolid, clarithromycin and moxifloxacin against clinical isolates of Mycobacterium kansasii. J Antimicrob Chemother 2005;55(6):950–3.

54. Luo J, Yu X, Jiang G, et al. In Vitro activity of clofazimine against nontuberculous mycobacteria isolated in Beijing, China. Antimicrob Agents Chemother 2018;62(7):000722. e118.

55. Kim DH, Jhun BW, Moon SM, et al. In vitro activity of bedaquiline and delamanid against nontuberculous mycobacteria, including macrolide-resistant clinical isolates. Antimicrob Agents Chemother 2019;63(8): 006655. e719.

56. Diel R, Ringshausen F, Richter E, et al. Microbiological and clinical outcomes of treating non-*Mycobacterium Avium* complex nontuberculous mycobacterial pulmonary disease: a systematic review and meta-analysis. Chest 2017;152(1):120–42.

57. Cowman S, Burns K, Benson S, et al. The antimicrobial susceptibility of non-tuberculous mycobacteria. J Infect 2016;72(3):324–31.

58. van Ingen J, van der Laan T, Dekhuijzen R, et al. In vitro drug susceptibility of 2275 clinical nontuberculous *Mycobacterium* isolates of 49 species in The Netherlands. Int J Antimicrob Agents 2010; 35(2):169–73.

59. Jenkins PA, Campbell IA. Pulmonary disease caused by *Mycobacterium xenopi* in HIV-negative patients: five year follow-up of patients receiving standardised treatment. Respir Med 2003;97(4):439–44.

60. Andréjak C, Lescure FX, Pukenyte E, et al. *Mycobacterium xenopi* pulmonary infections: a multicentric retrospective study of 136 cases in north-east France. Thorax 2009;64(4):291–6.

61. Jenkins PA, Campbell IA, Banks J, et al. Clarithromycin vs ciprofloxacin as adjuncts to rifampicin and ethambutol in treating opportunist mycobacterial lung diseases and an assessment of *Mycobacterium vaccae* immunotherapy. Thorax 2008;63(7):627–34.

62. Andrejak C, Veziris N, Lescure X, et al. Évaluation de l'efficacité de deux schémas thérapeutiques (inoculant Clarithromycine versus Moxifloxacine) sur la négativation des cultures à 6 mois au cours des infections pulmonaires à Mycobacterium xenopi. L'essai CaMoMy. Rev Malad Respir Actual 2021;13(1):25.

63. Andréjak C, Almeida DV, Tyagi S, et al. Improving existing tools for *Mycobacterium xenopi* treatment: assessment of drug combinations and characterization of mouse models of infection and chemotherapy. J Antimicrob Chemother 2013;68(3):659–65.

64. Haworth CS, Banks J, Capstick T, et al. British Thoracic Society guidelines for the management of non-tuberculous mycobacterial pulmonary disease (NTM-PD). Thorax 2017;72(Suppl 2):ii1–64.

65. Griffith DE, Eagle G, Thomson R, et al. Amikacin liposome inhalation suspension for treatment-refractory lung disease caused by *Mycobacterium avium* complex (CONVERT). A prospective, open-label, randomized study. Am J Respir Crit Care Med 2018;198(12):1559–69.

66. Hoefsloot W, van Ingen J, de Lange WCM, et al. Clinical relevance of *Mycobacterium malmoense* isolation in The Netherlands. Eur Respir J 2009;34(4):926–31.

67. Pulmonary disease caused by M. malmoense in HIV negative patients: 5-yr follow-up of patients

receiving standardised treatment. Eur Respir J 2003;21(3):478–82.

68. Henry MT, Inamdar L, O'Riordain D, et al. Nontuberculous mycobacteria in non-HIV patients: epidemiology, treatment and response. Eur Respir J 2004; 23(5):741–6.

69. Murray MP, Laurenson IF, Hill AT. Outcomes of a standardized triple-drug regimen for the treatment of nontuberculous mycobacterial pulmonary infection. Clin Infect Dis 2008;47(2):222–4.

70. van Ingen J, Totten SE, Heifets LB, et al. Drug susceptibility testing and pharmacokinetics question current treatment regimens in *Mycobacterium simiae* complex disease. Int J Antimicrob Agents 2012;39(2):173–6.

71. Akrami S, Dokht khosravi A, Hashemzadeh M. Drug resistance profiles and related gene mutations in slow-growing non-tuberculous mycobacteria isolated in regional tuberculosis reference laboratories of Iran: a three year cross-sectional study. Pathog Glob Health 2022;0(0):1–11.

72. Moghaddam S, Nojoomi F, Dabbagh Moghaddam A, et al. Isolation of nontuberculous mycobacteria species from different water sources: a study of six hospitals in Tehran, Iran. BMC Microbiol 2022;22:261.

73. Goswami B, Narang P, Mishra PS, et al. Drug susceptibility of rapid and slow growing non-

tuberculous mycobacteria isolated from symptomatics for pulmonary tuberculosis, Central India. Indian J Med Microbiol 2016;34(4):442–7.

74. Lu M, Fitzgerald D, Karpelowsky J, et al. Surgery in nontuberculous mycobacteria pulmonary disease. Breathe 2018;14(4):288–301.

75. Mitchell JD. Surgical approach to pulmonary nontuberculous mycobacterial infections. Clin Chest Med 2015;36(1):117–22.

76. Lang-Lazdunski L, Offredo C, Le Pimpec-Barthes F, et al. Pulmonary resection for *Mycobacterium xenopi* pulmonary infection. Ann Thorac Surg 2001;72(6): 1877–82.

77. Aznar ML, Zubrinic M, Siemienowicz M, et al. Adjuvant lung resection in the management of nontuberculous mycobacterial lung infection: a retrospective matched cohort study. Respir Med 2018;142:1–6.

78. Barclay J, Stanbridge TN, Doyle L. Pneumonectomy for drug resistant. Mycobacterium malmoense. Thorax 1983;38(10):796–7.

79. Ohno H, Matsuo N, Suyama N, et al. The first surgical treatment case of pulmonary *Mycobacterium malmoense* infection in Japan. Intern Med 2008;47(24): 2187–90.

80. Tsuyuguchi K, Amitani R, Matsumoto H, et al. A resected case of *Mycobacterium szulgai* pulmonary disease. Int J Tuberc Lung Dis 1998;2(3):258–60.

APPENDIX 1: LESS COMMON NTM APPENDIX

Clinical relevance estimates for respiratory isolates of less common nontuberculous mycobacterial species and *Mycobacterium avium*. Clinical relevance is defined as the proportion of patients meeting the contemporaneous American Thoracic Society diagnostic criteria for nontuberculous mycobacterial pulmonary disease (some studies provided estimates using only the microbiologic definition and these are indicated by grey shading). Estimates are based on a review of a limited selection of relevant publications, included if there were at least 15 patients evaluated for a given species.

Species	Clinically Significant Cases (A)	Number of Patients with Respiratory Isolates (B)	A/B in %	Source
M avium	4667	16,115	29	1
	24	59	41	2
	26	35	74	3
	10	19	53	4
	52	96	54	5
M kansasii	244	560	44	1
	12	17	71	2
	14	24	58	4
	86	105	82	6
M xenopi	9	28	32	1
	14	29	48	5
	36	98	37	4
	2	40	5	7
	41	147	28	3
M malmoense	5	58	9	8
	32	40	80	9
	30	41	73	10
M simiae	6	28	21	11
	21	97	22	12
	24	51	47	13
M szulgai	13	30	43	14
	11	15	73	15
	6	32	19	1
M gordonae	0	19	0	16
	1	48	2	2
	2	57	4	3
	1	56	2	5

Sources:
1. Morimoto K, Hasegawa N, Izumi K, et al. A Laboratory-based Analysis of Nontuberculous Mycobacterial Lung Disease in Japan from 2012 to 2013. *Ann Am Thorac Soc.* 2017;14(1):49-56.
2. Ingen J van, Bendien SA, Lange WCM de, et al. Clinical relevance of non-tuberculous mycobacteria isolated in the Nijmegen-Arnhem region, The Netherlands. *Thorax.* 2009;64(6):502-506.
3. Jankovic M, Sabol I, Zmak L, et al. Microbiological criteria in non-tuberculous mycobacteria pulmonary disease: a tool for diagnosis and epidemiology. *Int J Tuberc Lung Dis.* 2016;20(7):934-940.
4. Dakić I, Arandjelović I, Savić B, et al. Pulmonary isolation and clinical relevance of nontuberculous mycobacteria during nationwide survey in Serbia, 2010-2015. *PLoS One.* 2018;13(11):e0207751.
5. Vande Weygaerde Y, Cardinaels N, Bomans P, et al. Clinical relevance of pulmonary non-tuberculous mycobacterial isolates in three reference centres in Belgium: a multicentre retrospective analysis. *BMC Infect Dis.* 2019;19(1):1061.
6. Bakuła Z, Kościuch J, Safianowska A, et al. Clinical, radiological and molecular features of Mycobacterium kansasii pulmonary disease. *Respir Med.* 2018;139:91-100.
7. MENCARINI J, CRESCI C, SIMONETTI MT, et al. Non-tuberculous mycobacteria: epidemiological pattern in a reference laboratory and risk factors associated with pulmonary disease. *Epidemiol Infect.* 2017;145(3):515-522.
8. Buchholz UT, McNeil MM, Keyes LE, Good RC. Mycobacterium malmoense infections in the United States, January 1993 through June 1995. *Clin Infect Dis.* 1998;27(3):551-558.
9. Hoefsloot W, van Ingen J, de Lange WCM, Dekhuijzen PNR, Boeree MJ, van Soolingen D. Clinical relevance of Mycobacterium malmoense isolation in The Netherlands. *Eur Respir J.* 2009;34(4):926-931.
10. Böllert FG, Watt B, Greening AP, Crompton GK. Non-tuberculous pulmonary infections in Scotland: a cluster in Lothian? *Thorax.* 1995;50(2):188-190.
11. van Ingen J, Boeree MJ, Dekhuijzen PNR, van Soolingen D. Clinical relevance of Mycobacterium simiae in pulmonary samples. *Eur Respir J.* 2008;31(1):106-109.
12. Coolen-Allou N, Touron T, Belmonte O, et al. Clinical, Radiological, and Microbiological Characteristics of Mycobacterium simiae Infection in 97 Patients. *Antimicrob Agents Chemother.* 2018;62(7):e00395-18.
13. Hamieh A, Tayyar R, Tabaja H, et al. Emergence of Mycobacterium simiae: A retrospective study from a tertiary care center in Lebanon. *PLoS One.* 2018;13(4):e0195390.
14. Yoo H, Jeon K, Kim SY, et al. Clinical significance of Mycobacterium szulgai isolates from respiratory specimens. *Scand J Infect Dis.* 2014;46(3):169-174.
15. van Ingen J, Boeree MJ, de Lange WCM, de Haas PEW, Dekhuijzen PNR, van Soolingen D. Clinical relevance of Mycobacterium szulgai in The Netherlands. *Clin Infect Dis.* 2008;46(8):1200-1205.
16. Eckburg PB, Buadu EO, Stark P, Sarinas PS, Chitkara RK, Kuschner WG. Clinical and chest radiographic findings among persons with sputum culture positive for Mycobacterium gordonae: a review of 19 cases. *Chest.* 2000;117(1):96-102.

Medications and Monitoring in Treatment of Nontuberculous Mycobacterial Pulmonary Disease

Alice Sawka, MBBS, MPH, FRACP[a,b], Andrew Burke, MBBS, MPH, FRACP[c,d],*

KEYWORDS

• Nontuberculous mycobacteria • *Mycobacterium avium* • Aminoglycoside
• Therapeutic drug monitoring • *Mycobacterium abscessus*

KEY POINTS

- Treatment of nontuberculous mycobacteria (NTM) pulmonary disease requires prolonged administration of multiple antibiotics, during which adverse effects commonly occur.
- Data documenting the frequency, severity, and reversibility of adverse effects in the NTM patient population are lacking. Many recommendations for monitoring are based on expert consensus.
- Amikacin and linezolid therapeutic drug monitoring is important to optimize bactericidal killing and minimize toxicity; however, the optimal targets are yet to be determined.
- All patients should be counseled about adverse effects before commencing NTM treatment. Clinicians should develop an individualized monitoring plan for each patient based on toxicity profile of the selected drug, the presence of comorbidities, and perceived risk of adverse effects.
- Monitoring disease progress relies on assessment of clinical response together with frequent mycobacterial culture of respiratory samples.

INTRODUCTION

Treatment of nontuberculous mycobacteria (NTM) is lengthy and requires multiple antibiotics some of which have specific toxicity concerns such as optic neuritis with ethambutol and ototoxicity with aminoglycosides.[1,2] Use of a multidrug NTM regimen in patients with comorbid conditions may result in heightened susceptibility to gastrointestinal side effects with subsequent anorexia, weight loss, and worsening frailty. Treatment options may be limited by potential drug interactions with non-NTM drugs such as cystic fibrosis (CF) transmembrane conductance regulator modulator therapies and other cytochrome P450 mediated drugs.

Treatment toxicity is common with NTM treatment often requiring dose modification or drug discontinuation. In a retrospective study of 58 Japanese patients with *Mycobacterium avium* complex (MAC) treated with daily triple drug therapy as per American Thoracic Society (ATS) guidelines, 70% had an adverse event with 7% of these being grade 3 or 4.[3] The most frequent events were gastrointestinal disorders (17%) followed by hepatic dysfunction (13.8%). Seventeen percent discontinued all initial drugs with 32% discontinuing at least one initial drug. A systemic review of published MAC treatment outcomes in heterogeneous studies showed that 17% did not complete therapy due to a combination of side effects and loss to follow-up.[4] A more focused review

a Department of Thoracic Medicine, Royal Adelaide Hospital, Adelaide, South Australia, Australia; b University of Adelaide, Adelaide, South Australia, Australia; c University of Queensland Centre for Clinical Research, Faculty of Medicine, The University of Queensland, Brisbane, Australia; d Department of Thoracic Medicine, The Prince Charles Hospital, Brisbane, Queensland, Australia
* Corresponding author. The Prince Charles Hospital, 627 Rode Road, Chermside, Queensland 4032, Australia.
E-mail address: andrew.burke@health.qld.gov.au

Clin Chest Med 44 (2023) 815–828
https://doi.org/10.1016/j.ccm.2023.06.012
0272-5231/23/© 2023 Elsevier Inc. All rights reserved.

comprising 1462 patients restricted to 16 macrolide containing studies showed a 16% default rate with daily therapy dropping to 12% with thrice weekly therapy.[5] Dose modification or discontinuation of macrolides occurred in 6% most commonly due to decreased auditory acuity.

In the phase 3 studies for liposomal amikacin for inhalation in treatment refractory patients, those randomized to oral guideline based triple therapy had a discontinuation rate of only 3%.[6] In the arm of the study which was not receiving inhalation amikacin (and would therefore reflect current ATS guidelines) 4% had diarrhea, and 3% nausea. These lower rates of adverse events than in retrospective MAC studies may reflect more robust reporting mechanisms, better medical care, or also the fact that patients in clinical trials may differ in characteristics from less selective patient cohorts.[7] As these patents had been on chronic NTM therapy for an average of 4 years before commencement of the trial the study population may have selected out those patients who had been previously intolerant of guideline-based oral regimens.

There are fewer studies published on *Mycobacterium abscessus* (MABS) compared with MAC. *Mycobacterium abscessus* treatment regimens are more heterogeneous given the requirement for an intensive intravenous phase followed by a prolonged oral continuation phase often combined with inhaled amikacin.[8,9] The larger studies have not reported adverse event or drug discontinuation rates.[10] A review of 107 patients treated in the USA showed 65% of patients stopped an antibiotic because of adverse effects including 35% of those who received amikacin.[1] More contemporary studies showed a tigecycline dose adjustment or discontinuation rate of 57%.[11]

Treatment monitoring includes not only an awareness of side effects but also measures of clinical response. These include clinical outcomes such as symptoms, radiology, and sputum microbiology. Evidence suggests high rates of adverse events with NTM treatment leading to drug discontinuation. We aim to describe the current evidence for medication monitoring to prevent and manage side effects as well as strategies for dose optimization.

Clarithromycin and Azithromycin

Clarithromycin, a semisynthetic macrolide, and azithromycin, a member of the azalide group, are key drugs in the treatment of most NTM.[9,12] Macrolide antibiotics inhibit protein synthesis by binding to the 23S ribosomal RNA subunit. Given the paucity of studies that directly compare the treatment impact of azithromycin with clarithromycin in NTM-PD,[13] several drug factors summarized in **Table 4** influence macrolide selection.[14]

Gastrointestinal side effects and hepatotoxicity

Nausea, abdominal pain, and diarrhea frequently complicate macrolide use.[15] Superior tolerability with azithromycin relative to clarithromycin has been observed, and recent guidelines recommend an azithromycin-based regimen, in part due to expert perception of superior tolerability relative to clarithromycin-based regimens.[12,13] Metallic taste is most notable with clarithromycin. Switching between clarithromycin and azithromycin is appropriate when gastrointestinal adverse effects are encountered. Medication administration immediately prior to sleep, changing macrolides and pre-dosing with anti-emetic are strategies that can be trialed to address gastrointestinal disturbance. Minor serum aminotransferase derangement occurs more commonly with clarithromycin, but rarely with azithromycin.[16] Fulminant hepatitis is rare.[17]

QTc prolongation

In the majority of documented individual cases, arrhythmia complicating macrolide use has occurred in the presence of coexisting risk factors for QTc prolongation or sudden cardiac death.[18] Although there is no agreed threshold beyond which QT prolonging agents must be withheld, a QT interval of greater than 450 milliseconds in men and 470 ms in women has been linked with an increased risk of sudden cardiac death in adults over 55 years of age.[19] A QTc greater than 500 ms or greater than 60 ms over baseline has been proposed as a threshold that should prompt drug discontinuation.[20]

Recommendations from current NTM treatment guidelines vary from electrocardiogram (ECG) monitoring in selected patients with concurrent exposure to other QTc prolonging drugs,[12] to monthly ECG for all patients on macrolides.[21] Given the lack of evidence to guide recommendations, we suggest an ECG should be performed prior to macrolide commencement and a repeat ECG reviewed after 2 to 4 weeks of treatment. Patients with additional risk factors for macrolide-induced arrhythmia[18] should have ongoing ECG monitoring.

Ototoxicity

Population-based studies have reported increased frequency of sensorineural hearing loss[22] and tinnitus[23] among patients who have received a macrolide but meta-analyses have not confirmed this association.[15,24] One study assessing patients with chronic obstructive pulmonary disease (COPD) demonstrated a small statistically significant increase in the frequency of audiogram-confirmed hearing decrement in the azithromycin group (25% azithromycin group vs 20% placebo group; $P = 0.04$).[25] Recovery to baseline hearing was infrequent, regardless of whether azithromycin was discontinued or continued (34% among those who continued vs 32% among those who discontinued the drug). Among patients with non-CF bronchiectasis randomized to receive azithromycin 500 mg 3 times per week for 6 months[26] or 250 mg daily for 12 months,[27] no individuals reported a change in hearing, though the protocols did not include audiometry that may have detected subclinical change.

There is insufficient evidence to recommend regular audiometric testing for all patients with NTM taking a macrolide; however, obtaining a baseline audiogram is reasonable. Patients should be counseled to notify their clinician if they experience in hearing, impaired balance, vertigo, or tinnitus.

Rifampicin

Rifampicin and rifabutin are rifamycin antibiotics that inhibit DNA-dependent RNA polymerase suppressing protein synthesis. Nausea, diarrhea, and obstructive liver function tests derangement are common. A "flu-like" syndrome of myalgias, fevers, malaise, and weakness may develop, within weeks of treatment commencement, but may also emerge after months of therapy. Blood dyscrasias including lymphopenia, neutropenia, and occasionally thrombocytopenia may occur but rarely necessitate treatment interruption. Patients should be forewarned about the harmless orange discoloration of urine and tears.

Combination of rifabutin with clarithromycin results in elevated rifabutin levels which has resulted in anterior uveitis.[28] Otherwise, rifabutin has a similar safety profile to rifampicin. Relative to rifampicin, rifabutin is a less potent inducer of the CYP 3A4 enzyme system but medication lists should still be comprehensively reviewed for potential interactions.

Clofazimine

The antimycobacterial activity of clofazimine (CFZ) is thought to be multiple; enzymatic reduction of CFZ by type 2 NADH:quinone oxidoreductase generates reactive oxygen species,[29] whereas CFZ also disrupts the mycobacterial cell membrane.[30] CFZ is gradually sequestered as crystal-like aggregates in the cytoplasm of macrophages,[31] and the free base form accumulates in subcutaneous fat. Increased pigmentation of the skin and oral mucosa are common,[32] and brown mucosal discoloration of may be seen at bronchoscopy or colonoscopy after prolonged use. Skin pigmentation usually resolves following treatment cessation, though this may take several months due to the long half-life and concentration of CFZ in fatty tissue. Patients should be warned about these side effects before commencing. Rarely, polychromatic corneal and conjunctival crystal deposition can occur. Despite the sometimes significant psychological impact of skin discoloration, dryness, and itch.[33] CFZ is generally well tolerated, though gastrointestinal side effects and fatigue have been reported.[34]

CFZ accumulation in the small bowel lamina prior has resulted in CFZ enteropathy (**Figs. 1** and **2**). Patients develop abdominal pain, diarrhea, and malnutrition, usually following several months of drug exposure.[35]

Ethambutol

Ethambutol (ETO) inhibits the polymerization of arabinose, therefore interfering with biosynthesis of mycobacterial cell wall component arabinogalactan.[36] ETO is renally cleared; dose adjustment is required when creatinine clearance is less than 30 mL/min.[37]

Ethambutol optic neuropathy

Clinical manifestations Ethambutol optic neuropathy (EON) usually manifests clinically as painless, subacute, and symmetrical reduction in central visual acuity, usually following several months of medication exposure, though earlier onset has also been described.[38] Less common manifestations include color vision disturbance and bitemporal hemianopia. Visual loss is often reversible, but permanent visual loss can occur (**Table 2**).

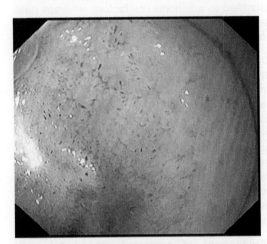

Fig. 1. Ileum of a patient with NTM-PD receiving clofazimine; demonstrating mucosal edema, altered vascularity, and speckled appearance secondary to innumerable purple-brown clofazimine deposits.

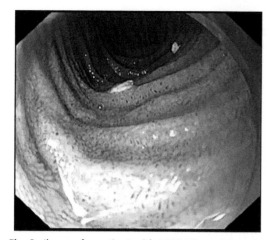

Fig. 2. Ileum of a patient with NTM-PD receiving clofazimine; demonstrating mucosal edema, altered vascularity, and speckled appearance secondary to innumerable purple-brown clofazimine deposits.

Frequency and risk factors for ethambutol optic neuropathy Patients with NTM pulmonary disease (PD) appear to be at greater risk for EON relative to tuberculosis (TB) patient cohorts, probably due to extended duration of use, and older average age of patients with NTM. In retrospective studies of patients who received ETO for NTM-PD, the incidence of symptomatic EOT either confirmed or suspected was 5% to 6.8%, with a median onset of 9.2 months post drug commencement.[39,40] Griffith and colleagues[41] reported that patients receiving daily ethambutol were more likely to develop ETO toxicity (6%), relative to those receiving 25 mg/kg 3 times per week (0%). Higher ethambutol dose,[42] advanced age[39] hypertension,[43] and reduced renal function[43] have been identified as additional risk factors, whereas peak serum ethambutol concentration does not appear to correlate with risk.[39]

Ocular monitoring In one large analysis of prospectively collected data from patients receiving treatment for MAC NTM lung disease,[41] all patients who were later confirmed to have developed EON reported ocular symptoms between clinic visits rather than being first detected on routine screening. This highlights the importance of counseling patients about manifestations of EON. Current guidelines[9,12] suggest visual acuity and color vision testing during treatment, though an alternative approach is to perform testing at baseline, and subsequently as clinically indicated.[44]

Management of suspected ethambutol optic neuropathy Early referral for detailed objective ophthalmology assessment to confirm EON and exclude alternative ocular pathology is important,

given the clear association between exclusion of ethambutol from a macrolide containing NTM regimen and heightened risk of macrolide resistance.[45,46]

Once EON is confirmed, there is no known effective intervention other than drug cessation, though the reported rate of recovery of visual function following drug cessation varies widely (42.2%–100%).[47,48] Recovery may be more likely in patients who are less than 60 years of age, but no other predictors of recovery have been identified. Where patients have developed EON in the context of a daily regimen but have gone on to fully recover after cessation of ETO, some specialists consider re-challenge with a 3 times a week dosing regimen in conjunction with close ophthalmologic monitoring.[41]

Other Other possible adverse effects of ETO include headache, hyperuricemia, and nausea; however, as part of a multidrug NTM regimen, it tends to be well tolerated relative to other commonly prescribed drugs. Desensitization via graduated dosing may successfully address headache and rash in some patients.[49]

Aminoglycosides

Amikacin is the preferred aminoglycoside for mycobacterial infection, with the exception of tobramycin for *Mycobacterium chelonae* infection. The aminoglycoside specific concerns for amikacin relate to nephrotoxicity, vestibular toxicity, and ototoxicity. Amikacin may be administered intravenously or nebulized. Nebulized amikacin solution may be used as a liposomal formulation as is currently approved for refractory MAC infection or by nebulizing the solution used for IV administration.

Intravenous amikacin The optimal dosing regimens for IV amikacin in NTM are unknown and there are differences in reported toxicity. A study of 45 patients with NTM, 84% of whom had 3 times a week dosing, reported an ototoxicity incidence of 18% with 7% having persistent hearing loss at 6 months.[50] Another study of 107 patients receiving amikacin for a median interquartile range (IQR) of 7(4–11) months had ototoxicity in 39%.[51] Female sex and the total cumulative dose of amikacin were predictors of ototoxicity. Most studies assessing different amikacin dosing techniques are short duration for non-mycobacterial infection and there is a lack of data to inform optimal dosing for longer NTM regimens.[52] A study of 28 patients with multidrug-resistant (MDR) TB showed that the area under the curve (AUC) of amikacin concentrations and cumulative drug dose per kilogram of body weight predicted ototoxicity whereas peak and trough levels did not.[53] Vestibular toxicity is

Table 1
Medications used in the treatment of nontuberculous mycobacteria pulmonary disease, notable adverse effects, suggested baseline studies and monitoring

Medication	Frequent and/or Important Adverse Effects	Suggested Baseline Studies	Suggested Monitoring Modality and Frequency
Azithromycin Clarithromycin	Gastrointestinal and hepatic disturbance	Baseline LFT	Repeat LFT at 1 mo and thereafter as indicated based on individual patient risk profile.
	QTc interval prolongation	Baseline ECG	Monthly ECG if additional risk factors for QTc prolongation or cardiac arrhythmia,[18] or in the setting of co-administration of other QTc prolonging drugs (including but not limited to the drugs in **Table 3**).
	Tinnitus and hearing loss	Audiometry	Repeat audiometry and dedicated vestibular assessment if hearing loss, tinnitus, or balance disturbance develop.
Rifampicin	Lymphopenia Neutropenia Thrombocytopenia	CBC	Repeat CBC and LFT at 1 month and then 3 monthly thereafter unless indicated based on individual patient factors.
	Liver enzyme derangement (classically obstructive pattern; less frequently hepatocellular)	LFT	Low threshold to repeat liver enzyme testing if anorexia or gastrointestinal disturbance develop.
Medication	Frequent and/or important adverse effects	Suggested baseline studies	Suggested monitoring modality and frequency.
Rifampicin *Cont.*	Headache Rash Flu-like syndrome Orange discoloration of urine and tears		
Rifabutin	As for rifampicin	As for rifampicin	Withhold drug pending urgent ophthalmology assessment if pain, redness, photophobia or blurred vision develop
	Uveitis Gastrointestinal disturbance Rash Headache		

(continued on next page)

Table 1
(continued)

Medication	Frequent and/or Important Adverse Effects	Suggested Baseline Studies	Suggested Monitoring Modality and Frequency
Ethambutol	Optic neuropathy	Baseline visual acuity and color vision assessment (Ishihara plates) Consider formal ophthalmology assessment prior to commencement ± ongoing regular ophthalmology review for patients with pre-existing ocular conditions	Ask about vision at each review visit. 1–3 monthly[a] visual acuity and Ishihara screening assessment. Withhold ethambutol pending urgent ophthalmology assessment if new visual blurring, deterioration in color vision, central scotoma, or impaired peripheral vision is reported between clinic assessments.
	Brown discoloration of skin, cornea and conjunctiva, and body fluids		
Clofazimine	Skin dryness and itch	Baseline CMP	Repeat CMP as required. Referral for comprehensive visual assessment if new ocular symptoms develop. Visual assessment if related symptoms
	Nausea, diarrhea, vomiting, abdominal pain Clofazimine enteropathy Dysphonia Hoarseness		
Amikacin (ALIS)[b,c]	Tinnitus	Patient education	Spirometry at baseline and with symptoms of bronchospasm
	Fatigue Dyspnea Hemoptysis Cytopenia	Baseline CBC	TDM after 3–5 d therapy Twice weekly EUC and CBC first month
Linezolid	Peripheral and optic neuropathy	Baseline examination for pre-existing PN and visual impairment	Ask about symptoms of neuropathy at each visit
	Lactic acidosis	Consider potential drug interactions	
Bedaquiline	QTc prolongation	Baseline ECG	Repeat ECG at 2 and 4 wk and then as clinically indicated
Tigecycline	Nausea Vomiting Diarrhea Pancreatitis (rare)	Baseline LFT and CBC	Nil specific

(continued on next page)

Medication	Frequent and/or Important Adverse Effects	Suggested Baseline Studies	Suggested Monitoring Modality and Frequency
Table 1 *(continued)*			
Cefoxitin	Nausea Vomiting Diarrhea Hepatitis Neutropenia, thrombocytopenia Rash	Baseline LFT and CBC	Weekly LFT and CBC
Imipenem	Nausea Vomiting Diarrhea Rash	Baseline LFT and CBC	Weekly LFT and CBC

CBC, complete blood count; CMP, comprehensive metabolic panel; ECG, electrocardiogram; LFT, liver function tests; QTc, corrected QT interval; TDM, therapeutic drug monitoring; UEC, urea electrolytes and creatinine.
[a] Author opinion, in absence of comprehensive evidence base.
[b] See other table for IV amikacin monitoring.
[c] In addition to comprehensive counseling about potential side effects of NTM medications.

uncommon and does not appear predictable with therapeutic drug monitoring (TDM).[54,55] Nephrotoxicity appears to be transient in most patients although data is lacking for older patients with NTM.[54] **Table 1** outline some TDM strategies for amikacin that are commonly used acknowledging that the optimal dosing strategy is still to be determined.

One of the roles of amikacin TDM is to optimize bactericidal killing and not just avoid toxicity. The optimal PK-PD target has been suggested as a C_{max}:MIC of 4 at the site of the infection, that is, the alveolar epithelial lining fluid.[56,57] Given the reduced penetration of aminoglycosides into the lung and macrophages, significantly higher plasma C_{max} may be necessary to achieve this.[54,58] The Clinical and Laboratory Standards Institute (CLSI) define amikacin resistance as a minimum inhibitory concentration (MIC) of $\geq$ 64 for both MAC and MABS mmol/L (intravenous use). For MAC only an additional resistance breakpoint of $\geq$128 mmol/L is stated if using inhaled liposomal amikacin.[59] Even for isolates with lower MIC, it is generally not possible to achieve such high peak concentrations to meet this target without incurring significant toxicity. Nevertheless, it does suggest that aiming for a higher C_{max} may be necessary, relative to other Gram-negative infections, although clinical outcomes supporting the safety of this approach are lacking. Given the post antibiotic effect of aminoglycosides, aiming for a higher peak with 3 times a week dosing is likely to achieve better PK-PD targets than a lower daily dosing.[54] Solely relying on trough levels to guide dosing may result in underdosing and not predict toxicity.[52]

Table 2
Amikacin therapeutic drug monitoring

TDM Methods	Suggested Target Concentration	References
C_{max}(peak)[a] target	35–45 mg/L (for daily dosing)[c] 65–80 mg/L (for 3 times per week dosing)[b]	9,12,63
C_{min} (trough)	< 5 mmol/L	9,12
AUC	Cumulative AUC may predict ototoxicity	53
Bayesian software	Measure C_{max} and C_{mid} (measure 6–14 h post dose). Individualize dosing with MIC, target C_{max}, C_{min}, AUC	60,64

[a] Suggested time of measuring Cmax is 1 h after start of a 30 min infusion.
[b] May aim for a lower Cmax if amikacin MIC is at lower range.
[c] Other studies have used higher C_{max} targets 55 to 65 mg/L for daily dosing.[65]

Table 3
Medication factors that may influence choice of macrolide in treatment of nontuberculous mycobacteria pulmonary disease

	Azithromycin	Clarithromycin
Dosing schedule	Daily or 3 times a week	Twice a day, either every day or 3 times a week
Adverse effect profile	Potentially better tolerated with fewer gastrointestinal adverse effects[12]	Thought to be less well tolerated with greater burden of gastrointestinal adverse effects
Interaction with CF modulator drugs	No dose adjustment required in patients taking elexacaftor/tezacaftor/ivacaftor.	Interaction with CF modulator drugs including elexacaftor/tezacaftor/ivacaftor and lumacaftor/ivacaftor; modulator dose adjustment required
Interaction with rifampicin	Lesser impact on peak azithromycin concentration (estimated 23% reduction C_{max})[14]	Greater impact on peak clarithromycin concentration (estimated 68% reduction C_{max})[14]
Predicted impact on QTc	Less likely to prolong QTc, in patients with additional risk factors for QT interval prolongation	More likely to prolong QTc, in patients with additional risk factors for QT interval prolongation
Other medication interactions	Weak inhibitor of cytochrome P450 (CYP) 3A4 enzyme system	Strong inhibitor of cytochrome P450 (CYP) 3A4 enzyme system

Bayesian software improves the likelihood of precision dosing and should be implemented where possible.[60] Optimal use requires knowing the pathogen MIC and target C_{max} and/or AUC.

The American Academy of Audiology monitoring guidelines highlight the need for baseline audiometry to allow interpretation of subsequent on-treatment testing given the high rates of pre-existing hearing loss in the population.[61] Ototoxicity is first manifest in the outer hair cells of the basal cochlear turn. High frequency audiometry comprises air-conduction threshold testing for frequencies above 8000 Hz and allows for detection of early ototoxicity before it is subjectively apparent.[61]

The recommendations for baseline and ongoing vestibular and audiometric testing in NTM infection are presented in **Table 4**. Although there is variation between guidelines, the authors believe it is reasonable to perform baseline and follow-up audiometry testing in all patients receiving amikacin.[61] Formal surveillance vestibular monitoring could be given to those with a high cumulative exposure to aminoglycosides (eg, persons with CF) and those with pre-existing balance problems.[62]

Independent of what formal testing process is used the most important factor is to educate patients of risks, and the need for immediate reporting of any change in hearing or balance. Patients should be asked of these symptoms at every visit.

Inhaled amikacin In the main study of amikacin liposome inhalation suspension (ALIS) for refractory MAC side effects were common. In those patients in the ALIS arm side effects included dysphonia (45%), cough (37%), hemoptysis (17%), and dyspnea (21%).[6] Most of these were in the first month and were often temporary and only rarely led to drug cessation. There was no difference in audiometry in subjects receiving ALIS or standard therapy at 3 or 6 months and no cases of vestibular toxicity.

Tigecycline
Tigecycline, a parenteral glycylcycline, is commonly used in MABS and has demonstrated *in vitro* efficacy although the optimum dosing is unclear.[66] A review of 35 treatment experienced patients receiving tigecycline for MABS showed a discontinuation rate in 46% of patients and dose reduction in an additional 11%.[11] The most common adverse reactions were gastrointestinal with 85% experiencing nausea, vomiting, and diarrhea despite high rates of anti-emetic pre-medication. In an earlier study of 52 patients, 30% of patients discontinued tigecycline due to adverse events.[67] Other less common side effects attributable to tigecycline in this population have included pancreatitis, hepatitis, and anemia.[11,67] Dosing strategies to minimize nausea with tigecycline and other IV antibiotics may include anti-emetic premedication and extended duration infusions.

Table 4
Summary of guideline recommendations for monitoring for aminoglycoside ototoxicity

Guideline Recommendations for Monitoring	Target Population	Ototoxicity	Vestibulotoxicity
American Academy of Audiology, 2009[61]	General population	• Routine questionnaire • Baseline audiometry pre-AG and repeat within 3 mo of treatment completion • Weekly or biweekly on AG treatment	• Routine questionnaire (dizziness handicap inventory) • Targeted formal vestibular testing based on symptoms
BTS NTM guideline, 2007[9]	NTM	• Routine questionnaire • Baseline audiometry pre-AG and repeat 2 mo after treatment completion • Monthly audiometry while on AG	• Routine questionnaire • Formal testing not specified
ATS/ERS/ESCMID /IDSA NTM guidelines, 2020[12]	NTM	• Routine questionnaire • Audiometry, frequency not specified (tailor to risk profile)	• Routine questionnaire • Formal testing not specified
International Ototoxicity Management Working Group (IOMG), 2021[62]	Pw CF including pediatrics	• Routine questionnaire • Baseline audiometry pre-AG and repeat within 3 mo of treatment completion • Targeted POC testing while on treatment[a] • Annual audiometry	• Routine questionnaire • Targeted vestibular POC testing on treatment[a] • Annual vestibular assessment

AG, aminoglycoside; ATS, American Thoracic Society ; BTS, British Thoracic Society; ERS, European Respiratory Society ; ESCMID, European Society of Clinical Microbiology and Infectious Diseases; IDSA, Infectious Diseases Society of America; POC, point of care; pwCF, people with cystic fibrosis.
[a] POC testing includes head impulse test, otoacoustic emissions, dynamic visual acuity, etc.

Amylase should be measured if the patient develops symptoms suggestive of pancreatitis, a rare complication.

Imipenem and cefoxitin

Imipenem and cefoxitin are the only β-lactams currently listed in guidelines for MABS. In a prospective study of cefoxitin, its use was associated with a higher rate of hepatotoxicity and neutropenia when used for 4 weeks (61%) compared with 2 weeks (7%).[68] In another study comparing high- and low-dose cefoxitin (12 g/d vs 4 g/d) with or without linezolid in MABS, there were high rates of cefoxitin discontinuation in the high-dose group due to leukopenia and hepatitis.[69] The median time to cefoxitin discontinuation was 23 days with resolution of adverse reactions on cessation.

Oxazolidinones

Linezolid and tedizolid are both orally formulated oxazolidinones with demonstrated activity against MABS, although clinical studies

documenting outcomes and toxicity in NTM cohorts are lacking. Linezolid has not been licensed for extended duration, but in practice, long-term use is complicated by mitochondrial toxicity with peripheral neuropathy, optic neuritis, and cytopenias. Extrapolating from trials in MDR-TB—performed in a younger and less co-morbid population—a 1200 mg daily dose of linezolid was associated with a 38% risk of peripheral neuropathy and myelosuppression in 22%.[70] We suggest a detailed baseline upper and lower limb and eye examination to assess for preexisting neuropathy and visual impairment prior to commencement of linezolid. Additionally, the drug list should be reviewed for potential interactions.

Clinicians should perform linezolid TDM to decrease the risk of toxicity if available. Dose adjustment should be performed if there is renal impairment.[71] Trough concentrations greater than 2 mg/L are associated with higher rates of neuro and myelotoxicity in a TB cohort.[72] A study of 37 patients receiving shorter course linezolid mostly for non-mycobacterial infection suggested a target range of 2 to 7 mg/L with initial plasma sampling on days 3 to 5.[73] There was a high association of thrombocytopenia with plasma concentrations above 7 mg/L. Linezolid induced mitochondrial toxicity can lead to lactic acidosis and can be detected on venous lactate. .

Bedaquiline

Bedaquiline is a diarylquinoline antibiotic developed for the treatment of MDR-TB that acts by inhibiting ATP synthase. There is *in vitro* evidence that both rapid and slow growing NTM may be susceptible to bedaquiline.[74] Given the lack of oral options for NTM infection, it is sometimes considered in refractory disease.[75] Because of the lack of published use in NTM to date, safety data are taken from MDR-TB cohorts. The main adverse reaction of concern for bedaquiline is that of QTc prolongation. In a large MDR-TB real world cohort there was an incidence of clinically significant QTc prolongation of 2.2%.[76] This was defined as a QTc greater than 500 milliseconds or a 60 milliseconds increase and symptoms (Torsade de pointes or polymorphic ventricular tachycardia, or signs/symptoms of serious arrhythmia). Other predisposing factors such as electrolyte imbalance, thyroid function, and concomitant drugs need to be considered and modified where possible. The low rates of QTc prolongation seen in TB populations should be interpreted cautiously as they are frequently a younger, less co-morbid population than would be expected in NTM cohorts. It is likely that some patients with NTM are at higher risk of QTc prolongation from bedaquiline than suggested in TB studies. The optimal frequency of ECG monitoring is unknown.

Monitoring Nontuberculous Mycobacteria Lung Disease During Treatment

Frequent sputum sampling is required to guide treatment duration, allow timely identification of treatment failure, identify infection with a second species, and may also assist prognostication. In patients with NTM-PD secondary to MAC, improvement in semiquantitative culture results by 2 or 3 months and improvement in cough were predictive of culture conversion by 12 months of treatment.[77] Monthly sputum sampling should be performed until there is evidence of culture conversion, which is defined as the collection date of the first of 3 consecutive negative acid-fast bacilli (AFB) cultures from respiratory samples collected at least 4 weeks apart.[78] Although there is a paucity of evidence to guide optimal frequency of ongoing sputum monitoring, the authors suggest that following culture conversion sputum should continue to be collected at 2 to 3 month intervals. New mycobacterial isolates detected following earlier culture conversion should be fully speciated and not assumed to be the initial pathogen given the possibility of co-infection with multiple NTM.

It is common for patients to become nonproductive of sputum as they respond to treatment. The role of sputum induction and bronchoscopy to confirm culture negativity in the setting of an apparent clinical response to therapy is unclear. Before undertaking a clinician should determine how the result will change treatment choice or duration.

The optimal frequency of computed tomography (CT) imaging during NTM treatment is not known. Current guidelines suggest CT imaging at the start and end of treatment.[9] Griffith and colleagues reported that among patients with NTM lung disease, improvement in appearance of a repeat CT performed an average of 59 ($\pm$34) days into treatment predicted culture conversion within 12 months.[77] Nevertheless, there is currently a lack of evidence to suggest that routine CT scans performed during treatment alter the clinician's management plan. If there has been an early clinical and microbiological response to treatment additional CT scans may be unnecessary. Alternatively, if there is a deterioration in symptoms, new hemoptysis or pulmonary nodules that require lung cancer surveillance then more frequent CT scans should be conducted.

SUMMARY

Most patients who are treated for NTM-PD will experience a treatment related adverse event. Adverse effects are the most frequently cited reason for alteration of a regimen away from guideline-based therapy and inappropriate treatment regimens are a strong risk factor for macrolide resistance.[46] When intolerances or adverse events occur, the patient and clinician must review the perceived risks of ongoing administration, weighed up against the likely benefit of continued treatment. There is often limited data to guide shared decision making. In an attempt to identify the causative agent of a non-severe side effect, stopping all medications followed by rechallenge in a staggered fashion is often necessary. An understanding of the common toxicity profiles of NTM antibiotics allows the prescriber to minimize risk, manage side effects as they arise, and increase the likelihood of successful treatment outcomes.

CLINICS CARE POINTS

- Although adverse reactions are common in NTM treatment many side effects can be managed without treatment cessation.

- clinicians should tailor treatment regimens based upon an individuals risk to specific adverse reactions and the goals of therapy.

- careful monitoring including direct questioning of patient is required throughout treatment especially for those drugs with uncommon but potentially severe side effects (amikacin, ethambutol, linezolid).

DISCLOSURE

A. Sawka: no financial or commercial conflicts of interest to declare. A. Burke has received research support from Merck Sharp and Dohme.

REFERENCES

1. Jarand J, Levin A, Zhang L, et al. Clinical and microbiologic outcomes in patients receiving treatment for *Mycobacterium abscessus* pulmonary disease. Clin Infect Dis 2011;52(5):565–71.

2. Ando T, Kage H, Matsumoto Y, et al. Lower dose of ethambutol may reduce ocular toxicity without radiological deterioration for *Mycobacterium avium* complex pulmonary disease. Respir Inv 2021;59(6):777–82.

3. Mori Y, Ito Y, Takeda N, et al. Tolerability, adverse events, and efficacy of treatment for *Mycobacterium avium* complex pulmonary disease in elderly patients. J Infect Chemother 2022;28(9):1255–60.

4. Amlabu V, Mulligan C, Jele N, et al. Isoniazid/acetylisoniazid urine concentrations: markers of adherence to isoniazid preventive therapy in children. Int J Tuberc Lung Dis 2014;18(5):528–30.

5. Kwak N, Park J, Kim E, et al. Treatment outcomes of *Mycobacterium avium* complex lung disease: a systematic review and meta-analysis. Clin Infect Dis 2017;65(7):1077–84.

6. Griffith DE, Eagle G, Thomson R, et al. Amikacin liposome inhalation suspension for treatment-refractory lung disease caused by *Mycobacterium avium* complex (CONVERT). A prospective, open-label, randomized study. Am J Respir Crit Care Med 2018;198(12):1559–69.

7. Metersky M, Chalmers J. Bronchiectasis insanity: Doing the same thing over and over again and expecting different results? F1000Research 2019;8.

8. Kwak N, Dalcolmo MP, Daley CL, et al. *Mycobacterium abscessus* pulmonary disease: individual patient data meta-analysis. Eur Resp J 2019;54(1).

9. Haworth CS, Banks J, Capstick T, et al. British Thoracic Society guidelines for the management of non-tuberculous mycobacterial pulmonary disease (NTM-PD). Thorax 2017;72(Suppl 2):ii1–64.

10. Koh WJ, Jeong BH, Kim SY, et al. Mycobacterial characteristics and treatment outcomes in *Mycobacterium abscessus* lung disease. Clin Infect Dis 2017;64(3):309–16.

11. Kwon YS, Levin A, Kasperbauer SH, et al. Efficacy and safety of tigecycline for *Mycobacterium abscessus* disease. Resp Med 2019;158:89–91.

12. Daley CL, Iaccarino JM, Lange C, et al. Treatment of nontuberculous mycobacterial pulmonary disease: an official ATS/ERS/ESCMID/IDSA clinical practice guideline. Eur Respir J 2020;56(1).

13. Field SK, Cowie RL. Treatment of *Mycobacterium avium-intracellulare* complex lung disease with a macrolide, ethambutol, and clofazimine. Chest 2003;124(4):1482–6.

14. van Ingen J, Egelund EF, Levin A, et al. The pharmacokinetics and pharmacodynamics of pulmonary *Mycobacterium avium* complex disease treatment. Am J Respir Crit Care Med 2012;186(6):559–65.

15. Hansen MP, Scott AM, McCullough A, et al. Adverse events in people taking macrolide antibiotics versus placebo for any indication. Cochrane Database Syst Rev 2019;1(1):Cd011825.

16. Macrolide Antibiotics. LiverTox: Clinical and Research Information on Drug-Induced Liver Injury 2012; Available at: https://www.ncbi.nlm.nih.gov/books/NBK548398/. Accessed September 15, 2022.

17. Bjornsson E, Olsson R. Suspected drug-induced liver fatalities reported to the WHO database. Dig Liver Dis 2006;38(1):33–8.

18. Albert RK, Schuller JL, Network CCR. Macrolide antibiotics and the risk of cardiac arrhythmias. Am J Respir Crit Care Med 2014;189(10):1173–80.

19. Straus SM, Kors JA, De Bruin ML, et al. Prolonged QTc interval and risk of sudden cardiac death in a population of older adults. J Am Coll Cardiol 2006;47(2):362–7.

20. Food, Drug Administration HHS. International Conference on Harmonisation; guidance on E14 clinical Evaluation of QT/QTc interval prolongation and Proarrhythmic potential for non-Antiarrhythmic drugs; availability. Notice. Fed Regist 2005;70(202):61134–5.

21. Kon OM, Beare N, Connell D, et al. BTS clinical statement for the diagnosis and management of ocular tuberculosis. BMJ Open Resp Res 2022;9(1):e001225.

22. Henkle E, Daley CL, Curtis JR, et al. Comparative safety of inhaled corticosteroids and macrolides in

Medicare enrolees with bronchiectasis. ERJ Open Res 2022;8(1). 00786-2020.

23. Vanoverschelde A, Oosterloo BC, Ly NF, et al. Macrolide-associated ototoxicity: a cross-sectional and longitudinal study to assess the association of macrolide use with tinnitus and hearing loss. J Antimicrob Chemother 2021;76(10):2708–16.

24. Alsowaida YS, Almulhim AS, Oh M, et al. Sensorineural hearing loss with macrolide antibiotics exposure: a meta-analysis of the association. Int J Pharm Pract 2021;29(1):21–8.

25. Albert RK, Connett J, Bailey WC, et al. Azithromycin for prevention of exacerbations of COPD. N Engl J Med 2011;365(8):689–98.

26. Wong C, Jayaram L, Karalus N, et al. Azithromycin for prevention of exacerbations in non-cystic fibrosis bronchiectasis (EMBRACE): a randomised, double-blind, placebo-controlled trial. Lancet 2012; 380(9842):660–7.

27. Altenburg J, de Graaff CS, Stienstra Y, et al. Effect of azithromycin maintenance treatment on infectious exacerbations among patients with non-cystic fibrosis bronchiectasis: the BAT randomized controlled trial. JAMA 2013;309(12):1251–9.

28. Hafner R, Bethel J, Power M, et al. Tolerance and pharmacokinetic interactions of rifabutin and clarithromycin in human immunodeficiency virus-infected volunteers. Antimicrob Agents Chemother 1998;42(3):631–9.

29. Yano T, Kassovska-Bratinova S, Teh JS, et al. Reduction of clofazimine by mycobacterial type 2 NADH: quinone oxidoreductase: a pathway for the generation of bactericidal levels of reactive oxygen species. J Biol Chem 2011;286(12):10276–87.

30. Cholo MC, Mothiba MT, Fourie B, et al. Mechanisms of action and therapeutic efficacies of the lipophilic antimycobacterial agents clofazimine and bedaquiline. J Antimicrob Chemother 2017; 72(2):338–53.

31. Baik J, Rosania GR. Molecular imaging of intracellular drug-membrane aggregate formation. Mol Pharm 2011;8(5):1742–9.

32. Carey G.B., Tebas P., Vinnard C., et al., Clinical outcomes of clofazimine use for rapidly growing mycobacterial infections, Open Forum Infect Dis, 6 (11), 2019, ofz456. https://doi.org/10.1093/ofid/ofz456.

33. Dey T, Brigden G, Cox H, et al. Outcomes of clofazimine for the treatment of drug-resistant tuberculosis: a systematic review and meta-analysis. J Antimicrob Chemother 2013;68(2):284–93.

34. Martiniano SL, Wagner BD, Levin A, et al. Safety and effectiveness of clofazimine for primary and refractory nontuberculous mycobacterial infection. Chest 2017;152(4):800–9.

35. Pais AV, Pereira S, Garg I, et al. Intra-abdominal, crystal-storing histiocytosis due to clofazimine in a patient with lepromatous leprosy and concurrent carcinoma of the colon. Lepr Rev 2004;75(2):171–6.

36. Belanger AE, Besra GS, Ford ME, et al. The embAB genes of Mycobacterium avium encode an arabinosyl transferase involved in cell wall arabinan biosynthesis that is the target for the antimycobacterial drug ethambutol. Proc Natl Acad Sci U S A 1996; 93(21):11919–24.

37. Launay-Vacher V, Izzedine H, Deray G. Pharmacokinetic considerations in the treatment of tuberculosis in patients with renal failure. Clin Pharmacokinet 2005;44(3):221–35.

38. Chamberlain PD, Sadaka A, Berry S, et al. Ethambutol optic neuropathy. Curr Opin Ophthalmol 2017;28(6):545–51.

39. Yang S, Falardeau J, Winthrop KL, et al. Ethambutol-induced optic neuropathy in nontuberculous mycobacterial disease. Int J Tuberc Lung Dis 2021; 25(8):680–2.

40. Kamii Y, Nagai H, Kawashima M, et al. Adverse reactions associated with long-term drug administration in Mycobacterium avium complex lung disease. Int J Tuberc Lung Dis 2018;22(12):1505–10.

41. Griffith DE, Brown-Elliott BA, Shepherd S, et al. Ethambutol ocular toxicity in treatment regimens for Mycobacterium avium complex lung disease. Am J Respir Crit Care Med 2005;172(2):250–3.

42. Talbert Estlin KA, Sadun AA. Risk factors for ethambutol optic toxicity. Int Ophthalmol 2010;30(1): 63–72.

43. Chen HY, Lai SW, Muo CH, et al. Ethambutol-induced optic neuropathy: a nationwide population-based study from Taiwan. Br J Ophthalmol 2012;96(11):1368–71.

44. Milburn H, Ashman N, Davies P, et al. Guidelines for the prevention and management of Mycobacterium tuberculosis infection and disease in adult patients with chronic kidney disease. Thorax 2010;65(6): 557–70.

45. Griffith DE, Brown-Elliott BA, Langsjoen B, et al. Clinical and molecular analysis of macrolide resistance in Mycobacterium avium complex lung disease. Am J Respir Crit Care Med 2006;174(8): 928–34.

46. Morimoto K, Namkoong H, Hasegawa N, et al. Macrolide-resistant Mycobacterium avium complex lung disease: analysis of 102 consecutive cases. Annals of the American Thoracic Society 2016;13(11): 1904–11.

47. Kumar A, Sandramouli S, Verma L, et al. Ocular ethambutol toxicity: is it reversible? J Clin Neuro Ophthalmol 1993;13(1):15–7.

48. Tsai RK, Lee YH. Reversibility of ethambutol optic neuropathy. J Ocul Pharmacol Therapeut 1997; 13(5):473–7.

49. Ban GY, Jeong YJ, Lee SH, et al. Efficacy and tolerability of desensitization in the treatment of delayed

drug hypersensitivities to anti-tuberculosis medications. Resp Med 2019;147:44–50.

50. Ellender CM, Law DB, Thomson RM, et al. Safety of IV amikacin in the treatment of pulmonary nontuberculous mycobacterial disease. Respirology 2016;21(2):357–62.

51. Aznar ML, Marras TK, Elshal AS, et al. Safety and effectiveness of low-dose amikacin in nontuberculous mycobacterial pulmonary disease treated in Toronto, Canada. BMC pharmacology & toxicology 2019;20(1):37.

52. Jenkins A, Thomson AH, Brown NM, et al. Amikacin use and therapeutic drug monitoring in adults: do dose regimens and drug exposures affect either outcome or adverse events? A systematic review. J Antimicrob Chemother 2016;71(10): 2754–9.

53. Modongo C, Pasipanodya JG, Zetola NM, et al. Amikacin concentrations predictive of ototoxicity in multidrug-resistant tuberculosis patients. Antimicrobial agents and chemotherapy 2015;59(10):6337–43.

54. Sturkenboom MGG, Simbar N, Akkerman OW, et al. Amikacin dosing for MDR Tuberculosis: a systematic review to establish or revise the current recommended dose for tuberculosis treatment. Clin Infect Dis 2018;67(suppl_3):S303–7.

55. Fu TS, Carr SD, Douglas-Jones P, et al. Gentamicin Vestibulotoxicity: Further Insights from a large clinical Series. Otol Neurotol 2020;41(7): e864–72.

56. Raaijmakers J, Schildkraut JA, Hoefsloot W, et al. The role of amikacin in the treatment of nontuberculous mycobacterial disease. Expet Opin Pharmacother 2021;22(15):1961–74.

57. Ferro BE, Srivastava S, Deshpande D, et al. Amikacin pharmacokinetics/pharmacodynamics in a novel hollow-fiber Mycobacterium abscessus disease model. Antimicrobial agents and chemotherapy 2015;60(3):1242–8.

58. Heffernan AJ, Sime FB, Lipman J, et al. Intrapulmonary pharmacokinetics of antibiotics used to treat nosocomial pneumonia caused by gram-negative bacilli: a systematic review. Int J Antimicrob Agents 2019;53(3):234–45.

59. Clinical and Laboratory Standards Institute (CLSI). CLSI. Performance Standards for Susceptibility Testing of Mycobacteria, Nocardia spp., and Other Aerobic Actinomycetes. 2018.

60. Ryan AC, Carland JE, McLeay RC, et al. Evaluation of amikacin use and comparison of the models implemented in two Bayesian forecasting software packages to guide dosing. Br J Clin Pharmacol 2021;87(3):1422–31.

61. Durrant JCK, Fausti S, O'Neil G, et al. American Academy of Audiology Position statement and clinical practice guidelines: ototoxicity monitoring. American Academy of Audiology 2009;1–25.

62. Garinis AC, Poling GL, Rubenstein RC, et al. Clinical considerations for routine auditory and vestibular monitoring in patients with cystic fibrosis. Am J Audiol 2021;30(3s):800–9.

63. Peloquin CA, Berning SE, Nitta AT, et al. Aminoglycoside toxicity: daily versus thrice-weekly dosing for treatment of mycobacterial diseases. Clin Infect Dis 2004;38(11):1538–44.

64. Sturkenboom MGG, Märtson AG, Svensson EM, et al. Population pharmacokinetics and Bayesian dose adjustment to advance TDM of anti-TB Drugs. Clin Pharmacokinet 2021;60(6): 685–710.

65. Lee H, Sohn YM, Ko JY, et al. Once-daily dosing of amikacin for treatment of Mycobacterium abscessus lung disease. Int J Tuberc Lung Dis 2017;21(7): 818–24.

66. Ferro BE, Srivastava S, Deshpande D, et al. Tigecycline is highly efficacious against Mycobacterium abscessus pulmonary disease. Antimicrobial agents and chemotherapy 2016;60(5):2895–900.

67. Wallace RJ Jr, Dukart G, Brown-Elliott BA, et al. Clinical experience in 52 patients with tigecycline-containing regimens for salvage treatment of Mycobacterium abscessus and Mycobacterium chelonae infections. J Antimicrob Chemother 2014;69(7): 1945–53.

68. Koh WJ, Jeong BH, Jeon K, et al. Oral Macrolide therapy following short-term combination Antibiotic treatment for Mycobacterium massiliense lung disease. Chest 2016;150:1211–21.

69. Li H, Tong L, Wang J, et al. An intensified regimen containing linezolid could improve treatment response in Mycobacterium abscessus lung disease. BioMed Res Int 2019;2019:8631563.

70. Conradie F, Bagdasaryan TR, Borisov S, et al. Bedaquiline-pretomanid-linezolid Regimens for drug-resistant tuberculosis. N Engl J Med 2022;387(9): 810–23.

71. Crass RL, Cojutti PG, Pai MP, et al. Reappraisal of linezolid dosing in renal impairment to improve safety. Antimicrobial agents and chemotherapy 2019;63(8).

72. Eimer J, Fréchet-Jachym M, Le Dû D, et al. Increased linezolid plasma concentrations are associated with the development of severe toxicity in MDR-TB treatment. Clin Infect Dis 2023;76(3): e947–56.

73. Komatsu T, Nakamura M, Uchiyama K, et al. Initial trough concentration may be beneficial in preventing linezolid-induced thrombocytopenia. J Chemother 2022;34(6):375–80.

74. Kim DH, Jhun BW, Moon SM, et al. In vitro activity of bedaquiline and delamanid against nontuberculous mycobacteria, including macrolide-resistant clinical isolates. Antimicrobial agents and chemotherapy 2019;63(8).

75. Philley JV, Wallace RJ Jr, Benwill JL, et al. Preliminary results of bedaquiline as salvage therapy for patients with nontuberculous mycobacterial lung disease. Chest 2015;148(2):499–506.

76. Hewison C, Khan U, Bastard M, et al. Safety of treatment regimens containing bedaquiline and delamanid in the end TB Cohort. Clin Infect Dis 2022;75(6): 1006–13.

77. Griffith DE, Adjemian J, Brown-Elliott BA, et al. Semi-quantitative culture analysis during therapy for *Mycobacterium avium* complex lung disease. Am J Respir Crit Care Med 2015;192(6):754–60.

78. van Ingen J, Aksamit T, Andrejak C, et al. Treatment outcome definitions in nontuberculous mycobacterial pulmonary disease: an NTM-NET consensus statement. Eur Respir J 2018;51(3).

Nontuberculous Mycobacterial Pulmonary Disease in the Immunocompromised Host

Cara D. Varley, MD, MPH[a,b,]*, Amber C. Streifel, PharmD[c],
Amanda M. Bair, PharmD[c], Kevin L. Winthrop, MD, MPH[a,b]

KEYWORDS

- Nontuberculous mycobacteria • Mycobacterium infections • Nontuberculous
- Immunocompromised host • HIV • Transplant recipients • Organ transplantation
- Immunosuppressive agents

KEY POINTS

- Those with reduced cell mediated immunity and exposure to immunosuppressive agents, especially TNF-alpha inhibitors, are at increased risk for pulmonary and extrapulmonary NTM infections.
- Mycobacterium avium complex and Mycobacterium abscessus are the most common species causing infections.
- Prior to starting therapy for NTM disease, providers should ensure diagnostic criteria are met as colonization is common.
- Treatment is long, requiring 2-4 agents, and is often associated with significant drug interactions, side effects and toxicities.
- Whenever possible, immunosuppression should be reduced or changed, particularly in the setting of TNF-alpha inhibitors.

BACKGROUND

We review the current data on nontuberculous mycobacterial infections associated with the immunocompromised host published over the last 7 years.

EPIDEMIOLOGY

Prevalence and Incidence of Nontuberculous Mycobacterial Infections

Nontuberculous mycobacteria (NTM) are commonly found in water and soil and are ubiquitous in the environment. Inhalation or aspiration leads to pulmonary disease, which is the most common site of infection, in susceptible hosts.[1,2]

Pulmonary NTM disease incidence and prevalence are increasing, with more than 100,000 prevalent cases, the majority due to *Mycobacterium avium complex* (MAC) with more than 80,000 pulmonary cases estimated in the United States in 2014.[3–12] A large national managed care claims database including 27 million people in the United States (US) identified an annual incidence and prevalence in 2015 at 4.73 per 100,000 person-years (95% confidence interval, 4.43–5.05) and 11.70 per 100,000 persons (95% confidence interval, 11.26–12.16), respectively.[13] They found a statistically significant average annual increase in incidence of 5.2% (95% confidence interval, 4.0%-6.4%) and prevalence of 7.5% (95%

a Department of Medicine, Division of Infectious Diseases, Oregon Health & Science University; b Program in Epidemiology, Oregon Health & Science University-Portland State University School of Public Health; c Department of Pharmacy Services, Oregon Health & Science University
* Corresponding author. OHSU Division of Infectious Diseases, 3181 Southwest Sam Jackson Park Road L457, Portland, OR 97239-3098.
E-mail address: varleyc@ohsu.edu

Clin Chest Med 44 (2023) 829–838
https://doi.org/10.1016/j.ccm.2023.06.007
0272-5231/23/© 2023 Elsevier Inc. All rights reserved.

confidence interval, 6.7%-8.2%) between 2008 and 2015.[13] Most (87.2%) cases occur in those older than age 50, with 55% of all cases in adults more than age 65.[6,7,12] Outside the United States, pulmonary NTM prevalence varies with an estimate of 6.2 per 100,000 people in 5 European countries (Spain, Italy, France, Germany, United Kingdom), 24.9 per 100,000 people in Japan, and 1.17 per 100,000 people in New Zealand with increases in annual incidence observed in many countries.[14-18] NTM disease disproportionately affects those with chronic underlying lung disease such as chronic obstructive pulmonary disease (COPD), bronchiectasis, and cystic fibrosis.[10,12] More recent studies have also found higher all-cause mortality for patients with NTM disease compared to their counterparts of similar age and gender without pulmonary NTM.[8,19-21]

Extrapulmonary NTM disease is commonly associated with surgical interventions, injections, penetrating trauma or the case of immuno-compromised hosts where exposures can lead to either localized infection of the skin and soft tissue, lymph nodes, bones, joints, implanted hardware or in some cases, to disseminated disease via gastrointestinal tract inoculation and spread.[22-25] In a study evaluating inpatient admissions between 2009 and 2014 through Cerner Health Facts Electronic Health Record (EHR) database, 6-year prevalence of extrapulmonary NTM infections was 11 infections per 100,000 inpatients with skin and soft tissue identified as the most common site (4.4 infections per 100,000 inpatients) and 20% of the population with prior exposure to immunosuppressive agents.[23] Disease surveillance by the Oregon Health Authority identified 134 extrapulmonary NTM cases between 2014 and 2016 (11 per 1,000,000 persons per year) with 34% immuno-compromised.[24] Wentworth, and colleagues evaluated the incidence of cutaneous NTM infections in Olmsted County, Minnesota between 1980 and 2009 and found a statistically significant increase in incidence from 0.7 per 100.000 person-years in 1980 to 1999 to 2.0 per 100,000 person-years in 2000 to 2009 with a substantial increase in the proportion caused by rapidly growing mycobacteria species.[25] Similar to other studies, 23% were classified as immunosuppressed.[25]

IMMUNOSUPPRESSIVE STATES
Human Immunodeficiency Virus/Acquired Immune Deficiency Syndrome

Early in the Human Immunodeficiency Virus (HIV) pandemic, disseminated MAC was a common opportunistic infection, diagnosed in nearly a quarter of those with Acquired Immune Deficiency Syndrome (AIDS) in the late 1980s and early 1990s.[26] However, the incidence of disseminated MAC infection declined significantly after combined antiretroviral therapy (ART) became available.[26,27] Typically observed in those with CD4 T lymphocyte (CD4) counts less than 50 cells/mm^3, disseminated MAC can cause fevers, night sweats, fatigue, weight loss and diarrhea with hepatomegaly, splenomegaly, and lymphadenopathy.[28] Laboratory abnormalities include profound anemia and elevated alkaline phosphatase levels.[28,29] Symptoms can often be unmasked or worsen with the initiation of ART in the setting of immune reconstitution inflammatory syndrome (IRIS).[30] Diagnosis is confirmed with the isolation of MAC by culture or molecular techniques from blood, bone marrow, lymph nodes or other sterile sites.[29]

Azithromycin or clarithromycin prophylaxis has been previously recommended if CD4 counts fall less than 50 cells/mm^3, however in 2019 guidance changed to not recommending primary prophylaxis for disseminated MAC if patients are initiated on ART.[29] In those who have CD4 counts less than 50 cells/mm^3, who are not receiving ART or do not have options for a suppressive ART regimen, and disseminated MAC has been ruled out, prophylaxis should be initiated with azithromycin 1200 mg PO once weekly or clarithromycin 500 mg PO BID.[26,29,31-36]

Treatment for disseminated MAC disease includes the initiation of ART and 2 to 4 antibiotics consisting of a macrolide (azithromycin preferred over clarithromycin due to fewer drug interactions and improved tolerability) and ethambutol plus a rifamycin or amikacin.[29] Poor absorption due to underlying HIV or disseminated MAC is sometimes observed in this population and, if concern exists, serum therapeutic drug monitoring (TDM) should be performed with the consideration of transition to intravenous antibiotics. Drug susceptibility testing should be obtained from a reliable laboratory for all MAC isolates, especially prior to pursuing second-line therapy, as resistance to fluoroquinolones and linezolid is common.[37,38] Therapy should be continued until CD4 counts are above 100 cells/mm^3 for 6 months and the patient has received MAC therapy for at least 12 months.[29]

Solid Organ Transplant

Patients who undergo solid organ transplantation (SOT) are largely at risk for NTM infection due to he various immunosuppressive agents given to prevent organ rejection including steroids, calcineurin inhibitors (tacrolimus and cyclosporine), mammalian target of rapamycin (mTOR) inhibitors (sirolimus, everolimus), and more recently lymphocyte depleting antibodies. The reported incidence is highest in lung transplant recipients (0.46%-3.0%), followed by heart (0.24%-2.8%), kidney (0.16%-0.38%) and liver (0.04%) recipients with MAC and *M abscessus* the most frequent NTM species.[39–45] The risk of NTM infection in SOT is often associated with the intensity of immunosuppression, structural abnormalities, and environmental exposure, which results in lung transplantation being associated with the highest risk.[39] In one case-control study evaluating 34 SOT recipients, both lung transplantation (OR = 11.5) and acute rejection (OR = 4) were statistically significantly associated with NTM infection.[46] In addition, diagnosis and management become more challenging in this population given nonspecific symptoms, more diverse sites of infection, drug interactions and toxicity. Similarly, in a larger, multinational case-control study including 85 SOT cases with NTM infections between 2008 and 2018, receipt of lymphocyte-specific antibodies (OR = 7.73; 95% CI, 1.07–56.14), antifungals (OR = 5.35; 95% CI, 1.7–16.91), hospital admission within 90 days (OR = 3.14; 95% CI, 1.41–6.98) and older age at SOT (OR = 1.04; 95% CI, 1.01–1.07), were statistically associated with NTM infection in a multivariable analysis.[47]

Longworth and colleagues published a retrospective, single-center cohort study evaluating 3-year mortality in 33 patients following SOT with NTM infection, with a focus on *M abscessus* versus other NTM species.[48] Time to infection following transplantation was bimodal, with approximately half the patients diagnosed with NTM within the first year.[48] No statistically significant difference in survival was observed between NTM species, however for those diagnosed with NTM disease within the first year post-SOT, 50% had died at 3 years compared to only 13% of those without diagnosed NTM disease.[48] In an evaluation of 375 lung transplant recipients at the University of Alberta, 5-year mortality was higher in those diagnosed with NTM disease post-transplantation ($P = .016$), but no statistically significant difference was seen with regards to allograft dysfunction.[49] In contrast, a meta-analysis noted both increased chronic lung allograft dysfunction (HR 2.11, 95% CI 1.03–4.35) and mortality (HR 2.69, 95% CI 1.70–4.26) in lung transplant recipients identified with NTM disease.[50]

Hematopoietic Stem Cell Transplant

Allogeneic hematopoietic stem cell transplant (HSCT) recipients are at an increased risk of opportunistic infections due to impaired cellular immunity from their underlying disease, myeloablative conditioning regimens, and graft-versus-host disease (GVHD).[51,52] The incidence of NTM infections in HSCT recipients is 50 to 600 times greater than the general population.[53,54] A 2018 retrospective study from Canada found the incidence to be 2.8% at 5 years post-HSCT.[51] The majority of patients in this study, 28/30 (93.3%), had a pulmonary site of infection while 2/30 (6.7%) had disseminated disease.[51] The significant risk factors were chronic GVHD and Cytomegalovirus (CMV) viremia.[51] While *Mycobacterium avium* complex is the most commonly reported species in HSCT recipients, other species commonly identified are *Mycobacterium fortuitum, M abscessus, Mycobacterium haemophilum*, and *Mycobacterium chelonae*.[42,43,51,55,56] Lung, skin, and catheter-related sites are the most common sites of infection.[42,56] The median time for an NTM infection to occur is 5 months (range, 3–11 months) following HSCT.[42,54] NTM infection should be considered in the differential diagnosis of HSCT recipients with central venous catheters (CVCs), skin lesions, pulmonary, joint and bone, or gastrointestinal disease.[42] Recent studies have identified NTM infections resulting from a contaminated water supply in the pediatric HSCT population.[53,57,58] Rapid growing mycobacteria were identified and traced back to the hospital drinking water/ice machines and inappropriate CVC care.[53,58] These incidences led to extra precautionary measures in patients with HSCT such as drinking bottled water and semi-permeable dressings to protect the CVC while patients are showering/bathing at home.[53,57] The reported mortality varies greatly in those with NTM disease post-HSCT, ranging from 7.5% to 50%.[43,51,52,59]

Primary Immunodeficiency Diseases

A variety of primary immunodeficiency diseases can increase the risk for NTM disease including chronic granulomatous disease, common variable immune deficiency, and hypogammaglobulinemia and other errors in the function of GATA2, IL-12, IFN gamma and TNF-alpha.[60–64] These are commonly associated with recurrent and disseminated NTM infections earlier in life.[63] Disseminated NTM disease in adults without HIV or immunosuppressive exposure should raise the suspicion for autoantibodies directed against IFN gamma or TNF-alpha.[65–70]

IMMUNOSUPPRESSIVE THERAPIES
Corticosteroids

Both systemic and inhaled corticosteroids (ICS) are used to treat a variety of inflammatory conditions, such as rheumatoid arthritis (RA), asthma, and COPD. Patients treated with oral corticosteroids are found to be at increased risk for both TB infection, with as much as a 5-fold increase in risk compared to those not receiving corticosteroids, and NTM infections, with a multicenter study case-control reporting use of oral prednisone was 8-fold higher in patients with MAC lung disease than those without.[71,72] ICS have also been shown to increase risk of NTM pulmonary infection.[73–75] In a case-control study of patients with either asthma, COPD or bronchiectasis, use of ICS was associated with significant increase in risk for pulmonary NTM infection (OR 2.51; 95% CI 1.40–4.49, $P < .01$).[73] Additionally, in a retrospective review of 268 patients with Sjögren's Syndrome, those treated with ICS resulted in higher rates of pulmonary NTM disease, although this difference did not reach statistical significance (45.0% vs 31.3%, $P = .07$).[75] In a study of patients with asthma, those with severe limitation in airflow, older age and higher doses of inhaled corticosteroids were at increased risk for NTM infections.[73]

Tumor Necrosis Factor Alpha Inhibitors

Tumor necrosis factor (TNF) alpha is a proinflammatory cytokine primarily produced by activated macrophages and is required for granuloma formation. Granuloma formation is key to the sequestration of mycobacterium and prevention of further dissemination.[76] Further, TNF-alpha induces endoplasmic reticulum stress response leading to apoptosis of mycobacterium infected macrophages.[77] Current US Food and Drug Administration (FDA) approved TNF-alpha inhibitors used in the treatment of various autoimmune diseases include adalimumab, certolizumab, etanercept, golimumab, and infliximab. In a review of more than 200 FDA MedWatch database reports, NTM infections were associated with a variety of these therapies, although most patients were receiving corticosteroids and methotrexate concurrently with the TNF-alpha inhibitor. Most commonly associated was MAC (50%) and extrapulmonary involvement was higher than in the general population at 44%.[78] Among a Kaiser Permanente Northern California cohort, TNF-alpha inhibitor exposure was associated with a higher incidence of NTM infection (74 per 100,000 person-years, 95% CI 37–111) compared to unexposed patients with rheumatoid arthritis (19.2 per 100,000 person-years, 95% CI 14.2–25.0) and the general

population (4.1 per 100,000 person-years, 95% CI 3.9–4.4).[79] A retrospective review of patients receiving TNF-alpha inhibitors in South Korea reported a rate of NTM infection higher than in the general population (230.7 per 100,000 patients per year).[80] Another retrospective review from South Korea identified a similar rate of NTM infection in those patients exposed to TNF-alpha inhibitors but found all of these cases to be pulmonary and the majority in patients with RA (83.3%).[81] A more recent retrospective cohort study conducted in South Korea compared rates of NTM disease in patients with untreated rheumatoid arthritis versus those receiving treatment with anti-TNF-alpha agents. For the more than 5400 patients included, rates of NTM were higher in those patients receiving TNF-alpha inhibitors than those with untreated RA (328.1 vs 187.4 per 100,000 patient years; adjusted HR 1.751, 95%CI 1.105–2.774).[82] Further, the risk of NTM was higher after anti-TNF-alpha therapy for patients aged 50 to 65 (aHR 2.018, 95% CI 1.062–3.833) and for females (aHR 2.108, 95% CI 1.287–3.453). The median duration from the start of anti-TNF-alpha therapy to the development of NTM infection was 29.4 months.[82]

Anti-interleukin 6 Monoclonal Antibody, Anti-interleukin 12/23 Monoclonal Antibody

A number of other biologic agents are commonly used in the treatment of autoimmune diseases, such as anti-interleukin 6 monoclonal antibody (tocilizumab) and anti-interleukin 12/23 monoclonal antibody (ustekinumab). While there is theoretic risk for infection and case reports of the development of NTM infections of patients on these biologics have been published, the literature is lacking any observational data to suggest the rate at which these agents increase risk of NTM infection.[83–85] However, several publications have suggested elevated rates of *Mycobacterium tuberculosis* (TB) with these agents, indicating ongoing evaluation is needed.[86,87]

Janus Kinase Inhibitors

Janus kinase (JAK) inhibitors such as tofacitinib, baricitinib, upadacitinib, and fligotinib are oral medications used in the treatment of rheumatoid arthritis. JAK1, JAK2, and JAK3 play complex roles in targeting various cytokine pathways in the JAK-STAT signaling pathway. Inhibition of JAK, especially more than one of these proteins, impacts immune responses.[88] Tofacitinib has been shown in mouse models to reduce the containment of TB.[89] A review of available RCTs assessing active TB occurrence during treatment with these four JAK inhibitors found a relatively low rate (0.25%) of active TB, although patients were screened for TB prior trial entry.[88] The majority of the identified TB cases occurred in countries with intermediate or high risk for TB and rates were higher than the background rate for the country.[88] While the rate of TB infection appears low, data on rates of NTM infection during treatment with JAK inhibitors is limited and larger studies are needed. Several case reports, however, have been reported in the literature.[90–92]

Immune Checkpoint Inhibitors

Used for many types of malignancies, programmed cell death-1/programmed cell death ligand-1 (PD-1/PD- L1) inhibitors, including nivolumab, pembrolizumab, atezolizumab, durvalumab and avelumab, have been implicated as risk factors for mycobacterial infections, initially with a case report of tuberculosis in 2016.[93–99] In a retrospective review of the FDA Adverse Events Reporting System (FAERS) between 2015 and 2020, Anand and colleagues identified 72 cases of tuberculosis and 13 cases of nontuberculous mycobacterial infections with an elevated odds ratio for exposure to PD-1/PD-L1 inhibitors compared to all other drugs (TB OR 1.79, NTM OR 5.49).[92] Sites of NTM infections included pulmonary, endocrine, gastrointestinal, and skin and soft tissue.[93] In 2 large studies evaluating the relationship between PD-1/PD-L1 exposure and active TB in South Korea, incidence was higher in the PD-1/PD-L1 group but did not reach statistical significance.[100,101] Additional case reports of NTM infections have been reported, primarily with MAC, however published data also suggest augmented IFN-gamma in the setting of PD-1 inhibition.[102–108] Data from larger controlled studies evaluating NTM in the setting of PD-1/PD-L1 inhibitor exposure are not available and are needed to fully assess the risk and potential benefits.

MANAGEMENT IN THE SETTING OF IMMUNOSUPPRESSION

Overall, treatment is NTM species-specific and antibiotics should be chosen based on antimicrobial susceptibilities. Some basic principles are important to consider given the long duration of therapy and increased potential for drug interactions, side effects, and toxicity in many of these populations.

1. Given NTM are often colonizers and ubiquitous in the environment, it is important to ensure criteria for NTM disease are met prior to initiating therapy. For extrapulmonary disease, diagnostic samples should be obtained from a sterile site and pathology, along with cultures and molecular testing should be sent if skin and soft tissue infection is suspected. For pulmonary disease, patients should meet microbiologic, radiographic and symptom criteria per American Thoracic Society (ATS)/Infectious Disease Society of America (IDSA) guidelines for NTM pulmonary disease.[1] Of note, at least one single-center study in Arizona identified that among lung transplant recipients, only 34.5% of NTM pulmonary infections and 50% of NTM pulmonary infections that were treated at their institution met ATS/IDSA criteria with 90% of the treated group experiencing adverse events and drug-drug interactions.[109] Similarly, a study evaluating NTM isolation following predominantly lung SOT in St. Louis, MO, found 41.8% with NTM isolation were treated but only 13.9% met ATS/IDSA disease criteria.[41] NTM isolation was not associated with increased mortality, however mortality was higher in those who met ATS/IDSA disease criteria (hazard ratio, 7.0; 95% CI, 1.5–31.5).[41] Similar results were observed in a meta-analysis, where NTM disease but not isolation was associated with mortality and chronic lung allograft dysfunction among lung transplant recipients.[50]

2. Antimicrobial therapy should be guided by culture results and antimicrobial susceptibilities and involve 2 or more agents to prevent the development of drug resistance.[1] In general, the selection of agents in the immunocompromised population is the same as treating a patient in the general population. However, some additional considerations, especially in transplant recipients or patients living with HIV, include the use of rifabutin instead of rifampin, and the use of azithromycin instead of clarithromycin due to drug interactions.[1,42,110,111] Rifamycins are potent cytochrome (CYP) P450 inducers and clarithromycin is a CYP450 inhibitor.[1,29,39,111] A drug interactions check should be completed before initiating these antimicrobials and close drug monitoring is needed, especially of calcineurin and mTOR inhibitors. In addition, gastrointestinal absorption may be reduced in the setting of underlying disease, oral intolerance due to chemotherapy or co-infections (eg, CMV gastroenteritis). If this is a concern, therapeutic drug monitoring and transition to intravenous antibiotics should be considered.[112,113]

3. Whenever feasible, immunosuppression should be reduced or changed, especially in the setting of TNF-alpha inhibitors or corticosteroids.[39,42,79,114] As with all mycobacterial infections, symptoms can often worsen 4 to 8 weeks

following therapy initiation due to an inflammatory response and this may be more pronounced or delayed depending on type of immunosuppression and timing of reduction in relation to antibiotic initiation.[112,115] If progression continues, especially if an acute change is seen, there should be a low threshold to evaluate for other contributing etiologies.

SUMMARY

Those with reduced cell mediated immunity and exposure to immunosuppressive agents, especially TNF-alpha inhibitors are at increased risk for pulmonary and extrapulmonary NTM infections with MAC and *M abscessus* the most common species. Where data are available in these specific populations, increased mortality is observed with NTM disease. Prior to starting therapy for NTM disease, providers should ensure diagnostic criteria are met as treatment is long and often associated with significant side effects and toxicities. Treatment should involve 2 to 4 agents and be guided by cultures and antimicrobial susceptibilities. Drug interactions are important to consider, especially in those with HIV or transplant recipients. Whenever possible, immunosuppression should be reduced or changed, particularly in the setting of TNF-alpha inhibitors.

CLINICS CARE POINT

- Prior to starting therapy for NTM disease, providers should ensure diagnostic criteria are met as colonization is common.
- Treatment is long, requiring 2-4 agents, and is often associated with significant drug interactions, side effects and toxicities.
- Whenever possible, immunosuppression should be reduced or changed, particularly in the setting of TNF-alpha inhibitors.

POTENTIAL CONFLICTS OF INTEREST

Dr K.L. Winthrop has research funding from Insmed, United States, Paratek Pharmaceuticals, Inc., Red Hill Biopharma, AN2 Therapeutics, Renovion, Inc., NTM Info and Research Inc. and serves as a consultant for Insmed Inc., Paratek Pharmaceuticals, Inc., Red Hill Biopharma, AN2 Therapeutics, Renovion, Inc. Dr C.D. Varley has research funding from NTM Info and Research Inc. Dr A.C. Streifel and Dr A.M. Bair report no conflicts of interest.

REFERENCES

1. Daley CL, Iaccarino JM, Lange C, et al. Treatment of Nontuberculous mycobacterial pulmonary disease: an Official ATS/ERS/ESCMID/IDSA clinical practice fuideline. Clin Inf Dis 2020;71(4):e1–36.
2. Griffith DE, Aksamit T, Brown-Elliott BA, et al. An official ATS/IDSA statement: diagnosis, treatment, and prevention of nontuberculous mycobacterial diseases. Am J Respir Crit Care Med 2007; 175(4):367–416.
3. Adjemian J, Olivier KN, Seitz AE, et al. Prevalence of nontuberculous mycobacterial lung disease in U.S. Medicare beneficiaries. Am J Respir Crit Care Med 2012;185(8):881–6.
4. Billinger ME, Olivier KN, Viboud C, et al. Nontuberculous mycobacteria-associated lung disease in hospitalized persons, United States, 1998-2005. Emerg Infect Dis 2009;15(10):1562–9.
5. Bodle EE, Cunningham JA, Della-Latta P, et al. Epidemiology of nontuberculous mycobacteria in patients without HIV infection, New York City. Emerg Infect Dis 2008;14(3):390–6.
6. Cassidy PM, Hedberg K, Saulson A, et al. Nontuberculous mycobacterial disease prevalence and risk factors: a changing epidemiology. Clin Infect Dis 2009;49(12):e124–9.
7. Henkle E, Hedberg K, Schafer S, et al. Population-based incidence of pulmonary nontuberculous mycobacterial disease in Oregon 2007 to 2012. Ann Am Thorac Soc 2015;12(5):642–7.
8. Marras TK, Vinnard C, Zhang Q, et al. Relative risk of all-cause mortality in patients with nontuberculous mycobacterial lung disease in a US managed care population. Respir Med 2018;145:80–8.
9. O'Brien RJ, Geiter LJ, Snider DE Jr. The epidemiology of nontuberculous mycobacterial diseases in the United States. Results from a national survey. Am Rev Respir Dis 1987;135(5):1007–14.
10. Prevots DR, Shaw PA, Strickland D, et al. Nontuberculous mycobacterial lung disease prevalence at four integrated health care delivery systems. Am J Respir Crit Care Med 2010;182(7):970–6.
11. Ringshausen FC, Wagner D, de Roux A, et al. Prevalence of nontuberculous mycobacterial pulmonary disease, Germany, 2009-2014. Emerg Infect Dis 2016;22(6):1102–5.
12. Winthrop KL, McNelley E, Kendall B, et al. Pulmonary nontuberculous mycobacterial disease prevalence and clinical features: an emerging public health disease. Am J Respir Crit Care Med 2010;182(7):977–82.
13. Winthrop KL, Marras TK, Adjemian J, et al. Incidence and prevalence of nontuberculous mycobacterial lung disease in a large U.S. managed care health plan, 2008-2015. Ann Am Thorac Soc 2020;17(2):178–85.

14. Prevots DR, Marras TK. Epidemiology of human pulmonary infection with nontuberculous mycobacteria: a review. Clin Chest Med 2015;36(1):13–34.

15. Schildkraut JA, Gallagher J, Morimoto K, et al. Epidemiology of nontuberculous mycobacterial pulmonary disease in Europe and Japan by Delphi estimation. Respir Med 2020;173:106164.

16. Wagner D, van Ingen J, Adjemian J, et al. Annual prevalence and treatment estimates of nontuberculous mycobacterial pulmonary disease in Europe: a NTM-NET collaborative study. Eur Respir J 2014; 44(Suppl 58):P1067.

17. Thomson RM, Furuya-Kanamori L, Coffey C, et al. Influence of climate variables on the rising incidence of nontuberculous mycobacterial (NTM) infections in Queensland, Australia 2001–2016. Sci Total Environ 2020;740:139796.

18. Freeman J, Morris A, Blackmore T, et al. Incidence of nontuberculous mycobacterial disease in New Zealand, 2004. NZMJ 2007;120(1256):50–6.

19. Marras T, Campitelli M, Lu H, et al. Pulmonary nontuberculous mycobacteria–associated deaths, Ontario, Canada, 2001–2013. Emerging Infectious Disease journal 2017;23(3):468.

20. Novosad SA, Henkle E, Schafer S, et al. Mortality after respiratory isolation of nontuberculous mycobacteria. A Comparison of patients who did and did not meet disease criteria. Ann Am Thorac Soc 2017;14(7):1112–9.

21. Vinnard C, Longworth S, Mezochow A, et al. Deaths related to nontuberculous mycobacterial infections in the United States, 1999–2014. Annals of the American Thoracic Society 2016;13(11): 1951–5.

22. Piersimoni C, Scarparo C. Extrapulmonary infections associated with nontuberculous mycobacteria in immunocompetent persons. Emerg Infect Dis 2009;15(9):1351–8 [quiz: 544].

23. Ricotta EE, Adjemian J, Blakney RA, et al. Extrapulmonary nontuberculous mycobacteria infections in hospitalized patients, United States, 2009-2014. Emerg Infect Dis 2021;27(3):845–52.

24. Shih DC, Cassidy PM, Perkins KM, et al. Extrapulmonary nontuberculous mycobacterial disease surveillance - Oregon, 2014-2016. MMWR Morbidity and mortality weekly report 2018;67(31):854–7.

25. Wentworth AB, Drage LA, Wengenack NL, et al. Increased incidence of cutaneous nontuberculous mycobacterial infection, 1980 to 2009: a population-based study. Mayo Clin Proc 2013;88(1):38–45.

26. Karakousis PC, Moore RD, Chaisson RE. Mycobacterium avium complex in patients with HIV infection in the era of highly active antiretroviral therapy. Lancet Infect Dis 2004;4(9):557–65.

27. Varley CD, Ku JH, Henkle E, et al. Disseminated nontuberculous mycobacteria in HIV-infected patients, Oregon, USA, 2007-2012. Emerg Infect Dis 2017;23(3):533–5.

28. Gordin FM, Cohn DL, Sullam PM, et al. Early manifestations of disseminated Mycobacterium avium complex disease: a prospective evaluation. The Journal of infectious diseases 1997;176(1):126–32.

29. Panel on Guidelines for the Prevention and Treatment of Opportunistic Infections in Adults and Adolescents with HIV: National Institutes of Health CfDCaP, HIV Medicine Association, and Infectious Diseases Society of America. Guidelines for the Prevention and Treatment of Opportunistic Infections in Adults and Adolescents with HIV. 2019 12/16/2022. Available at: https://clinicalinfo.hiv.gov/en/guidelines/adult-and-adolescent-opportunistic-infection.

30. Phillips P, Bonner S, Gataric N, et al. Nontuberculous mycobacterial immune reconstitution syndrome in HIV-infected patients: spectrum of disease and long-term follow-up. Clin Infect Dis 2005;41(10):1483–97.

31. Currier JS, Williams PL, Koletar SL, et al. Discontinuation of Mycobacterium avium complex prophylaxis in patients with antiretroviral therapy-induced increases in CD4+ cell count. A randomized, double-blind, placebo-controlled trial. AIDS Clinical Trials Group 362 Study Team. Annals of internal medicine 2000;133(7):493–503.

32. Dworkin MS, Hanson DL, Kaplan JE, et al. Risk for preventable opportunistic infections in persons with AIDS after antiretroviral therapy increases CD4+ T lymphocyte counts above prophylaxis thresholds. The Journal of infectious diseases 2000;182(2):611–5.

33. El-Sadr WM, Burman WJ, Grant LB, et al. Discontinuation of prophylaxis against Mycobacterium avium complex disease in HIV-infected patients who have a response to antiretroviral therapy. Terry Beirn Community Programs for Clinical Research on AIDS. N Engl J Med 2000;342(15):1085–92.

34. Havlir DV, Dube MP, Sattler FR, et al. Prophylaxis against disseminated Mycobacterium avium complex with weekly azithromycin, daily rifabutin, or both. California Collaborative Treatment Group. N Engl J Med 1996;335(6):392–8.

35. Pierce M, Crampton S, Henry D, et al. A randomized trial of clarithromycin as prophylaxis against disseminated Mycobacterium avium complex infection in patients with advanced acquired immunodeficiency syndrome. N Engl J Med 1996; 335(6):384–91.

36. Yangco BG, Buchacz K, Baker R, et al. Is primary mycobacterium avium complex prophylaxis necessary in patients with CD4 <50 cells/muL who are virologically suppressed on cART? AIDS patient care and STDs 2014;28(6):280–3.

37. Tarashi S, Siadat SD, Fateh A. Nontuberculous mycobacterial resistance to antibiotics and Disinfectants: Challenges Still Ahead. BioMed Res Int 2022;2022:8168750.

38. Gardner EM, Burman WJ, DeGroote MA, et al. Conventional and molecular epidemiology of macrolide resistance among new Mycobacterium avium complex isolates recovered from HIV-infected patients. Clin Infect Dis 2005;41(7):1041–4.

39. Abad CL, Razonable RR. Non-tuberculous mycobacterial infections in solid organ transplant recipients: an update. J Clin Tuberc Other Mycobact Dis 2016;4:1–8.

40. Anjan S, Morris MI. Nontuberculous mycobacteria in solid organ transplant. Curr Opin Organ Transplant 2019;24(4):476–82.

41. George IA, Santos CA, Olsen MA, et al. Epidemiology and outcomes of nontuberculous mycobacterial infections in solid organ transplant recipients at a Midwestern center. Transplantation 2016;100(5):1073–8.

42. Knoll BM. Update on nontuberculous mycobacterial infections in solid organ and hematopoietic stem cell transplant recipients. Curr Infect Dis Rep 2014;16(9):421.

43. Pena T, Klesney-Tait J. Mycobacterial infections in solid organ and hematopoietic stem cell transplantation. Clin Chest Med 2017;38(4):761–70.

44. Yoo JW, Jo KW, Kim SH, et al. Incidence, characteristics, and treatment outcomes of mycobacterial diseases in transplant recipients. Transpl Int 2016;29(5):549–58.

45. Longworth SA, Daly JS, Practice ASTIDCo. Management of infections due to nontuberculous mycobacteria in solid organ transplant recipients-Guidelines from the American Society of Transplantation Infectious Diseases Community of Practice. Clin Transplant 2019;33(9):e13588.

46. Longworth SA, Vinnard C, Lee I, et al. Risk factors for nontuberculous mycobacterial infections in solid organ transplant recipients: a case-control study.2014. Transpl Infect Dis 2014;16(1):76–83.

47. Mejia-Chew C, Carver PL, Rutjanawech S, et al. Risk factors for nontuberculous mycobacteria infections in solid organ transplant recipients: a multinational case-control study. Clin Infect Dis 2023;76(3):e995-e1003.

48. Longworth SA, Blumberg EA, Barton TD, et al. Non-tuberculous mycobacterial infections after solid organ transplantation: a survival analysis. Clin Microbiol Infection 2015;21(1):43–7.

49. Friedman DZP, Cervera C, Halloran K, et al. Non-tuberculous mycobacteria in lung transplant recipients: prevalence, risk factors, and impact on survival and chronic lung allograft dysfunction. Transpl Infect Dis 2020;22(2):e13229.

50. Marty PK, Yetmar ZA, Gerberi DJ, et al. Risk factors and outcomes of non-tuberculous mycobacteria infection in lung transplant recipients: a systematic review and meta-analysis. J Heart Lung Transplant 2023;42(2):264–74.

51. Beswick J, Shin E, Michelis FV, et al. Incidence and risk factors for nontuberculous mycobacterial infection after allogeneic hematopoietic cell transplantation. Biol Blood Marrow Transplant 2018;24(2):366–72.

52. Hirama T, Brode SK, Beswick J, et al. Characteristics, treatment and outcomes of nontuberculous mycobacterial pulmonary disease after allogeneic haematopoietic stem cell transplant. Eur Respir J 2018;51(5):05.

53. Habermann S, Ferran E, Hatcher J, et al. Outbreak of non-tuberculous mycobacteria in a paediatric bone marrow transplant unit associated with water contamination of needle-free connectors and literature review. Bone Marrow Transplant 2021;56(9):2305–8.

54. Wobma H, Chang AK, Jin Z, et al. Low CD4 count may be a risk factor for non-tuberculous mycobacteria infection in pediatric hematopoietic cell transplant recipients. Pediatr Transplant 2021;25(4):e13994.

55. Karri PV, Torres CA, Dailey Garnes NJ, et al. Disseminated atypical mycobacterial infection in an allogeneic stem cell transplant recipient. Dermatol Online J 2021;27(6):15.

56. Moreno-Bonilla G, Choy B, Fernandez-Penas P. Cutaneous non-tuberculous mycobacterial infection in patients with chronic graft-versus-host disease: a case series. Australas J Dermatol 2015;56(2):124–7.

57. Guspiel A, Menk J, Streifel A, et al. Management of risks from water and ice from ice machines for the Very immunocompromised host: a Process Improvement Project Prompted by an Outbreak of rapidly growing mycobacteria on a pediatric hematopoietic stem cell transplant (Hsct) Unit. Infect Control Hosp Epidemiol 2017;38(7):792–800.

58. Iroh Tam PY, Kline S, Wagner JE, et al. Rapidly growing mycobacteria among pediatric hematopoietic cell transplant patients traced to the hospital water supply. Pediatr Infect Dis J 2014;33(10):1043–6.

59. Kang JY, Ha JH, Kang HS, et al. Clinical significance of nontuberculous mycobacteria from respiratory specimens in stem cell transplantation recipients. Int J Hematol 2015;101(5):505–13.

60. Haverkamp MH, van de Vosse E, van Dissel JT. Nontuberculous mycobacterial infections in children with inborn errors of the immune system. J Infect 2014;68(Suppl 1):S134–50.

61. Marciano BE, Olivier KN, Folio LR, et al. Pulmonary manifestations of GATA2 deficiency. Chest 2021;160(4):1350–9.

62. Mika T, Vangala D, Eckhardt M, et al. Case report: Hemophagocytic Lymphohistiocytosis and nontuberculous Mycobacteriosis caused by a Novel GATA2 variant. Front Immunol 2021;12:682934.

63. Lee WI, Huang JL, Yeh KW, et al. Immune defects in active mycobacterial diseases in patients with primary immunodeficiency diseases (PIDs). J Formos Med Assoc 2011;110(12):750–8.

64. Sexton P, Harrison AC. Susceptibility to nontuberculous mycobacterial lung disease. Eur Respir J 2008;31(6):1322–33.

65. Kampmann B, Hemingway C, Stephens A, et al. Acquired predisposition to mycobacterial disease due to autoantibodies to IFN-gamma. J Clin Invest 2005;115(9):2480–8.

66. Lin YF, Lee TF, Wu UI, et al. Disseminated Mycobacterium chimaera infection in a patient with adult-onset immunodeficiency syndrome: case report. BMC Infect Dis 2022;22(1):665.

67. Yeh Y-K, Ding J-Y, Ku C-L, et al. Disseminated *Mycobacterium avium* complex infection mimicking malignancy in a patient with anti-IFN-γ autoantibodies: a case report. BMC Infect Dis 2019;19(1):909.

68. Harada M, Furuhashi K, Karayama M, et al. Subcutaneous injection of interferon gamma therapy could be useful for anti–IFN-γ autoantibody associated disseminated nontuberculous mycobacterial infection. J Infect Chemother 2021;27(2):373–8.

69. Kireev FD, Lopatnikova JA, Laushkina ZA, et al. Autoantibodies to tumor necrosis factor in patients with active pulmonary tuberculosis. Front Biosci (Landmark Ed) 2022;27(4):133.

70. Browne SK, Burbelo PD, Chetchotisakd P, et al. Adult-Onset immunodeficiency in Thailand and Taiwan. N Engl J Med 2012;367(8):725–34.

71. Dirac MA, Horan KL, Doody DR, et al. Environment or host? Am J Respir Crit Care Med 2012;186(7):684–91.

72. Jick SS, Lieberman ES, Rahman MU, et al. Glucocorticoid use, other associated factors, and the risk of tuberculosis. Arthritis Rheum 2006;55(1):19–26.

73. Hojo M, Iikura M, Hirano S, et al. Increased risk of nontuberculous mycobacterial infection in asthmatic patients using long-term inhaled corticosteroid therapy. Respirology 2012;17(1):185–90.

74. Liu VX, Winthrop KL, Lu Y, et al. Association between inhaled corticosteroid Use and pulmonary nontuberculous mycobacterial infection. Ann Am Thorac Soc 2018;15(10):1169–76.

75. Weingart MF, Li Q, Choi S, et al. Analysis of non-TB mycobacterial lung disease in patients with primary Sjögren's syndrome at a Referral center. Chest 2021;159(6):2218–21.

76. Gardam MA, Keystone EC, Menzies R, et al. Antitumour necrosis factor agents and tuberculosis risk: mechanisms of action and clinical management. Lancet Infect Dis 2003;3(3):148–55.

77. Oh SM, Lim YJ, Choi JA, et al. TNF-α-mediated ER stress causes elimination of Mycobacterium fortuitum reservoirs by macrophage apoptosis. Faseb j 2018;32(7):3993–4003.

78. KL W, E C, S Y, et al. Nontuberculosis mycobacteria infections and anti-tumor necrosis factor-alpha therapy. Emerg Infect Dis 2009;1556–61.

79. Winthrop KL, Baxter R, Liu L, et al. Mycobacterial diseases and antitumour necrosis factor therapy in USA. Annals of the rheumatic diseases 2013;72(1):37–42.

80. Lee SK, Kim SY, Kim EY, et al. Mycobacterial infections in patients treated with tumor necrosis factor antagonists in South Korea. Lung 2013;191(5):565–71.

81. Yoo JW, Jo KW, Kang BH, et al. Mycobacterial diseases developed during anti-tumour necrosis factor-alpha therapy. Eur Respir J 2014;44(5):1289–95.

82. Park DW, Kim YJ, Sung YK, et al. TNF inhibitors increase the risk of nontuberculous mycobacteria in patients with seropositive rheumatoid arthritis in a mycobacterium tuberculosis endemic area. Sci Rep 2022;4003.

83. Kobayashi D, Ito S, Hirata A, et al. *Mycobacterium abscessus* pulmonary infection under treatment with tocilizumab. Intern Med 2015;54(10):1309–13.

84. Novosad SA, Winthrop KL. Beyond tumor necrosis factor inhibition: the Expanding Pipeline of biologic therapies for inflammatory diseases and their associated infectious Sequelae. Clin Infect Dis 2014;58(11):1587–98.

85. Shim HH, Cai SCS, Chan W, et al. Mycobacterium abscessus infection during Ustekinumab treatment in Crohn's disease: a case report and review of the literature. J Crohns Colitis 2018;12(12):1505–7.

86. Jung SM, Han M, Kim EH, et al. Comparison of developing tuberculosis following tumor necrosis factor inhibition and interleukin-6 inhibition in patients with rheumatoid arthritis: a nationwide observational study in South Korea, 2013–2018. Arthritis Res Ther 2022;24(1):157.

87. Koike T, Harigai M, Inokuma S, et al. Postmarketing surveillance of tocilizumab for rheumatoid arthritis in Japan: interim analysis of 3881 patients. Annals of the rheumatic diseases 2011;70(12):2148.

88. Cantini F, Blandizzi C, Niccoli L, et al. Systematic review on tuberculosis risk in patients with rheumatoid arthritis receiving inhibitors of Janus Kinases. Expet Opin Drug Saf 2020;19(7):861–72.

89. Maiga M, Ahidjo BA, Maiga MC, et al. Efficacy of Adjunctive tofacitinib therapy in mouse models of tuberculosis. EBioMedicine 2015;2(8):868–73.

90. Kerschbaumer A, Smolen JS, Nash P, et al. Points to consider for the treatment of immune-mediated inflammatory diseases with Janus kinase inhibitors: a systematic literature research. RMD Open 2020;6(3).

91. Winthrop KL, Harigai M, Genovese MC, et al. Infections in baricitinib clinical trials for patients with active rheumatoid arthritis. Annals of the rheumatic diseases 2020;79(10):1290–7.

92. Winthrop KL, Park SH, Gul A, et al. Tuberculosis and other opportunistic infections in tofacitinib-treated patients with rheumatoid arthritis. Annals of the rheumatic diseases 2016;75(6):1133–8.

93. Anand K, Sahu G, Burns E, et al. Mycobacterial infections due to PD-1 and PD-L1 checkpoint inhibitors. ESMO Open 2020;5(4):e000866.

94. Anastasopoulou A, Ziogas DC, Samarkos M, et al. Reactivation of tuberculosis in cancer patients following administration of immune checkpoint inhibitors: current evidence and clinical practice recommendations. Journal for immunotherapy of cancer 2019;7(1):239.

95. Barber DL, Mayer-Barber KD, Feng CG, et al. CD4 T cells promote rather than control tuberculosis in the absence of PD-1-mediated inhibition. J Immunol 2011;186(3):1598–607.

96. Chu Y-C, Fang K-C, Chen H-C, et al. Pericardial Tamponade caused by a Hypersensitivity response to tuberculosis reactivation after anti-PD-1 treatment in a patient with advanced pulmonary Adenocarcinoma. J Thorac Oncol 2017;12(8):e111–4.

97. Fujita K, Terashima T, Mio T. Anti-PD1 antibody treatment and the development of acute pulmonary tuberculosis. J Thorac Oncol 2016;11(12):2238–40.

98. Lee JJX, Chan A, Tang T. Tuberculosis reactivation in a patient receiving anti-programmed death-1 (PD-1) inhibitor for relapsed Hodgkin's lymphoma. Acta oncologica (Stockholm, Sweden) 2016;55(4): 519–20.

99. Sirgiovanni M, Hinterleitner C, Horger M, et al. Long-term remission of small cell lung cancer after reactivation of tuberculosis following immune-checkpoint blockade: a case report. Thoracic cancer 2021;12(5):699–702.

100. Bae S, Kim Y-J, Kim M-J, et al. Risk of tuberculosis in patients with cancer treated with immune checkpoint inhibitors: a nationwide observational study. Journal for immunotherapy of cancer 2021;9(9).

101. Kim HW, Kim JS, Lee SH. Incidence of tuberculosis in advanced lung cancer patients treated with immune checkpoint inhibitors - a nationwide population-based cohort study. Lung cancer (Amsterdam, Netherlands) 2021;158:107–14.

102. Baba K, Yoshida T, Shiotsuka M, et al. Rapid development of pulmonary Mycobacterium avium infection during chemoradiotherapy followed by durvalumab treatment in a locally advanced NSCLC patient. Lung Cancer 2021;153:182–3.

103. Chi C-Y, Yeh Y-C, Pan S-W. Cavitary Mycobacterium avium complex lung disease developed after

Immunotherapy. Arch Bronconeumol 2022;58(2): 174.

104. Fujita K, Yamamoto Y, Kanai O, et al. Development of Mycobacterium avium complex lung disease in patients with lung cancer on immune checkpoint inhibitors. Open Forum Infect Dis 2020;7(3):067.

105. Koyama T, Funakoshi Y, Imamura Y, et al. Device-related Mycobacterium mageritense infection in a patient treated with nivolumab for Metastatic Breast cancer. Internal Medicine 2021;60(21):3485–8.

106. Lombardi A, Gramegna A, Ori M, et al. Nontuberculous mycobacterial infections during cancer therapy with immune checkpoint inhibitors: a systematic review. ERJ Open Research 2022;8(4): 00364–2022.

107. Yamaba Y, Takakuwa O, Tomita Y, et al. Mycobacterium avium complex lung disease in a patient treated with an immune checkpoint inhibitor: a case report. Mol Clin Oncol 2022;16(2):37.

108. Ratnatunga CN, Tungatt K, Proietti C, et al. Characterizing and correcting immune dysfunction in nontuberculous mycobacterial disease. Front Immunol 2022;13:1047781.

109. Grimes R, Cherrier L, Nasar A, et al. Outcomes of nontuberculous mycobacteria isolation among lung transplant recipients: a matched case-control with retrospective cohort study. Am J Health Syst Pharm 2022;79(5):338–45.

110. Doucette K, Fishman JA. Nontuberculous mycobacterial infection in hematopoietic stem cell and solid organ transplant recipients. Clin Infect Dis 2004;38(10):1428–39.

111. Kendall BA, Varley CD, Choi D, et al. Distinguishing tuberculosis from nontuberculous mycobacteria lung disease, Oregon, USA. Emerg Infect Dis 2011;17(3):506–9.

112. Luke C, Strand KLW. Mycobacterium avium complex. In: John E, Bennett M, Raphael Dolin MD, et al, editors. Mandell, Douglas, and Bennett's principles and practice of infectious diseases. 9th edition. Philadelphia, PA: Elsevier; 2020. p. 3035–48.

113. Peloquin C. The role of therapeutic drug monitoring in mycobacterial infections. Microbiol Spectr 2017; 5(1).

114. Winthrop KL, Chiller T. Preventing and treating biologic-associated opportunistic infections. Nat Rev Rheumatol 2009;5(7):405–10.

115. Kobayashi M, Tsubata Y, Shiratsuki Y, et al. Nontuberculous Mycobacterium-associated immune reconstitution inflammatory syndrome in a non-HIV immunosuppressed patient. Respirology Case Reports 2022;10(3):e0918.

Host-Directed Therapy in Nontuberculous Mycobacterial Pulmonary Disease
Preclinical and Clinical Data Review

Ifeanyichukwu U. Anidi, MD, PhD[a],*, Kenneth N. Olivier, MD, MPH[b]

KEYWORDS

- Nontuberculous mycobacteria • *Mycobacterium avium* complex • *Mycobacterium abscessus*
- Host directed therapy

KEY POINTS

- Standard treatment of nontuberculous mycobacterial pulmonary disease (NTM-PD) involves a multi-drug antimicrobial regimen for at least 12 months.
- The length, complexity, and side effect profile of antibiotic therapy for NTM-PD pose significant difficulties for maintaining patient adherence.
- Physician adherence to NTM guidelines is also poor. Evaluation of physician NTM treatment practices has shown that only 13% of antibiotic regimens met ATS/IDSA guidelines.

INTRODUCTION

Standard treatment of nontuberculous mycobacterial pulmonary disease (NTM-PD) involves a multi-drug antimicrobial regimen for at least 12 months. The length, complexity, and side effect profile of antibiotic therapy for NTM-PD pose significant difficulties for maintaining patient adherence. Furthermore, physician adherence to NTM guidelines suffers for similar reasons to the extent that a study evaluating treatment approaches across multiple specialties found that only 13% of antibiotic regimens met ATS/IDSA guidelines.[1] For this reason, a great need exists for therapy that augments the current armamentarium of antimicrobial chemotherapeutics or provides an alternative approach for decreasing host mycobacterial burden. As our knowledge of the mechanisms driving protective responses to NTM-PD infections by mammalian hosts expand, these processes provide novel therapeutic targets. These agents, which are commonly referred to as host directed therapies (HDT) have the potential of providing the much-needed boost to the nontuberculous mycobacterial therapeutic pipeline. In this review, we will focus on translational research and clinical trial data that detail the creation of therapeutic modalities developed to improve host mechanical protection and immunologic responses to NTM-PD infection.

PREDOMINANT HOST DEFENSES TO PULMONARY MYCOBACTERIAL INFECTION
Mechanical

Mycobacterium avium complex (MAC), the most common NTM-PD organism, initiates respiratory infection when MAC bacilli adhere to human respiratory mucosa via the fibronectin attachment

a Pulmonary Division, National Heart, Lung and Blood Institute, National Institutes of Health, 33 North Drive, Room 1W10A, Bethesda, MD 20892, USA; b Division of Pulmonary Diseases and Critical Care Medicine, University of North Carolina School of Medicine, 125 Mason Farm Road, CB#7248, 7214 Marsico Hall, Chapel Hill, NC 27599-7248, USA
* Corresponding author.
E-mail address: ifeanyichukwu.anidi@nih.gov

Clin Chest Med 44 (2023) 839–845
https://doi.org/10.1016/j.ccm.2023.07.004
0272-5231/23/Published by Elsevier Inc.

protein (FAP) when the mucosa is damaged. FAP on the surface of MAC mediates this interaction by binding to integrin receptors on the surface bronchial epithelial cells.[2] Healthy adults produce between 10 and 100 mL of airway secretions per day in order to maintain the air-liquid interface of the lungs.[3] This airway lining fluid is made of a number of lipids, proteoglycans, glycoproteins (eg, mucins), secretory IgA immunoglobulins, surfactant, and other substances. Though the airway epithelium contains a diversity of cell populations contributing to the production of these mediators, only the ciliated columnar cells and secretory cells such as goblet cells contribute to mucociliary function. Airway cilia are spontaneously active and beat in a coordinated fashion with cycles of resting, followed by effective, then recovery strokes.[4] Thus, at the level of the bronchial epithelium, motile cilia transport airway lining fluid with trapped material, including bound bacteria, out of the lungs, serving as a frontline of defense against NTM-PD. For this reason, the repair or augmentation of host mucociliary clearance at the level of the bronchial epithelium has become a primary HDT strategy against NTM-PD.

Immunological

As with many infectious insults to the human lung, the coordinated immune response to nontuberculous mycobacteria can be generally subdivided into innate and adaptive phases. The initial identification of a NTM pulmonary infection by the human innate immune response often occurs via the recognition of mycobacterial pathogen-associated molecular patterns (PAMPs) by innate immune mediators. Many such PAMPs are opsonized with complement proteins or immunoglobulins. The glycolipid and glycopeptidolipid components of the mycobacterial cell wall conjugate pattern recognition receptors (PRRs) on monocytes and macrophages. Phagocytosis of NTM bacilli will subsequently occur by opsonized and non-opsonized mechanisms. IFN-γ serves as the main cytokine stimulus to monocytes and macrophages to proceed with phagolysosome and autophagosome maturation necessary for mycobacterial killing. Phagolysosome maturation leads to the production of potent bactericidal molecules such as nitric oxide (NO) and reactive oxygen species.[5] Intertwined with the innate immune response, incorporation of adaptive immune cell populations occurs when IL-12 produced from infected macrophages and other antigen-presenting cells activate T lymphocytes and natural killer (NK) cells to divide and produce IFN-γ. Furthermore, CD4 and CD8 T cells recognize

mycobacterial peptides presented on MHCII and MHCI respectively, which leads to the secretion of proinflammatory cytokines IFN-y and TNF-α. This Th1 polarized cytokine production by T and NK cells is critical for NTM infection control as it promotes macrophage activation and mycobacterial killing.[6] Though there exists much greater complexity in the human immune response to NTM-PD, the majority of immunological HDTs that have been developed focus on the interplay needed between myeloid cells and T lymphocytes to protect hosts both acutely and over the lifetime of the infection.

AUGMENTING HOST MECHANICAL DEFENSES TO NTM
CFTR modulators

Dysfunction of the cystic fibrosis transmembrane conductance regulator (CFTR) protein results in a decrease or loss of chloride secretion across epithelial cells leading to dysregulated mucus development and clearance in the lungs, GI tract, reproductive organs, and more. Due to this deficit at the air liquid interface of the bronchial epithelium, patients with cystic fibrosis (CF) have a significantly increased risk of NTM-PD, in addition to other pathogenic bacteria responsible for acute and chronic lung infections.[7] Beyond the lack of effective mucociliary clearance, there is evidence that CFTR impairment also leads to innate immunological defects such as reduced phagocyte reactive oxygen species production necessary for myeloid-mediated mycobacterial clearance or neutrophil chemotaxis to sites of infection.[8] The advent of the CFTR potentiator drug, ivacaftor, which increases the probability of CFTR channel opening at the cell surface to enhance ion transport, has been pivotal in decreasing airway epithelial dysfunction in CF lungs.[9] The combination of ivacaftor with corrector drugs, which enhance the cellular processing and trafficking of normal and mutated CFTR protein in order to increase the amount of functional CFTR at the cell surface (eg, lumacaftor, tezacaftor, elexacaftor), has led to significant improvement in lung function among patients with CF.[10,11] This improvement in endobronchial mucociliary clearance and pulmonary function by CFTR modulator use has been shown to be beneficial in reducing the burden of pathogenic bacteria commonly afflicting patients with CF including nontuberculous mycobacteria.[12] Furthermore, Ricotta and colleagues[13] demonstrated that CFTR modulator use, either Ivacaftor monotherapy or combination therapy, is associated with reduced NTM sputum culture positivity and delayed time to culture positivity as compared to individuals not receiving therapy. These data provide disease-specific evidence of the significant protective benefits obtained via chemotherapeutic augmentation of host mechanical mucociliary clearance as preventative treatment of NTM-PD. It is unknown whether these drugs may also have a beneficial role in patients with monoallelic mutations or no mutations in the *CFTR* gene.

Sildenafil

Apart from CF disease, patients with NTM-PD alone have been found to exhibit respiratory ciliary dysfunction. Infection of primary human bronchial epithelial cells with MAC or *Mycobacterium abscessus* (MAB) in vitro leads to the downregulation of genes related to ciliary movement, assembly, and organization.[14] Additionally, whole-exome sequencing of a cohort of patients with NTM-PD revealed significantly more cilia-related gene variants as compared to age-matched controls.[15] When evaluated more specifically, respiratory epithelium from patients with NTM-PD had consistently lower resting ciliary beat frequency (CBF) when compared to normal human bronchial epithelial cells. Patients with NTM-PD also display lower nasal levels of nitric oxide which has been linked to ciliary dysfunction and is important not only in pulmonary artery pressures but also tissue repair and direct toxic effects on respiratory pathogens. However, the low CBF found on the respiratory epithelium of patients with NTM-PD can be normalized with the augmentation of the NO-cylic guanosine monophosphate (cGMP) pathway in vitro.[16] This modulation of the NO-cGMP pathway can be accomplished with the drug, sildenafil, which increases intracellular concentrations of cGMP through selective inhibition of cGMP phosphodiesterase type 5. The stimulatory effect of sildenafil on respiratory cilia was further confirmed in vivo as oral administration of the drug to a small cohort of patients with NTM-PD led to increased CBF on collected primary human respiratory epithelial cells after one dose and was sustained with repeated dosing.[17] It is not known whether this increase in CBF correlates with the enhancement of airway clearance and in this cohort over a 30-day period there was no measured change in sputum production, nasal nitric oxide production or respiratory symptom questionnaires. It may be that the ciliary abnormalities in NTM-PD are modest in nature and do not contribute to disease on the level of patient symptoms or quality of life. Longer term studies in larger numbers of patients are needed to determine whether chemotherapeutic modulation of the NO-cGMP pathway results in any clinically significant change in the course of NTM-PD.

AUGMENTING HOST IMMUNOLOGIC DEFENSES TO NTM
IFN-γ

Throughout the history of evaluation of the mammalian host immune response during NTM disease several studies have detailed the importance of the proinflammatory cytokine, interferon-γ (IFN-γ), in both the innate and adaptive responses to mycobacterial infection. Mutations in the IFN-γ receptor that result in the dysfunction of the IL-12/IFN-γ axis lead to susceptibility to disseminated NTM disease.[18] Additionally, autoantibodies to IFN-γ have been isolated as the immunological culprit of disease in individuals with unusual presentations of disseminated and pulmonary NTM infection.[19,20] These data strongly suggest that the disruption of the IL-12/IFN-γ axis interferes with the natural immune response to mycobacterial infection. For this reason, systemic administration of IFN-γ in combination with antibiotics has been trialed and found to have some promise as adjuvant therapy in specific patients with disseminated and pulmonary NTM disease. When Squires and colleagues[21] treated 2 patients with HIV and disseminated MAC disease with intravenous or subcutaneous administration of recombinant IFN-γ in addition to anti-mycobacterial drugs, they noted a decrease in MAC CFU recovered from peripheral blood during treatment and a paradoxical increase in blood bacillary burden once the IFN-γ was discontinued. Holland and colleagues[22] subsequently demonstrated that subcutaneous administration of IFN-γ to 7 HIV-negative patients with refractory disseminated NTM disease resulted in the radiographic abatement of lesions and clinical improvement. In order to evaluate the role of systemic IFN-γ in NTM-PD, Milanes-Virelles and colleagues. assessed the efficacy of intramuscular IFN-γ as adjuvant therapy to antimicrobial drugs in 18 patients with NTM-PD. Though they found that IFN-γ administration led to earlier improvement in respiratory symptoms and radiographic reduction of pulmonary lesions compared to placebo, additional corroborative studies are needed to determine if this is a viable adjunctive therapy for NTM-PD.[23]

Despite these studies supporting the adoption of systemic IFN-γ as a NTM-PD HDT, there is conflicting evidence regarding the benefits of inhaled IFN-γ as an adjuvant treatment. A case report of the effect of IFN-γ therapy via nebulization in an individual with pulmonary MAB disease refractory to antibiotic therapy demonstrated sputum culture conversion and mild improvement in pulmonary function post inhalational administration.[24] However, a randomized double-blind placebo-controlled trial of 91 patients with pulmonary MAC disease revealed that inhalational IFN-γ treatment was not related to any improvement in sputum culture conversion, radiographic disease or symptoms.[25] Though there is clear immunologic mechanistic clarity that IFN-y and its downstream mediators are essential components to mammalian host responses to pulmonary NTM infection, the complexity of innate and adaptive responses to mycobacterial antigens in NTM-PD appears to dilute any benefit that may be derived from the singular administration of this proinflammatory cytokine as adjuvant therapy. However, benefit does remain for systemic delivery of IFN-γ in patients with genetic defects of IL-12/IFN-γ signaling that result in disseminated NTM disease.

GM-CSF

Monocytes and macrophages are essential for the cell-mediated immune response to pulmonary NTM infection as they are the primary cell type to perform intracellular killing of mycobacterial bacilli. The alveolar macrophage specifically remains at the frontline of the local pulmonary immune response to NTM bacilli after infection is initiated upon the binding of NTM to bronchial epithelial cells. For these reasons, alveolar macrophages provide an intuitive target for enhancing the host response to pulmonary NTM infection.

Granulocyte-macrophage colony-stimulating factor (GM-CSF) is a glycoprotein produced by a variety of cell types including fibroblasts, endothelial cells, epithelial cells, mesothelial cells, T cells, and macrophages. It acts as a potent growth factor that stimulates the proliferation of myeloid progenitor cells and maturation of granulocytes (neutrophils and eosinophils) and monocytes/macrophages.[26] In light of its myeloid stimulatory effects, GM-CSF has been assessed and found to serve as a potentiator of macrophage antimycobacterial function in ex vivo settings. Human-derived alveolar macrophages stimulated with GM-CSF are able to restrict intracellular growth of MAC more so than when exposed to TNF-α, IFN-γ or IL-2.[27] Providing GM-CSF to monocytes derived from a patient infected with M. kansasii resulted in improved ex vivo inhibition of intracellular mycobacterial growth.[28] Similarly, the addition of GM-CSF to mycobacterial antibiotics augments the intracellular killing of MAC bacilli by human-derived macrophages.[29]

Despite the above ex vivo data, systemic administration of GM-CSF has yielded mixed results when used as an adjunct for the treatment of NTM-PD. A randomized trial in which 8 patients with HIV with disseminated MAC disease received azithromycin with or without subcutaneous GM-CSF revealed no difference in bacteremia between groups despite confirming increased reactive oxygen species production and monocyte-mediated suppression of MAC intracellular growth within the GM-CSF group.[30] However, there are selected case reports cataloguing patients with disseminated MAC disease who have derived clinical benefit from systemic GM-CSF augmentation of antibiotic therapy.[31,32] Despite the conflicting nature of the results, these findings paved the way for the evaluation of inhalational delivery of GM-CSF to provide more direct activation of alveolar macrophages interfacing with NTM bacilli during infection. In a small study of two patients with CF with MAB pulmonary infection Scott and colleagues[33] found that aerosolized GM-CSF in addition to antibiotics or alone led to clinical improvement (ie, an increase in forced expiratory volume in the first second (FEV1) and forced vital capacity (FVC)) and earlier sputum culture conversion after 4 to 6 months of therapy. Of note, an open-label phase 2 trial of the efficacy and safety of inhaled GM-CSF in 32 refractory NTM infections (both MAC and MAB) has been completed and finalized results are pending publication.[34] Overall, given the inconsistency in results supporting the use of systemic or inhalational GM-CSF as treatment for NTM infection, it will require continued investigation to determine which specific NTM-PD populations are most likely to benefit.

NTM-PD HDT PIPELINE
Inhaled nitric oxide

Nitric Oxide (NO) plays a multi-faceted role in the lungs, involved not only in the relaxation of smooth muscle lining pulmonary vessels and airways leading to vasodilation and bronchodilation but it is also produced by lung macrophages to act as a cytostatic and cytotoxic mediator against various pathogenic organisms.[35] In the CF population, studies have demonstrated that patients with CF have lower levels of exhaled NO as compared to age-matched controls and that these lower levels correlate with worsening severity of disease.[36–38] Additionally, evidence exists to suggest that the inhalation of the NO synthase substrate, L-arginine, can lead to transient improvement in pulmonary function in treated patients with CF.[39] Administration of inhaled NO at levels similar to what is found physiologically in the airways of normal individuals had no effect on lung function in a cohort of 13 patients with CF as measured by spirometry.[40] However, in order to test the direct antimicrobial activity of inhaled NO in NTM-PD, Bentur and colleagues administered

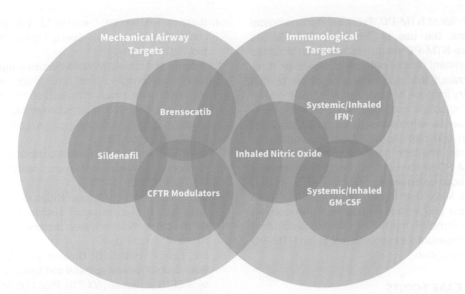

Fig. 1. Venn diagram of pulmonary NTM-PD HDT therapies.

intermittent high dose inhaled NO to 9 patients with CF and pulmonary MAB infection. In this pilot study they found that though this dose of inhaled NO (iNO) was well tolerated and led to significant increases in FEV1 and six-minute walk distance, there was only a modest increase in culture time to positivity and decrease in bacterial load.[41] Furthermore, preliminary results from a recently completed clinical trial, evaluating the use of iNO as adjunctive therapy for treatment-refractory NTM-PD, has also added much needed data regarding the tolerability and effectiveness of this HDT approach. In this multicenter pilot study of 15 individuals with and without CF, high-dose intermittent iNO was administered in addition to standard antimicrobial therapy for 84 days (NCT04685720). NO was again well-tolerated with minimal serious adverse events noted. Interestingly, in this study, early data demonstrated no significant change in spirometry or six-minute walk distance post therapy. Yet, there was an improvement in patient-reported quality of life measures and a trend towards reduction in microbial load after iNO treatment.[42] These data as a whole point to the potential of inhaled NO as an adjunctive NTM-PD therapy that is in much need of additional study, specifically addressing suitability to a broader range of NTM-PD patient populations.

Brensocatib

It is well known to the field that bronchiectasis is commonly associated with NTM-PD as a risk factor for succumbing to infection or as a downstream consequence of bronchial inflammation and destruction mediated by NTM bacilli. Targeting mechanisms involved in the pathogenesis of bronchiectasis will be directly beneficial to patients with NTM-PD as it will mitigate some of the downstream clinical manifestations of this bronchial destruction while also slowing down insults to the mucociliary machinery needed to expel bacilli. The inflammation of bronchiectasis is often predominated by neutrophils which secrete serine proteases (neutrophil elastase, cathepsin G, proteinase 3) that contribute to bronchial wall destruction and dilation.[43,44] Brensocatib is an oral potent selective inhibitor of dipeptidyl peptidase 1, a protease that activates neutrophil serine proteases in the bone marrow. In the phase 2 WILLOW trial Chalmers and colleagues evaluated the effect of brensocatib on the incidence of bronchiectasis exacerbations. In addition to confirming that brensocatib induced a dose-dependent decrease in sputum neutrophil-elastase concentration, they found that the drug prolonged the time to the first bronchiectasis exacerbation.[45] This early data suggests that brensocatib may be beneficial as a HDT for NTM-PD with bronchiectatic-predominant disease (**Fig. 1**).

SUMMARY

Upon the evaluation of translational and clinical trial data of HDTs for NTM-PD, it is clear that nearly all avenues of therapeutic intervention have not reached the level of efficacy to be considered a replacement to antibiotic treatment. Of the therapies directed at enhancing mechanical mucociliary clearance, CFTR modulators stand out as a class of drugs that effectively counteract genetic deficits that place patients with CF at higher risk of NTM-PD. From an immunological standpoint, the use of IFN-γ or GM-CSF as adjunctive NTM-PD treatment has been troubled by inconsistent clinical outcomes. However, it remains obvious that our knowledge of the human pulmonary immune response to NTM, at the level of the alveolus and accompanying airways is lacking. Deliberate efforts should be made to foster collection and banking of BAL cells, endobronchial tissue, and lung parenchyma from patients with NTM-PD to correct this deficit in knowledge of local host defenses to NTM bacilli. With that said, it is likely that the implementation of both mechanical and immunological HDTs in concert with antimicrobials may be required to precipitate clinically measurable improvement in the NTM-PD patient population.

CLINICS CARE POINTS

- HDTs have been developed to augment the antibiotic treatment of NTM-PD via improvement of host mechanical clearance and enhancement of immunologic responses to inhaled NTM.
- CFTR modulators are efficacious HDTs that reduce the burden of pulmonary NTM infection in patients with cystic fibrosis.
- Clinical studies of a majority of NTM-PD HDTs have demonstrated conflicting results over time that point to the need for further investigation prior to widespread use.

DISCLOSURE

None.

ACKNOWLEDGMENTS

This work was supported by the Intramural Research Program of the DIR/NHLBI.

REFERENCES

1. Adjemian J, Prevots DR, Gallagher J, et al. Lack of adherence to evidence-based treatment guidelines for nontuberculous mycobacterial lung disease. Ann Am Thorac Soc 2014;11(1):9–16.
2. Middleton AM, Chadwick MV, Nicholson AG, et al. The role of Mycobacterium avium complex fibronectin attachment protein in adherence to the human respiratory mucosa. Mol Microbiol 2000;38:381–91.
3. Wanner A, Salathé M, O'Riordan TG. Mucociliary clearance in the airways. Am J Respir Crit Care Med 1996;154(6 Pt 1):1868–902.
4. Bustamante-Marin XM, Ostrowski LE. Cilia and mucociliary clearance. Cold Spring Harbor Perspect Biol 2017;9:a028241.
5. Shamaei M, Mirsaeidi M. Nontuberculous mycobacteria, macrophages, and host innate immune response. Infect Immun 2021;89(8):e0081220.
6. Wu UI, Holland SM. Host susceptibility to nontuberculous mycobacterial infections. Lancet Infect Dis 2015;15(8):968–80.
7. Martiniano SL, Nick JA, Daley CL. Nontuberculous mycobacterial infections in cystic fibrosis. Thorac Surg Clin 2019;29:95–108.
8. Bernut A, Dupont C, Ogryzko NV, et al. CFTR protects against Mycobacterium abscessus infection by fine-tuning host oxidative defenses. Cell Rep 2019;26(7):1828–40.e4.
9. Van Goor F, Hadida S, Grootenhuis PDJ, et al. Rescue of CF airway epithelial cell function in vitro by a CFTR potentiator, VX-770. Proc Natl Acad Sci U S A 2009;106:18825–30.
10. Taylor-Cousar JL, Munck A, McKone EF, et al. Tezacaftor–ivacaftor in patients with cystic fibrosis homozygous for Phe508del. N Engl J Med 2017;377:2013–23.
11. Rowe SM, Daines C, Ringshausen FC, et al. Tezacaftor–ivacaftor in residual-function heterozygotes with cystic fibrosis. N Engl J Med 2017;377:2024–35.
12. Frost FJ, Nazareth DS, Charman SC, et al. Ivacaftor is associated with reduced lung infection by key cystic fibrosis pathogens. A cohort study using national registry data. Ann Am Thorac Soc 2019;16:1375–82.
13. Ricotta EE, Prevots DR, Olivier KN. CFTR modulator use and risk of nontuberculous mycobacteria positivity in cystic fibrosis, 2011-2018. ERJ Open Res 2022;8(2):00724–2021.
14. Matsuyama M, Martins AJ, Shallom S, et al. Transcriptional response of respiratory epithelium to nontuberculous mycobacteria. Am J Respir Cell Mol Biol 2018;58(2):241–52.
15. Szymanski EP, Leung JM, Fowler CJ, et al. Pulmonary nontuberculous mycobacterial infection. a multisystem, multigenic disease. Am J Respir Crit Care Med 2015;192(5):618–28.
16. Fowler CJ, Olivier KN, Leung JM, et al. Abnormal nasal nitric oxide production, ciliary beat frequency, and Toll-like receptor response in pulmonary nontuberculous mycobacterial disease epithelium. Am J Respir Crit Care Med 2013;187(12):1374–81.
17. Fowler C, Wu UI, Shaffer R, et al. The effects of sildenafil on ciliary beat frequency in patients with pulmonary non-tuberculous mycobacteria disease: phase I/II trial. BMJ Open Respir Res 2020;7(1):e000574.
18. Newport MJ, Huxley CM, Huston S, et al. A mutation in the interferon-g-receptor gene and susceptibility

to mycobacterial infection. N Engl J Med 1996;335: 1941e1949.

19. Kampmann B, Hemingway C, Stephens A, et al. Acquired predisposition to mycobacterial disease due to autoantibodies to IFN-gamma. J Clin Invest 2005; 115:2480–8.

20. Patel SY, Ding L, Brown MR, et al. Anti-IFN-gamma autoantibodies in disseminated nontuberculous mycobacterial infections. J Immunol 2005;175. 4769–7.

21. Squires KE, Murphy WF, Madoff LC, et al. Interferon-gamma and Mycobacterium avium-intracellulare infection. J Infect Dis 1989;159:599–600.

22. Holland SM, Eisenstein EM, Kuhns DB, et al. Treatment of refractory disseminated nontuberculous mycobacterial infection with interferon gamma. A preliminary report. N Engl J Med 1994;330:1348–55.

23. Milanés-Virelles MT, García-García I, Santos-Herrera Y, et al. Adjuvant interferon gamma in patients with pulmonary atypical Mycobacteriosis: a randomized, double-blind, placebo-controlled study. BMC Infect Dis 2008;8:17.

24. Hallstrand TS, Ochs HD, Zhu Q, et al. Inhaled IFN-gamma for persistent nontuberculous mycobacterial pulmonary disease due to functional IFN-gamma deficiency. Eur Respir J 2004;24:367–70.

25. Lam PK, Griffith DE, Aksamit TR, et al. Factors related to response to intermittent treatment of Mycobacterium avium complex lung disease. Am J Respir Crit Care Med 2006;173(11):1283–9.

26. Gasson JC. Molecular physiology of granulocyte-macrophage colony-stimulating factor. Blood 1991; 77(6):1131–45.

27. Bermudez LE, Young LS. Recombinant granulocyte-macrophage colony-stimulating factor activates human macrophages to inhibit growth or kill Mycobacterium avium complex. J Leukoc Biol 1990; 48(1):67–73.

28. Bermudez LE, Kemper CA, Deresinski SC. Dysfunctional monocytes from a patient with disseminated Mycobacterium kansasii infection are activated in vitro and in vivo by GM-CSF. Biotherapy 1994;8: 135–42.

29. Onyeji CO, Nightingale CH, Tessier PR, et al. Activities of clarithromycin, azithromycin, and ofloxacin in combination with liposomal or unencapsulated granulocyte-macrophage colony-stimulating factor against intramacrophage Mycobacterium avium-Mycobacterium intracellulare. J Infect Dis 1995; 172:810–6.

30. Kemper CA, Bermudez LE, Deresinski SC. Immunomodulatory treatment of Mycobacterium avium complex bacteremia in patients with AIDS by use of recombinant granulocyte-macrophage colony-stimulating factor. J Infect Dis 1998;177:914–20.

31. Nannini EC, Keating M, Binstock P, et al. Successful treatment of refractory disseminated Mycobacterium avium complex infection with the addition of linezolid and mefloquine. J Infect 2002;44(3):201–3.

32. de Silva TI, Cope A, Goepel J, et al. The use of adjuvant granulocyte-macrophage colony-stimulating factor in HIV-related disseminated atypical mycobacterial infection. J Infect 2007;54:e207–10.

33. Scott JP, Ji Y, Kannan M, et al. Inhaled granulocyte-macrophage colony-stimulating factor for Mycobacterium abscessus in cystic fibrosis. Eur Respir J 2018;51:1702127.

34. Thomson RM, Waterer G, Loebinger MR, et al. Use of inhaled GM-CSF in treatment-refractory NTM infection. An open-label, exploratory clinical trial. Eur Respir J 2021;58(Suppl. 65):OA1603.

35. Barnes PJ, Belvisi MG. Nitric oxide and lung disease. Thorax 1993 Oct;48(10):1034–43.

36. Grasemann H, Michler E, Wallot M, et al. Decreased concentration of exhaled nitric oxide (NO) in patients with cystic fibrosis. Pediatr Pulmonol 1997;24:173–7.

37. Ho LP, Innes JA, Greening AP. Exhaled nitric oxide is not elevated in the inflammatory airways diseases of cystic fibrosis and bronchiectasis. Eur Respir J 1998;12:1290–4.

38. Keen C, Gustafsson P, Lindblad A, et al. Low levels of exhaled nitric oxide are associated with impaired lung function in cystic fibrosis. Pediatr Pulmonol 2010;45:241–8.

39. Grasemann H, Kurtz F, Ratjen F. Inhaled L-arginine improves exhaled nitric oxide and pulmonary function in patients with cystic fibrosis. Am J Respir Crit Care Med 2006;174:208–12.

40. Ratjen F, Gartig S, Wiesemann HG, et al. Effect of inhaled nitric oxide on pulmonary function in cystic fibrosis. Respir Med 1999;93:579–83.

41. Bentur L, Gur M, Ashkenazi M, et al. Pilot study to test inhaled nitric oxide in cystic fibrosis patients with refractory Mycobacterium abscessus lung infection. J Cyst Fibros 2020;19(2):225–31.

42. Thomson RM, Morgan LC, Burke A, et al. Home-based treatment of nontuberculous mycobacteria pulmonary disease via a novel nitric oxide generator and delivery system. Chest 2022;162(4):A470–1.

43. Chalmers JD, Hill AT. Mechanisms of immune dysfunction and bacterial persistence in non-cystic fibrosis bronchiectasis. Mol Immunol 2013;55: 27–34.

44. Chalmers JD, Moffitt KL, Suarez-Cuartin G, et al. Neutrophil elastase activity is associated with exacerbations and lung function decline in bronchiectasis. Am J Respir Crit Care Med 2017;195:1384–93.

45. Chalmers JD, Haworth CS, Metersky ML, et al, WILLOW Investigators. Phase 2 trial of the DPP-1 inhibitor brensocatib in bronchiectasis. N Engl J Med 2020;383(22):2127–37.

Cystic Fibrosis-Related Nontuberculous Mycobacterial Pulmonary Disease

Timothy Baird, BSc, MBBS, DTM&H, FRACP[a,b,c,]*,
Scott Bell, MBBS, FRACP, MD[d,e,f,g]

KEYWORDS

- Cystic fibrosis • Non-tuberculous mycobacteria • NTM • *Mycobacterium avium* complex
- *Mycobacterium abscessus* complex

KEY POINTS

- Nontuberculous mycobacteria (NTM) is a major cause of morbidity in cystic fibrosis (CF) with rates increasing worldwide.
- *Mycobacterium avium* complex and *Mycobacterium abscessus* account for the majority of NTM infections in CF.
- Treatment guidelines are available to aid in the management of CF-related NTM infection.
- The management of NTM in CF is likely to evolve with improved diagnostics, emerging treatment options, and the widespread uptake of CFTR modulator therapy.

INTRODUCTION

Respiratory infections caused by nontuberculous mycobacteria (NTM) in people with cystic fibrosis (pwCF) are increasing globally and are a major cause of morbidity.[1] NTM pulmonary disease (NTM-PD) in pwCF is challenging to diagnose and treat due to difficulties in determining what is true infection (or disease), the requirement for complex and lengthy drug regimens, and suboptimal treatment outcomes. Importantly, not all pwCF develop NTM-PD, and it is not uncommon for transient infection to spontaneously clear.[1] The most common NTM pathogens in pwCF are *Mycobacterium avium* complex (MAC) and *Mycobacterium*

abscessus (Mabs). Mabs is the most virulent NTM in pwCF, possesses multiple intrinsic and acquired resistance mechanisms, is associated with accelerated pulmonary decline, and is more likely to be associated with NTM-treatment failure.[1,2] Recent consensus guidelines have been published to support management decisions of these pathogens in pwCF; however, new diagnostics and emerging therapies are being increasingly investigated to improve outcomes. This review explores the epidemiology of NTM in pwCF, illustrates the risk factors and acquisition of infection, outlines the current and future diagnostic and screening methods, and examines the current guidelines and emerging treatment strategies.

[a] Department of Respiratory Medicine, Sunshine Coast University Hospital, Sunshine Coast, Queensland, Australia; [b] Sunshine Coast Health Institute, Sunshine Coast, Queensland, Australia; [c] University of the Sunshine Coast, Sunshine Coast, Queensland, Australia; [d] Department of Thoracic Medicine, The Prince Charles Hospital, Brisbane, Queensland, Australia; [e] Children's Health Research Centre, Faculty of Medicine, The University of Queensland, Brisbane, Australia; [f] Translational Research Institute, Brisbane, Queensland, Australia; [g] Department of Thoracic Medicine, The Prince Charles Hospital, Chermside, Queensland, Australia
* Corresponding author. Respiratory Medicine Department, Sunshine Coast University Hospital, 6 Doherty Street, Birtinya, Queensland 4575, Australia.
E-mail address: timothy.baird@health.qld.gov.au

Clin Chest Med 44 (2023) 847–860
https://doi.org/10.1016/j.ccm.2023.06.008

EPIDEMIOLOGY

In parallel with the increasing prevalence of NTM reported globally, rates have also been rising in CF cohorts.[3,4] There are several factors likely to be contributing to this observation, including increased awareness of the potential of NTM infection (and its impact), implementation of screening programs as a part of clinical care, changes to laboratory methods, improved patient survival leading to increased lifetime NTM exposure, and the use of intensive mycobacterial therapy approaches.[5]

There is marked variability in prevalence rates of infection in CF populations, ranging from less than 5% in the UK and Europe to greater than 15% in the USA.[6,7] Registry data demonstrate that NTM is infrequent in young children, increases during adolescence, and rates are maintained in the adult population.[7–9] The dominant species that cause infection in pwCF are slow-growing mycobacteria, MAC and rapid-growing mycobacteria, Mabs group.[1,7] The relative proportion of Mabs and MAC are also variable between countries and even regions within countries. Mabs is responsible for most CF-associated infections in Europe and Australia (50%–80%), whereas MAC is dominant in the USA representing almost 60% of all NTM in pwCF. It is likely that the regional variations relate to climatic and environmental factors including humidity, proximity to water, and even differences in soil composition.[10]

RISK FACTORS FOR NONTUBERCULOUS MYCOBACTERIA ACQUISITION

NTM acquisition risk may be associated with host susceptibility (including the extent of lung damage and antibiotic exposure), airway microbiota diversity, and NTM pathogen characteristics. Higher rates of NTM infection overall have been reported in patients with clinical indicators of severe disease.[3,4] Rates of Pseudomonas aeruginosa infection have been reported to be both higher or lower in patients with Mabs infection in different cohorts, and further study is needed to better understand the interrelationship.[4] Gastroesophageal reflux has been associated with NTM risk and is also a common comorbidity in pwCF.[11,12] Patients with Mabs are usually younger and have poorer lung function than those with MAC.[13]

The composition of the lung microbiome in patients with CF has been shown to be related to these factors.[3,14,15] Such relationships reflect differences in airway environment and potentially influence the growth of specific bacterial, mycobacterial and fungal species. Increased rates of Staphylococcus aureus and Stenotrophomonas maltophilia, and higher prevalence of Aspergillus isolation (and a patient diagnosis of allergic bronchopulmonary aspergillosis [ABPA]) are seen in individuals with NTM infection.[1,9,14,16] Using 16S rRNA sequencing, differences in airway microbiota were seen in patients with NTM infection compared to those without.[17] The basis of these links may be indirect (whereby disease course and treatment history are associated with both airway microbiota diversity and risk of NTM acquisition), or direct, reflecting interactions between NTM species and the wider lung microbiota.[18]

In an in vitro study of macrophages, azithromycin adversely affected autophagy and intracellular killing of NTM.[19] Long-term macrolide therapy (specifically, azithromycin) is recommended for pwCF who have frequent pulmonary exacerbations; however, it has been observed that the increase in NTM infection rates has occurred in the era of increased macrolide use.[19] Despite this observation, most studies examining this risk in pwCF prescribed azithromycin suggest reduced risk (ie, a protective effect) rather than increased risk.[13,19–21]

The impact of the introduction of CFTR modulators on the risk of NTM acquisition is not well understood and in part relates to the limited timeframes since their widespread availability.[22] In the single published study to assess the impact of modulator drugs on risk of NTM suggested reduced risk of positive cultures (hazard ratio = 0.88). Careful interpretation of studies examining this question in the future will be required.

ACQUISITION OF NONTUBERCULOUS MYCOBACTERIA

Environmental exposure and, in some instances, cross-transmission can be sources of NTM infection in pwCF.[23–26] Significant spatial clustering of NTM has been reported in the USA, with particularly high prevalence in the West and Southeast (>20%) where humidity is high.[27] Increasing incidence of NTM isolation was found in Queensland between 1999 and 2005 and clusters of high relative risk for MAC and Mabs were identified differentially in regions across Queensland.[28] Several socioecological, economic, and environmental factors were found to be associated with NTM infection risk, including higher income/education levels, higher water evaporation, and soil copper and sodium levels.[27]

NTM are ubiquitous in the natural and built environments including drinking water and its system, soil, water pipes, showerheads, and in some situations form biofilm structures.[29] Susceptible individuals may acquire infection from drinking water in their home.[29] Municipal water sampling showed widespread contamination of the drinking water supply in the city of Brisbane (Australia), with Mabs isolates that clustered using molecular typing methods with patients' isolates.[29,30] The origin of MAC is less well understood but is known to be present in soil and dust, including households. Inhalation of aerosols of viable NTM directly into the lower respiratory tract is likely to be a key mode of acquisition in susceptible hosts, although ingestion of contaminated water and microaspiration in patients with gastroesophageal reflux has also been proposed.[31,32]

Until recently, person to person transmission was not considered an acquisition pathway for NTM. In an outbreak report at the Seattle lung transplant center, several post-transplant pwCF demonstrated identical strains of Mabs when compared by whole genome sequencing (WGS).[25] In a study following this, investigators at the adult CF center in Cambridge (UK) identified clonal strains in pwCF and found that patients had overlapping inpatient episodes suggesting the potential for transmission.[26] Subsequently, an international collaborative study examined a large cohort of Mabs isolates derived from pwCF from the UK, Europe, the USA, and Australia, with most isolates (74%) grouped within 1 of 3 clonally related Mabs clusters (called dominant circulating clones).[30] However, other studies examining relatedness of Mabs isolates from pwCF attending the same treatment center have failed to demonstrate clonal infections.[31,33–35] The US multicenter study, health care-associated links in transmission of NTM (HALT-NTM), aims to systemically analyze health care outbreaks of NTM using evidence-based epidemiologic investigation tools.[36]

DIAGNOSIS AND SCREENING
Nontuberculous Mycobacteria Criteria

Although the criteria for the diagnosis of NTM-PD have been well established, their utility in pwCF has several limitations.[37,38] Although the microbiological criteria can be applied as for non-CF populations, the clinical and imaging criteria are challenging—pwCF can have symptoms (eg, cough, sputum production, weight loss, night sweats, etc.) which might be suggestive of NTM infection, but such symptoms could also result from the emergence of a new airway bacterial pathogen or an exacerbation of a chronic infection.[12]

Similarly, the cardinal features of NTM-PD on high-resolution CT scans of bronchiolectasis and tree-in-bud changes lack specificity in pwCF where these features can be related to the CF airway pathology itself and also related to a range of non-mycobacterial pathogens.[39] Therefore, the microbiological criteria take on even more importance in deciding if a pwCF has NTM-PD with careful consideration regarding the type of NTM sample, number of positive samples, and changes in clinical status.

Diagnostic Challenges

The presence of bacterial pathogens in the sample (ie, P. aeruginosa) can directly impact the ability to detect NTM in the laboratory. Overgrowth of gram-negative bacteria can be problematic in some patients; this requires close collaboration and communication between the CF team and the microbiology laboratory. An important consequence of decontamination of sputum samples is the adverse impact on the viability of NTM and resultant reduction in culture yield.[40] To attempt to address overgrowth and the need for specific decontamination steps in sample processing, selective mycobacterial media and methods have been developed, and validated in CF samples.[40–42]

Laboratories vary in the approach undertaken to speciate cultured NTM, and a range of molecular techniques are now used. In recent years, matrix-assisted laser desorption/ionization time-of-flight mass spectrometry identification has been applied to NTM isolates to confirm identification and WGS is increasingly being used for NTM species confirmation and especially when an outbreak is suspected.[43]

Direct detection of NTM from samples to allow earlier diagnosis has been reported using real-time PCR approaches and has demonstrated some promise.[44] Serologic approaches (IgG- and IgA-based enzyme-linked immunosorbent assay [ELISA] assays) have also shown potential in detecting patients with known NTM, and in the future, may be useful to support more intensive respiratory sampling and monitoring (eg, imaging) of patients identified.[2,45,46] Validated non-pulmonary screening approaches will be important in the era where the majority of pwCF are prescribed CFTR modulator drugs.

Screening Approaches

In 2016, the Cystic Fibrosis Foundation (CFF) / European Cystic Fibrosis Society (ECFS) NTM guidelines were published and recommended annual NTM culture screening of sputum for all spontaneously expectorating pwCF.[47] Upper airway sampling approaches (eg, cough or oropharyngeal swabs) or induced sputum or bronchoscopy in those patients who were not productive were not recommended for use to screen for NTM. In a study to determine annual screening rates in US CF centers, screening rates were suboptimal with reported samples collected in 46% (median, range 9%–73%) of suitable patients.[48] Improved health in patients on CFTR modulators will further impact the ability of clinics to screen for NTM and more invasive approaches (including sputum induction, bronchoscopy) may need to be considered in the non-productive patient whose symptoms could be explained by NTM.

TREATMENT

The decision to treat or observe a pwCF and NTM-PD remains a challenge. Despite a patient having a confirmed diagnosis of NTM-PD, this does not necessitate commencement of antimicrobial therapy.[37] Treatment decisions should remain individualized and determined by the NTM species, severity of disease, desired treatment outcomes, and patient preference. For example, a pwCF and MAC infection with minimal symptoms, stability of lung function, and non-progressive radiology can be reasonably observed. Conversely, a pwCF and Mabs infection with progressive symptoms, smear-positive, or cavitary changes on radiology and or declining lung function should be promptly offered mycobacterial therapy.[38,47,49]

Mycobacterial Therapy for Mycobacterium avium Complex

Antimicrobial treatment of MAC-PD typically comprises a macrolide (azithromycin or clarithromycin), rifampicin, and ethambutol (**Table 1**).[38,47,49,50] Azithromycin is the preferred macrolide in CF due to equal efficacy with better tolerance, less drug interactions, and single daily dosing.[38] Although a thrice weekly dosing regimen is recommended for some patients with MAC and non-CF bronchiectasis, a daily dosing regimen is preferred in CF.[38,47,49] Current guidelines recommend that drug-susceptibility testing for macrolide (clarithromycin) resistance should be performed prior to treatment commencement, and performed again in cases of refractory treatment or relapsed infection.[38,47,50]

In cavitary MAC-PD, the addition of an injectable aminoglycoside (amikacin or streptomycin) to the above 3-drug regimen for at least 4 to 12 weeks

Table 1
Suggested antimicrobial regimens for *Mycobacterium avium* complex in cystic fibrosis[38,47,49]

M. avium Complex	Treatment Regimen	Frequency and Duration
Nodular bronchiectatic non-cavitary disease	3 Agents consisting of: Macrolide (azithromycin or clarithromycin) Ethambutol Rifamycin (rifampicin or rifabutin); or clofazimine[b]	Daily[a] 12 mo post culture conversion
Cavitary or severe disease	At least 3 agents consisting of: Macrolide (azithromycin or clarithromycin) Ethambutol Rifamycin (rifampicin or rifabutin); and/or clofazimine Systemic aminoglycoside (amikacin or streptomycin)	Daily (or thrice weekly for parenteral aminoglycosides) 12 mo post culture conversion
Treatment refractory disease	At least 4 agents consisting of: Macrolide (azithromycin or clarithromycin) Ethambutol Rifamycin (rifampicin or rifabutin); and/or clofazimine[b] Amikacin liposome inhalation solution (ALIS); or systemic aminoglycoside (amikacin or streptomycin)	Daily (or thrice weekly for parenteral aminoglycosides) 12 mo post culture conversion

[a] Thrice weekly dosing not recommended in cystic fibrosis.
[b] Consider clofazimine in place of the rifamycins to minimize drug interactions with CFTR modulators and the "azole" antifungals.

Table 2
Suggested antimicrobial regimens for *Mycobacterium abscessus* complex in cystic fibrosis[38,47,49,50,54]

M. abscessus Complex	Treatment Regimen	Frequency and Duration

Macrolide susceptible	Intensive phase
	At least 3 agents of:
	  1–2 parenteral: amikacin;
	    imipenem (or cefoxitin);
	    tigecycline plus 1–2 oral:
	    macrolide (azithromycin or
	    clarithromycin); clofazimine;
	    linezolid
	Continuation phase
	At least 2 agents of:
	  Oral macrolide (azithromycin or
	    clarithromycin); clofazimine;
	    linezolid; moxifloxacin;
	    minocycline; plus Inhaled
	    amikacin
	  Consider other oral options:[b]
	  Rifabutin; omadacycline; tedizolid;
	    bedaquiline
		Daily (or thrice weekly for
		  parenteral aminoglycosides)
		4–12 wk
		Daily
		12 mo post culture conversion

Inducible or mutational
  macrolide resistance
	Intensive phase
	At least 4 agents of:
	  1–2 parenteral: amikacin;
	    imipenem (or cefoxitin);
	    tigecycline plus:
	  1–2 oral: macrolide (azithromycin
	    or clarithromycin);[a] clofazimine;
	    linezolid
	Continuation phase
	At least 2 agents of:
	  Oral macrolide (azithromycin or
	    clarithromycin);[a] clofazimine;
	    linezolid; moxifloxacin;
	    minocycline; plus inhaled
	    amikacin
	  Consider other oral options[b]
	  Rifabutin; omadacycline; tedizolid;
	    bedaquiline
		Daily (or thrice weekly for
		  parenteral aminoglycosides)
		4–12 wk
		Daily
		12 mo post culture conversion

[a] Azithromycin and clarithromycin are unlikely to be active and should not be counted as one of the active drugs in the regimen, but can be given as an immune modulator.
[b] Not recommended in current guidelines; however, it may be considered in view of emerging *in vitro* and *in vivo* evidence, clinical experience, and expert opinion.

should be considered.[38,47,49,50] In treatment refractory MAC-PD, defined as persistent culture positivity at 6 months, the addition of amikacin liposome inhaled suspension (ALIS) is suggested due to recent results of the CONVERT Study that demonstrated a significantly higher rate of culture conversion in this cohort with ALIS plus guideline based treatment (GBT) compared to GBT alone.[50,51] Although there is minimal evidence for additional or alternative agents, some centers not uncommonly will use clofazimine as a third or fourth agent, due to its attractive *in vitro* efficacy against MAC, and due to the critical rifamycin-CFTR modulator drug-interactions.[52]

Mycobacterial Therapy for *Mycobacterium abscessus* Complex

The treatment of Mabs-PD remains highly problematic due to antimicrobial resistance, treatment-related toxicity, and low rates of treatment success.[47,50,53,54] Current guidelines recommend that drug regimens consist of an intensive phase, including multidrug intravenous therapy for a number of months, followed by a continuation phase with oral plus inhaled antibiotics for 12 months post culture conversion (**Table 2**).[38,47,54] The intensive phase should include a macrolide (preferably azithromycin) in conjunction with 4 to

Table 3
Antibiotic-dosing regimens used to treat *Mycobacterium avium* complex and *Mycobacterium abscessus* complex pulmonary disease in cystic fibrosis

Antibiotic	Route	Dose Suitable for Children/Adolescents	Dose Suitable for Adults
Amikacin	Intravenous	Children: 15–30 mg/kg/dose once daily Adolescents: 10–15 mg/kg/dose once daily Maximum dose 1500 mg daily	10–30 mg/kg once daily or 15 mg/kg/d in 2 divided doses Daily to 3 × weekly dosing
	Nebulized	250–500 mg/dose once or twice daily	250–500 mg once or twice daily
Azithromycin	Oral	Children: 10–12 mg/kg/dose once daily Adolescents: adult dosing regimen Maximum dose 500 mg	250–500 mg once daily
Cefoxitin	Intravenous	50 mg/kg/dose thrice daily (maximum dose 12 g/d)	200 mg/kg/d in 3 divided doses (maximum dose 12 g/d)
Clarithromycin	Oral	7.5 mg/kg/dose twice daily (maximum dose 500 mg)	500 mg twice daily[d,e]
	Intravenous	Not recommended	500 mg twice daily[d]
Clofazimine	Oral	1–2 mg/kg/dose once daily (maximum dose 100 mg)	50–100 mg once a day
Co-trimoxazole (sulfamethoxazole and trimethoprim)	Oral	10–20 mg/kg/dose twice daily	960 mg twice daily
	Intravenous	10–20 mg/kg/dose twice daily	1.44 g twice daily
Ethambutol	Oral	Infants and children: 15 mg/kg/dose once daily Adolescents: 15 mg/kg/dose once daily	15 mg/kg once daily
Imipenem-cilastatin	Intravenous	15–20 mg/kg/dose twice daily (maximum dose 1000 mg)	1 g twice daily
Linezolid[f]	Oral	<12 y old: 10 mg/kg/dose thrice daily 12 y and older: 10 mg/kg/dose once or twice daily (maximum dose 600 mg)	600 mg once or twice daily
Linezolid[f]	Intravenous	<12 y old: 10 mg/kg/dose thrice daily 12 y and older: 10 mg/kg/dose once or twice daily (maximum dose 600 mg)	600 mg once or twice daily
Moxifloxacin	Oral	7.5–10 mg/kg/dose once daily (maximum dose 400 mg daily)	400 mg once daily
Minocycline	Oral	2 mg/kg/dose once daily (maximum dose 200 mg)	100 mg twice daily
Rifampin (rifampicin)	Oral	10–20 mg/kg/dose once daily (maximum dose 600 mg)	<50 kg 450 mg once daily >50 kg 600 mg once daily

(continued on next page)

Table 3
(continued)

Antibiotic	Route	Dose Suitable for Children/ Adolescents	Dose Suitable for Adults
Rifabutin	Oral	5–10 mg/kg/dose once daily (maximum dose 300 mg)	150–300 mg once daily 150 mg if patient taking strong CYP3A4 inhibitor 450–600 mg if patient taking strong CYP3A4 inducer
Streptomycin[a]	Intramuscular/ intravenous	20–40 mg/kg/dose once daily (maximum dose 1000 mg)	15 mg/kg once daily (maximum dose 1000 mg)
Tigecycline[b,c,g]	Intravenous	8–11 y: 1.2 mg/kg/dose twice daily (maximum dose 50 mg) 12 y and older: 100 mg loading dose and then 50 mg once or twice daily	100 mg loading dose and then 50 mg once or twice daily

Abbreviations: FDA, Food and Drug Administration; IND, investigational new drug.

[a] Adjust dose according to levels. Usually, starting dose is 15 mg/kg aiming for a peak level of 20 to 30 μg/mL and trough levels of <5 to 10 μg/mL.

[b] As tolerated.

[c] Mixed with normal saline.

[d] For individuals under 55 kg, many practitioners recommend 7.5 mg/kg twice daily.

[e] Only available in the USA through an IND application to the FDA.

[f] Usually given with high dose (100 mg daily) pyridoxine (vitamin B_6) to reduce risk of cytopenia.

[g] Many practitioners recommend pre-dosing with one or more anti-emetics before dosing and/or gradual dose escalation from 25 mg daily to minimize nausea and vomiting.

Reproduced from [Thorax 2016] *with permission.*[47]

12 weeks of intravenous amikacin plus one or more of tigecycline, imipenem-cilastatin, and/or cefoxitin.[47] The continuation phase should include azithromycin and inhaled amikacin, in conjunction with 2 or 3 additional agents guided by *in vitro* susceptibility testing.[38,47,54]

It is now well recognized that treatment outcomes depend largely on the Mabs subspecies and the resultant presence of inducible or mutational macrolide resistance. In cases where an isolate demonstrates resistance to macrolides, it should not be considered an active drug in the overall regimen; however, inclusion is still suggested for its immunomodulatory effects.[38,50,54]

Cystic Fibrosis-Specific Treatment Considerations

Despite the absence of high-level evidence demonstrating direct efficacy in combating NTM-PD, the usual adjunct non-pharmacological therapies for pwCF remain important and include airway clearance, mucolytic therapies, optimization of vitamin and nutritional status, exercise, and avoidance of smoking.[47] Moreover, the introduction of the novel CFTR modulators has already lead to substantial clinical improvements in pwCF, with the proposition that restoration of CFTR function will result in a reduction in risk of chronic airway infection.[55]

Appropriate dosing of antibiotics in CF is challenging due to altered pharmacokinetics (PK), difficulty with lung tissue penetration, and high levels of antimicrobial resistance.[56,57] As such, an understanding of the potential altered PK of antibiotics used to treat NTM infections in pwCF is important with consideration of therapeutic drug monitoring recommended in complex cases.[56] Suggested dosing regimens for the common NTM antibiotics in pwCF are presented in **Table 3**.

Drug–drug interactions remain an important aspect of CF management and are particularly pertinent for NTM drugs.[52] Rifampicin and rifabutin are potent inducers of CYP3A4 and result in substantially reduced plasma concentration levels for the "azole" antifungals.[52] Additionally, the CFTR modulators are strong CYP3A4 inhibitors, largely due to the active drug ivacaftor. As such, when rifampicin or rifabutin is administered in combination with ivacaftor, these disease altering therapies are rendered ineffective.[52,58] With widespread uptake of CFTR modulators, the currently recommended NTM regimens in CF, particularly

Table 4
Emerging therapies to treat non-tuberculous mycobacteria in cystic fibrosis

Antibiotic (Class)	Suggested Adult Dose and (Route)	Evidence	References
Rifabutin (rifamycin)	300 mg q24 h (PO)	• *In vitro* bactericidal activity against *M. abscessus* • Synergistic activity with clarithromycin, tigecycline, imipenem, and tedizolid	50,59
Bedaquiline (diarylquinoline)	400 mg q24 h or 2 wk (PO); followed by 200 mg thrice weekly (PO)	• *In vitro* bacteriostatic activity against both MAC and *M. abscessus* • Synergy with clofazimine • May decrease the activity of cefoxitin and imipenem	50,59–61
Omadacycline (tetracycline)	300 mg q24 h (PO); or 100 mg q24 h (IV)	• *In vitro* activity against *M. abscessus* with similar MIC to tigecycline • Case reports and series demonstrating efficacy with minimal toxicity	62–65
Eravacycline (tetracycline)	1 mg/kg q12 h (IV)	Superior *in vitro* activity against *M. abscessus* with MICs lower than tigecycline and omadacycline	67
Tedizolid (oxazolidinone)	200 mg q24 h (PO or IV)	• Superior *in vitro* activity against *M. abscessus* compared with linezolid • Possible synergy against NTM when combined with imipenem and ethambutol	66,69

Dual Beta-lactams (possible options)
  Amoxycillin
  Cefoxitin
  Ceftaroline
  Ceftazidime/avibactam
  Imipenem-cilastatin
  Imipenem-cilastatin/ relebactam
	1 g q8h (PO)
	1–2g q6–8h (IV)
	600 mg q12 h (IV)
	2.5 g q8h (IV)
	0.5–1g q6–12h (IV)
	1.25 g q6h (IV)
		• *In vitro* synergy with amoxycillin and imipenem/cilastastin/ relebactam
		• *In vitro* synergy between imipenem and cefoxitin or and imipenem and ceftaroline
			59,68–70

Inhaled antibiotics
  Amikacin (ALIS)
  Tigecycline
  Clofazimine
  Imipenem-cilastatin
	590 mg/8.4 mL od (INH)
	Unknown
	Unknown
	250 mg q12 h (INH)
		• Recommended for continuation phase of treatment[a]
		• Reduction in pulmonary bacterial load in a GM-CSF knockout model
		• Improved bacterial elimination from the lungs in NTM-infected mouse models *(MAC and M. abscessus)*
			38,71–73

(*continued on next page*)

Table 4
(continued)

Antibiotic (Class)	Suggested Adult Dose and (Route)	Evidence	References
		• Well tolerated in 2 pediatric CF patients with *M. abscessus* with stabilization of lung function over 9 mo	

Non-antibiotic agents
  Inhaled NO
  IFN-γ
  GM-CSF
  Bacteriophage therapy
	150–250 ppm q6–24 h (INH)
	Unknown (INH)
	Unknown (INH)
	NA (IV or INH)
		• Potent *in vitro* activity against mycobacteria
		• Variable *in vivo* results in case series and reports series (reduction in sputum burden, improvement in symptoms, improvement in lung function and 6MWD, no sustained culture conversion)
		• Improved NTM clearance in patients with IFN-γ deficiency
		• Improvement in lung function and culture conversion in 2 CF patients with *M. abscessus*
		• Improvement in lung function, liver function, and skin lesions in a CF patient with disseminated *M. abscessus*
			74–79

Abbreviations: ALIS, amikacin liposome inhalation suspension; INH, inhaled; IV, intravenous (parenteral); MAC, *Mycobacterium avium* complex; PO, oral.

ᵃ 2020 ATS/ERS/ESCMID/IDSA Guidelines recommend inhaled amikacin use with no specification for ALIS versus the standard nebulized IV formulation.

for MAC-PD, will likely need further study, with clofazimine the current preferred alternative to the rifamycins.[58]

Given these complexities in CF pharmacokinetics and the high rates of drug interactions and treatment toxicity, expert pharmacist input and specialist NTM/CF physician collaboration is advised.[47,49,58]

EMERGING THERAPIES FOR NONTUBERCULOUS MYCOBACTERIA

As a result of the complex, lengthy, and toxic antibiotic regimens for Mabs-PD, interest in both new or "repurposed" antibiotics and non-antibiotic agents as therapeutic options is growing.[59] Bedaquiline has demonstrated *in vitro* activity against MAC and Mabs, with a small case series in 10 patients (2 with CF) reporting improvement in symptoms, radiology, and bacterial load.[60,61] Omadacycline and tedizolid have demonstrated

potent *in vitro* activity against MAC and Mabs, with case recent reports and small series demonstrating possible clinical efficacy.[62–66] Eravacycline has shown superior *in vitro* activity against Mabs with MIC's 2-fold lower than tigecycline and omadacycline; however, *in vivo* data are currently lacking.[67]

Recent *in vitro* studies exploring dual beta-lactam use suggest synergistic activity between a number of agents and lowered MICs through combination therapy with the new-age beta-lactamase inhibitors avibactam and relebactam.[68–70] "Repurposed" inhaled antibiotics (in addition to amikacin) may also have an increasing role due to delivery of higher concentration of drug and reduced systemic toxicity: Inhaled imipenem-cilastatin was well tolerated in 2 pediatric patients with CF with Mabs-PD with stabilization of lung function over 9 months; inhaled tigecycline demonstrated a reduction in pulmonary bacterial load in a granulocyte macrophage stimulating factor (GM-CSF) knockout model with Mabs infection; and inhaled clofazimine was shown to be well tolerated in a mouse-model with NTM-PD.[71–73]

Finally, early case reports and small case series using inhaled nitric oxide, inhaled interferon-gamma (IFN-γ), inhaled GM-CSF, and engineered bacteriophage therapy have all demonstrated therapeutic potential.[74–79] A summary of these antibiotic and non-antibiotic emerging therapies is outlined in **Table 4**.

LUNG TRANSPLANTATION AND SURGERY

Infection with NTM in pwCF is of relevance during assessment for lung transplantation. At some centers historically, NTM infection was considered an absolute contraindication for lung transplantation due to the increased risk of postoperative complications and the prolonged and complex antimicrobial regimens required.[80,81] However, a recent worldwide survey by Tissot and colleagues highlighted significant variation in practices across different CF centers.[80] Mabs provides CF clinicians with the greatest uncertainty as it has been shown to be associated with an increased risk of post-transplant skin, soft tissue, and disseminated infection.[81,82] Despite this, reported case series have still demonstrated successful transplantation in persons with CF and NTM-PD, inclusive of those with Mabs-PD, through aggressive pre- and post-transplant mycobacterial treatment.[81–84]

Current guidelines recommend that pwCF being considered for lung transplantation should be evaluated for NTM-PD, should commence treatment prior to transplant listing, and may be eligible for transplant listing if they have demonstrated sustained culture conversion.[47,49] However, it is recommended that these individuals be counseled about the high postoperative risk for developing invasive and disseminated NTM disease that may lead to significant morbidity.[47,49]

New NTM infection should also be considered in people with CF post-transplantation with rates of NTM isolation in this cohort reported to range between 1.5% and 22.4%.[85–87] Treatment should remain in line with the antimicrobial regimens outlined above; however, decisions around reduction of transplant-related immunosuppression and drug interactions need to be carefully navigated.[87]

Although current guidelines suggest that there may be a role for lung resection surgery in individuals with localized and treatment refractory NTM-PD, data, outcomes, and evidence-based recommendations for this approach in CF-associated NTM-PD are lacking.[47,49] As such, the 2016 CFF/ECFS Guidelines recommend that lung resection surgery only be considered under extraordinary circumstances and in consultation with experts on the treatment of NTM and CF.[47]

SUMMARY

NTM-PD is a major cause of morbidity in pwCF with rates of infection increasing worldwide. Accurate diagnosis and decisions surrounding best management remain challenging. Current treatment involves prolonged and complex mycobacterial regimens, often associated with significant toxicity. Established guidelines have been developed to assist physicians; however, evidence quality remains low, and outcomes suboptimal. Fortunately, there seems to be increasing enthusiasm internationally to better understand the risk factors and mechanisms for acquisition of infection, as well as to improve our current diagnostics and therapies to help combat disease if treatment is required. Whether the widespread uptake of the disease modifying CFTR modulators will impact on NTM-PD outcomes in pwCF is unknown. Ultimately, however, current management strategies need to evolve to reduce treatment-related burden and toxicity, and to improve outcomes for pwCF and NTM infection.

CLINICS CARE POINTS

- NTM infection in CF is increasing worldwide.
- MAC and Mabs account for the majority of NTM infections in CF.
- Treatment guidelines are available to assist with the management of NTM in CF; however, it involves prolonged and complex mycobacterial regimens, often associated with significant toxicity.
- CF-specific adjunctive treatments, pharmacokinetics, and drug interactions need consideration.
- The current management and outcomes of NTM in CF are likely to evolve due to improved understanding of disease acquisition, better diagnostics, emerging antimycobacterial therapies, and the widespread uptake of CFTR modulator therapies.

DISCLOSURE

Dr T. Baird holds an active research grant from MSD as a co-principal investigator, work of which is outside the scope of this article. Professor S. Bell has received institutional payments from Vertex for chairing and speaking at education events.

Prof. S. Bell is an investigator for a currently funded Merck, Sharp & Dohme (MSD); and Ataxia Telangiectasis Medical Research Future Fund trial, of which he receives no personal payment for activity. Prof. S. Bell is a non-executive director for the Gallipoli Medical Research Foundation and Health Translation Queensland, both of which are unpaid roles.

REFERENCES

1. Olivier KN, Weber DJ, Wallace RJ Jr, et al. Nontuberculous mycobacteria. I: multicenter prevalence study in cystic fibrosis. Am J Respir Crit Care Med 2003;167(6):828–34.

2. Esther CR Jr, Esserman DA, Gilligan P, et al. Chronic Mycobacterium abscessus infection and lung function decline in cystic fibrosis. J Cyst Fibros 2010;9(2):117–23.

3. Qvist T, Gilljam M, Jönsson B, et al. Epidemiology of nontuberculous mycobacteria among patients with cystic fibrosis in Scandinavia. J Cyst Fibros 2015;14(1):46–52.

4. Bar-On O, Mussaffi H, Mei-Zahav M, et al. Increasing nontuberculous mycobacteria infection in cystic fibrosis. J Cyst Fibros 2015;14(1):53–62.

5. Burke A, Thomsom R, Wainwright C, et al. Nontuberculous mycobacteria in cystic fibrosis in the era of cystic fibrosis Transmembrane Regulator modulators. Semin Respir Crit Care Med 2023;44(2):287–96.

6. Martiniano SL, Nick JA, Daley CL. Nontuberculous mycobacterial infections in cystic fibrosis. Clin Chest Med 2022;43(4):697–716.

7. Adjemian J, Olivier KN, Prevots DR. Epidemiology of pulmonary nontuberculous mycobacterial sputum positivity in patients with cystic fibrosis in the United States, 2010-2014. Ann Am Thorac Soc 2018;15(7):817–26.

8. Hatziagorou E, Orenti A, Drevinek P, et al. Changing epidemiology of the respiratory bacteriology of patients with cystic fibrosis-data from the European cystic fibrosis society patient registry. J Cyst Fibros 2020;19(3):376–83.

9. Gardner AI, McClenaghan E, Saint G, et al. Epidemiology of nontuberculous mycobacteria infection in children and young people with cystic fibrosis: analysis of UK cystic fibrosis registry. Infect Dis 2019;68(5):731–7.

10. Prevots DR, Adjemian J, Fernandez AG, et al. Environmental risks for nontuberculous mycobacteria. Individual exposures and climatic factors in the cystic fibrosis population. Ann Am Thorac Soc 2014;11(7):1032–8.

11. Ward C, Al Momani H, Perry A, et al. Clonally related viable nontuberculous mycobacteria in gastric Juice and sputum in people with cystic fibrosis. Am J Respir Crit Care Med 2020;202(7):1061.

12. Bell SC, Mall MA, Gutierrez H, et al. The future of cystic fibrosis care: a global perspective. Lancet Respir Med 2020;8(1):65–124 [published correction appears in Lancet Respir Med. 2019;7(12):e40].

13. Catherinot E, Roux AL, Vibet MA, et al. Mycobacterium avium and Mycobacterium abscessus complex target distinct cystic fibrosis patient subpopulations. J Cyst Fibros 2013;12(1):74–80.

14. Saint GL, Thomas MF, Zainal Abidin N, et al. Treating nontuberculous mycobacteria in children with cystic fibrosis: a multicentre retrospective study. Arch Dis Child 2022;107(5):479–85.

15. Viviani L, Harrison MJ, Zolin A, et al. Epidemiology of nontuberculous mycobacteria (NTM) amongst individuals with cystic fibrosis (CF). J Cyst Fibros 2016;15(5):619–23.

16. Reynaud Q, Bricca R, Cavalli Z, et al. Risk factors for nontuberculous mycobacterial isolation in patients with cystic fibrosis: a meta-analysis. Pediatr Pulmonol 2020;55(10):2653–61.

17. Caverly LJ, Zimbric M, Azar M, et al. Cystic fibrosis airway microbiota associated with outcomes of nontuberculous mycobacterial infection. ERJ Open Res 2021;7(2):00578–2020.

18. Gannon AD, Darch SE. Same Game, different Players: emerging pathogens of the CF lung. mBio 2021;12(1):e01217–20.

19. Renna M, Schaffner C, Brown K, et al. Azithromycin blocks autophagy and may predispose cystic fibrosis patients to mycobacterial infection. J Clin Invest 2011;121(9):3554–63.

20. Binder AM, Adjemian J, Olivier KN, et al. Epidemiology of nontuberculous mycobacterial infections and associated chronic macrolide use among persons with cystic fibrosis. Am J Respir Crit Care Med 2013;188(7):807–12.

21. Cogen JD, Onchiri F, Emerson J, et al. Chronic azithromycin Use in cystic fibrosis and risk of treatment-Emergent respiratory pathogens. Ann Am Thorac Soc 2018;15(6):702–9.

22. Ricotta EE, Prevots DR, Olivier KN. CFTR modulator use and risk of nontuberculous mycobacteria positivity in cystic fibrosis, 2011-2018. ERJ Open Res 2022;8(2):00724–2021.

23. Halstrom S, Price P, Thomson R. Review: environmental mycobacteria as a cause of human infection. Int J Mycobacteriol 2015;4(2):81–91.

24. Hoefsloot W, van Ingen J, Andrejak C, et al. The geographic diversity of nontuberculous mycobacteria isolated from pulmonary samples: an NTM-NET collaborative study. Eur Respir J 2013;42(6):1604–13.

25. Aitken ML, Limaye A, Pottinger P, et al. Respiratory outbreak of Mycobacterium abscessus subspecies massiliense in a lung transplant and cystic fibrosis center. Am J Respir Crit Care Med 2012;185(2):231–2.

26. Bryant JM, Grogono DM, Greaves D, et al. Whole-genome sequencing to identify transmission of

Mycobacterium abscessus between patients with cystic fibrosis: a retrospective cohort study. Lancet 2013;381(9877):1551–60.

27. Adjemian J, Olivier KN, Seitz AE, et al. Prevalence of nontuberculous mycobacterial lung disease in U.S. Medicare beneficiaries. Am J Respir Crit Care Med 2012;185(8):881–6.

28. Thomson RM, Furuya-Kanamori L, Coffey C, et al. Influence of climate variables on the rising incidence of nontuberculous mycobacterial (NTM) infections in Queensland, Australia 2001-2016. Sci Total Environ 2020;740:139796.

29. Thomson R, Tolson C, Carter R, et al. Isolation of nontuberculous mycobacteria (NTM) from household water and shower aerosols in patients with pulmonary disease caused by NTM. J Clin Microbiol 2013;51(9):3006–11.

30. Bryant JM, Grogono DM, Rodriguez-Rincon D, et al. Emergence and spread of a human-transmissible multidrug-resistant nontuberculous mycobacterium. Science 2016;354(6313):751–7.

31. Kim Y, Yoon JH, Ryu J, et al. Gastroesophageal reflux disease increases susceptibility to nontuberculous mycobacterial pulmonary disease. Chest 2022. https://doi.org/10.1016/j.chest.2022.08.2228. S0012-3692(22)03704-03707.

32. Gross JE, Caceres S, Poch K, et al. Investigating nontuberculous mycobacteria transmission at the Colorado adult cystic fibrosis program. Am J Respir Crit Care Med 2022;205(9):1064–74.

33. Lewin A, Kamal E, Semmler T, et al. Genetic diversification of persistent Mycobacterium abscessus within cystic fibrosis patients. Virulence 2021;12(1): 2415–29.

34. Davidson RM, Hasan NA, Epperson LE, et al. Population Genomics of Mycobacterium abscessus from U.S. Cystic fibrosis care centers. Ann Am Thorac Soc 2021;18(12):1960–9.

35. Tortoli E, Kohl TA, Trovato A, et al. Mycobacterium abscessus in patients with cystic fibrosis: low impact of inter-human transmission in Italy. Eur Respir J 2017;50(1):1602525.

36. Gross JE, Caceres S, Poch K, et al. Healthcare-associated links in transmission of nontuberculous mycobacteria among people with cystic fibrosis (HALT NTM) study: Rationale and study design. PLoS One 2021;16(12):e0261628.

37. Griffith DE, Aksamit T, Brown-Elliott BA, et al. An official ATS/IDSA statement: diagnosis, treatment, and prevention of nontuberculous mycobacterial diseases. Am J Respir Crit Care Med 2007;175(4):367–416.

38. Daley CL, Iaccarino JM, Lange C, et al. Treatment of nontuberculous mycobacterial pulmonary disease: an official ATS/ERS/ESCMID/IDSA clinical practice guideline. Clin Infect Dis 2020;71(4):e1–36.

39. Kwak N, Lee CH, Lee HJ, et al. Non-tuberculous mycobacterial lung disease: diagnosis based on computed tomography of the chest. Eur Radiol 2016;26(12):4449–56.

40. Stephenson D, Perry A, Nelson A, et al. Decontamination strategies used for AFB culture significantly reduce the viability of Mycobacterium abscessus complex in sputum samples from patients with cystic fibrosis. Microorganisms 2021;9(8):1597.

41. Rotcheewaphan S, Odusanya OE, Henderson CM, et al. Performance of RGM medium for isolation of nontuberculous mycobacteria from respiratory Specimens from non-cystic fibrosis patients. J Clin Microbiol 2019;57(2). 015199-18.

42. Scohy A, Gohy S, Mathys V, et al. Comparison of the RGM medium and the mycobacterial growth indicator tube automated system for isolation of nontuberculous mycobacteria from sputum samples of cystic fibrosis patients in Belgium. J Clin Tuberc Other Mycobact Dis 2018;13:1–4.

43. Toney NC, Zhu W, Jensen B, et al. Evaluation of MALDI Biotyper mycobacteria Library for identification of nontuberculous mycobacteria. J Clin Microbiol 2022;60(9):e0021722.

44. Bordin A, Pandey S, Coulter C, et al. Rapid macrolide and amikacin resistance testing for Mycobacterium abscessus in people with cystic fibrosis. J Med Microbiol 2021;70(4). https://doi.org/10.1099/jmm.0.001349.

45. Ravnholt C, Qvist T, Kolpen M, et al. Antibody response against Mycobacterium avium complex in cystic fibrosis patients measured by a novel IgG ELISA test. J Cyst Fibros 2019;18(4):516–21.

46. Le Moigne V, Roux AL, Mahoudo H, et al. IgA Serological response for the diagnosis of Mycobacterium abscessus infections in patients with cystic fibrosis. Microbiol Spectr 2022;10(3):e0019222.

47. Floto RA, Olivier KN, Saiman L, et al. US Cystic Fibrosis Foundation and European Cystic Fibrosis Society consensus recommendations for the management of non-tuberculous mycobacteria in individuals with cystic fibrosis. Thorax 2016;71(Suppl 1):i1–22.

48. Low D, Wilson DA, Flume PA. Screening practices for nontuberculous mycobacteria at US cystic fibrosis centers. J Cyst Fibros 2020;19(4):569–74.

49. Haworth CS, Banks J, Capstick T, et al. British Thoracic Society guidelines for the management of non-tuberculous mycobacterial pulmonary disease (NTM-PD). Thorax 2017;72(Suppl 2):ii1–64.

50. Kumar K, Daley CL, Griffith DE, et al. Management of Mycobacterium avium complex and Mycobacterium abscessus pulmonary disease: therapeutic advances and emerging treatments. Eur Respir Rev 2022;31(163):210212.

51. Griffith DE, Eagle G, Thomson R, et al. Amikacin liposome inhalation suspension for treatment-refractory lung disease caused by Mycobacterium avium complex (CONVERT). A Prospective, Open-Label, Randomized study. Am J Respir Crit Care Med 2018; 198(12):1559–69.

52. Jordan CL, Noah TL, Henry MM. Therapeutic challenges posed by critical drug-drug interactions in cystic fibrosis. Pediatr Pulmonol 2016;51(S44): S61–70.

53. Martiniano SL, Esther CR, Haworth CS, et al. Challenging scenarios in nontuberculous mycobacterial infection in cystic fibrosis. Pediatr Pulmonol 2020; 55(2):521–5.

54. Griffith DE, Daley CL. Treatment of Mycobacterium abscessus pulmonary disease. Chest 2022;161(1): 64–75.

55. Saluzzo F, Riberi L, Messore B, et al. CFTR modulator therapies: potential impact on airway infections in cystic fibrosis. Cells 2022;11(7):1243.

56. Akkerman-Nijland AM, Akkerman OW, Grasmeijer F, et al. The pharmacokinetics of antibiotics in cystic fibrosis. Expert Opin Drug Metab Toxicol 2021; 17(1):53–68.

57. Castagnola E, Cangemi G, Mesini A, et al. Pharmacokinetics and pharmacodynamics of antibiotics in cystic fibrosis: a narrative review. Int J Antimicrob Agents 2021;58(3):106381.

58. Martiniano SL, Wagner BD, Brennan L, et al. Pharmacokinetics of oral antimycobacterials and dosing guidance for Mycobacterium avium complex treatment in cystic fibrosis. J Cyst Fibros 2021;20(5): 772–8.

59. Laudone TW, Garner L, Kam CW, et al. Novel therapies for treatment of resistant and refractory nontuberculous mycobacterial infections in patients with cystic fibrosis. Pediatr Pulmonol 2021;56:S55–68.

60. Brown-Elliott BA, Philley JV, Griffith DE, et al. In Vitro susceptibility testing of Bedaquiline against Mycobacterium avium complex. Antimicrob Agents Chemother 2017;61(2). e01798-16.

61. Philley JV, Wallace RJ Jr, Benwill JL, et al. Preliminary results of Bedaquiline as Salvage therapy for patients with nontuberculous mycobacterial lung disease. Chest 2015;148(2):499–506.

62. Brown-Elliott BA, Wallace RJ Jr. In vitro susceptibility testing of omadacycline against nontuberculous mycobacteria. Antimicrob Agents Chemother 2021; 65(3). e01947-20.

63. Shoen C, Benaroch D, Sklaney M, et al. In Vitro Activities of omadacycline against rapidly growing mycobacteria. Antimicrob Agents Chemother 2019; 63(5). e02522-18.

64. Pearson JC, Dionne B, Richterman A, et al. Omadacycline for the treatment of Mycobacterium abscessus disease: a case series. Open Forum Infect Dis 2020;7(10):ofaa415.

65. Morrisette T, Alosaimy S, Philley JV, et al. Preliminary, real-world, multicenter experience with omadacycline for Mycobacterium abscessus infections. Open Forum Infect Dis 2021;8(2):ofab002.

66. Poon YK, La Hoz RM, Hynan LS, et al. Tedizolid vs Linezolid for the treatment of nontuberculous mycobacteria infections in Solid Organ transplant recipients. Open Forum Infect Dis 2021;8(4): ofab093.

67. Kaushik A, Ammerman NC, Martins O, et al. In vitro activity of new Tetracycline Analogs omadacycline and Eravacycline against drug-resistant clinical isolates of Mycobacterium abscessus. Antimicrob Agents Chemother 2019;63(6). e00470-19.

68. Dubée V, Bernut A, Cortes M, et al. β-Lactamase inhibition by avibactam in Mycobacterium abscessus. J Antimicrob Chemother 2015;70(4): 1051–8.

69. Le Run E, Arthur M, Mainardi JL. In Vitro and intracellular activity of imipenem combined with tedizolid, rifabutin, and avibactam against Mycobacterium abscessus. Antimicrob Agents Chemother 2019;63(4):e01915–8.

70. Story-Roller E, Galanis C, Lamichhane G. β-Lactam combinations that Exhibit Synergy against Mycobacteroides abscessus clinical isolates. Antimicrob Agents Chemother 2021;65(4). e02545-20.

71. Jones LA, Doucette L, Dellon EP, et al. Use of inhaled imipenem/cilastatin in pediatric patients with cystic fibrosis: a case series. J Cyst Fibros 2019;18(4):e42–4.

72. Pearce C, Ruth MM, Pennings LJ, et al. Inhaled tigecycline is effective against Mycobacterium abscessus in vitro and in vivo. J Antimicrob Chemother 2020;75(7):1889–94.

73. Banaschewski B, Verma D, Pennings LJ, et al. Clofazimine inhalation suspension for the aerosol treatment of pulmonary nontuberculous mycobacterial infections. J Cyst Fibros 2019;18(5):714–20.

74. Yaacoby-Bianu K, Gur M, Toukan Y, et al. Compassionate nitric oxide Adjuvant treatment of persistent Mycobacterium infection in cystic fibrosis patients. Pediatr Infect Dis J 2018;37(4):336–8.

75. Bentur L, Gur M, Ashkenazi M, et al. Pilot study to test inhaled nitric oxide in cystic fibrosis patients with refractory Mycobacterium abscessus lung infection. J Cyst Fibros 2020;19(2):225–31.

76. Hallstrand TS, Ochs HD, Zhu Q, et al. Inhaled IFN-gamma for persistent nontuberculous mycobacterial pulmonary disease due to functional IFN-gamma deficiency. Eur Respir J 2004;24(3):367–70.

77. Scott JP, Ji Y, Kannan M, et al. Inhaled granulocyte-macrophage colony-stimulating factor for Mycobacterium abscessus in cystic fibrosis. Eur Respir J 2018;51:1702127.

78. Dedrick RM, Guerrero-Bustamante CA, Garlena RA, et al. Engineered bacteriophages for treatment of a patient with a disseminated drug-resistant Mycobacterium abscessus. Nat Med 2019;25(5):730–3.

79. Nick JA, Dedrick RM, Gray AL, et al. Host and pathogen response to bacteriophage engineered against Mycobacterium abscessus lung infection. Cell 2022;185(11):1860–74.e12.

80. Tissot A, Thomas MF, Corris PA, et al. NonTuberculous Mycobacteria infection and lung transplantation in cystic fibrosis: a worldwide survey of clinical practice. BMC Pulm Med 2018;18(1):86.

81. Hamad Y, Pilewski JM, Morrell M, et al. Outcomes in lung transplant recipients with Mycobacterium abscessus infection: a 15-year experience from a large Tertiary care center. Transplant Proc 2019;51(6): 2035–42.

82. Raats D, Lorent N, Saegeman V, et al. Successful lung transplantation for chronic Mycobacterium abscessus infection in advanced cystic fibrosis, a case series. Transpl Infect Dis 2019;21(2):e13046.

83. Qvist T, Pressler T, Thomsen VO, et al. Nontuberculous mycobacterial disease is not a contraindication to lung transplantation in patients with cystic fibrosis: a retrospective analysis in a Danish patient population. Transplant Proc 2013;45(1):342–5.

84. Lobo LJ, Noone PG. Respiratory infections in patients with cystic fibrosis undergoing lung transplantation. Lancet Respir Med 2014;2(1):73–82.

85. Chernenko SM, Humar A, Hutcheon M, et al. Mycobacterium abscessus infections in lung transplant recipients: the international experience. J Heart Lung Transplant 2006;25(12):1447–55.

86. Knoll BM, Kappagoda S, Gill RR, et al. Non-tuberculous mycobacterial infection among lung transplant recipients: a 15-year cohort study. Transpl Infect Dis 2012;14(5):452–60.

87. Shah SK, McAnally KJ, Seoane L, et al. Analysis of pulmonary non-tuberculous mycobacterial infections after lung transplantation. Transpl Infect Dis 2016;18(4):585–91.

Surgical Resection in Nontuberculous Mycobacterial Pulmonary Disease

Lauren J. Taylor, MD[a], John D. Mitchell, MD[b],*

KEYWORDS

- Nontuberculous mycobacteria • Lung resection • Minimally invasive thoracic surgery

KEY POINTS

- Careful patient selection is critical and should include a multidisciplinary approach to ensure that the patient is medically and nutritionally optimized and has a disease burden amenable to resection.
- Surgery for nontuberculous mycobacterial pulmonary disease (NTM-PD) may commonly be performed using minimally invasive techniques but key differences exist compared to surgery for oncologic indications including density of adhesions, hypertrophied bronchial circulation, and obliteration of tissue planes requiring careful dissection.
- While a bronchopleural fistula is a feared complication, data demonstrate that pulmonary resection for NTM-PD is effective and may be performed with acceptable morbidity and mortality in experienced centers.

INTRODUCTION

Nontuberculous mycobacteria (NTM) represent hundreds of mycobacteria aside from the more well-known and contagious *Mycobacterium leprae* and *Mycobacterium tuberculosis* complex. These organisms are ubiquitous within our environment and cause no harm in most people. However, when symptomatic infection does occur in a susceptible host, the lungs are the predominant target of the disease.[1–7]

Long-term multidrug antibiotic therapy is the cornerstone of treatment for symptomatic nontuberculous mycobacterial pulmonary disease (NTM-PD), with duration of therapy commonly extending beyond 12 months.[8] Despite pharmacologic advancements, success rates are low and recurrence rates are high. Treatment success, measured by the rate of culture negative conversion, has been quoted in the literature between 34% and 65% depending on the causative mycobacterial species.[9–12] Similarly, recurrence rates after successful treatment have been reported as high as 48%.[13,14] Furthermore, these multidrug regimens are often poorly tolerated by patients, access to appropriate treatment may be challenging, and significant drug resistance may develop. These factors further contribute to treatment failure.

Due to these challenges, surgery has emerged as an adjunctive treatment modality for patients with NTM-PD to reduce disease burden and promote treatment success.[8] While there is variability in the literature regarding postoperative outcomes, adjunctive surgical resection is considered to be a viable option in the treatment armamentarium for patients with NTM-PD. In this article, we will review the indications for surgery, perioperative considerations, surgical techniques, and recent literature on surgical outcomes.

a Department of Surgery, Division of Cardiothoracic Surgery, University of Colorado, 12631 East 17th Avenue, C-310, Aurora, CO 80045, USA; b General Thoracic Surgery, Department of Surgery, Division of Cardiothoracic Surgery, University of Colorado, 12631 East 17th Avenue, C-310, Aurora, CO 80045, USA
* Corresponding author.
E-mail address: John.mitchell@cuanschutz.edu

Clin Chest Med 44 (2023) 861–868
https://doi.org/10.1016/j.ccm.2023.06.013
0272-5231/23/© 2023 Elsevier Inc. All rights reserved.

Indications for Surgery

In 2007, the American Thoracic Society (ATS) and the Infectious Diseases Society of America (IDSA) joined forces to publish an official statement guiding the treatment of NTM-PD.[1] These recommendations were updated in 2020 by international collaborative efforts from the ATS, IDSA, European Respiratory Society, and the European Society of Clinical Microbiology and Infectious Diseases.[8] Additionally, the British Thoracic Society reference surgical indications in the 2017 guideline statement.[15] Guidelines offer a conditional recommendation to proceed with surgical resection as adjuvant treatment in select patients who have failed medical management, acknowledging that careful examination of the risks and benefits of surgery and consultation with an experienced surgeon are essential.

Surgical resection in the setting of NTM-PD is indicated in 3 primary situations: failure of medical management, to slow disease progression, and provide symptom relief.[16] Failure of medical treatment is the most frequent scenario in which patients are referred for surgical evaluation; it is commonly defined as persistence or recurrence of positive cultures after 12 months of therapy.[17] Failure may be due to a variety of different reasons, including development of antibiotic resistance, intolerance to medical therapy, or recurrent infection. In these cases, the goal of surgery is typically cure and as such it is important to ensure that disease is localized to an area of lung amenable to resection with preservation of the remaining healthy parenchyma. In contrast, select patients may benefit from operative debulking. In these situations, diseased lung remains postoperatively rendering cure nearly impossible; however, removing the most severely damaged parenchyma may impede disease progression. This strategy is commonly employed in patients with a dominant cavitary lesion and mild parenchymal disease in other lobes. Finally, patients with persistent or potentially life-threatening symptoms such as chronic cough or hemoptysis may derive relief from surgery. In these situations, like patients who undergo operative debulking, residual disease often remains after surgery. It is important to note that patients may experience symptom benefit even if it is not possible to resect all areas of the disease.

Preoperative Considerations

For patients referred for surgical evaluation, a minority will go on to resection. A thorough preoperative evaluation is essential for optimal patient selection. In addition to the standard cardiopulmonary assessment to demonstrate that a patient will tolerate the planned resection from a physiologic standpoint, patients with NTM-PD require a multimodal approach to ensure treatment success.

Patients who are amenable for surgery typically demonstrate 1 of 3 common disease phenotypes, which dictate the optimal operative strategy. The first is referred to as "Lady Windermere syndrome" and consists of bronchiectasis localized to the lingula and right middle lobe (**Fig. 1**). This disease pattern has a strong female predominance and resection usually occurs in a staged fashion, with minimally invasive anatomic resections planned several weeks apart.[18] The second common pattern includes cavitary lung disease or focal bronchiectasis amenable to a lobar or segmental resection (**Fig. 2**). In these scenarios, if the problematic area is indeed focal, resection has the potential to render the patient culture negative if combined with effective antimicrobial treatment. It is important to note that many patients may have multiple areas of focal abnormality. The third pattern of presentation is the most severe. Patients with significant to complete unilateral lung destruction from NTM-PD may require pneumonectomy (**Fig. 3**).

A comprehensive multidisciplinary review is essential in the evaluation of patients with NTM-PD prior to surgery. Representation should include thoracic surgery, pulmonology, and infectious disease providers with expertise in mycobacterial disease. The committee reviews all radiologic, physiologic, nutritional, and culture data before determining candidacy for surgery.

High-resolution computed tomography (HRCT) is an important initial test to assess the underlying burden of the disease and determine the extent of surgical resection. A computed tomography (CT) scan can also shed light on the likelihood that

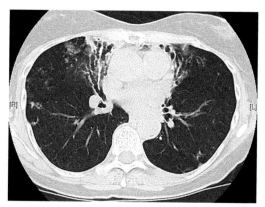

Fig. 1. Computed tomography image of right middle lobe and lingula bronchiectasis, commonly referred to as Lady Windermere Syndrome.

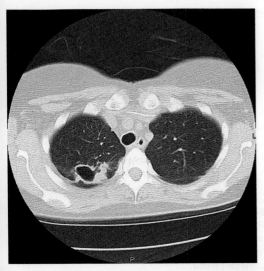

Fig. 2. Computed tomography image of a patient with NTM-PD and a cavitary lesion amenable to minimally invasive surgical resection.

surgery may be successful in a minimally invasive fashion.[19] Once this is known, workup proceeds to establish if a patient has sufficient cardiopulmonary reserve to tolerate the planned resection. Similar to a cancer patient preparing for lung resection, evaluation includes pulmonary function tests, ventilation perfusion scans, and exercise testing when appropriate.

In addition to cardiopulmonary status, a complete preoperative nutritional assessment is conducted. While feeding tubes are generally not necessary in patients who present with focal disease, many are initiated on dietary supplementation in the weeks before surgery. Optimization of the patient's nutritional status is critical, particularly if an extended resection is anticipated. All patients are also evaluated for gastroesophageal reflux disease, as this may contribute to underlying chronic pulmonary disease.

Unique to the NTM-PD population is preoperative sputum analysis to identify causative organisms. In some cases, bronchoscopy may be advantageous to obtain a bronchoalveolar lavage

specimen and may help localize endobronchial pathology and the source of hemoptysis, if present. Based on in vitro susceptibility testing, patients are initiated on multidrug regimens, often consisting of 3 to 4 drugs. Treatment commonly involves a combination of intravenous and inhaled antibiotics and is typically administered for 8 to 12 weeks preoperatively. The timing of surgery may be delayed if issues with drug intolerance arise necessitating trial of an alternative regimen. Ideally, surgery should occur when mycobacterial counts are at a nadir, as this is thought to minimize the incidence of perioperative complications.[20]

All patients should return for multidisciplinary evaluation after completion of preoperative antibiotics. As treatment response is variable, it is prudent to obtain an updated CT scan in close proximity to the operative date to ensure there has not been a significant change in the disease burden that would warrant alteration of the operative plan. The patient's overall nutritional status and state of other relevant comorbidities should also be reevaluated at this time. Attempts should be made to render patients' sputum negative prior to surgery; however, this is not always possible and should not be an absolute contraindication to resection.

Surgical Technique

Pulmonary resection for NTMPD may be performed through a thoracotomy or in a minimally invasive fashion. Anatomic resections—whether they be segmentectomies, lobectomies, or pneumonectomies—are preferred to wedge resections both to minimize the risk of complications and to ensure complete resection of the involved parenchyma. The choice of technique varies based on the extent of disease and surgeon experience.

Open resections are typically performed via a posterolateral thoracotomy. While minimally invasive surgery is becoming more commonplace for NTM-PD, patients with extensive disease necessitating a pneumonectomy or reoperative surgery still commonly require an open approach. For those who have previously undergone pulmonary

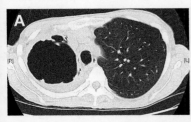
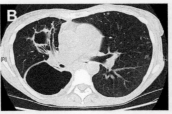
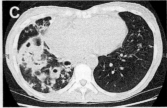

Fig. 3. (A–C): Three computed tomography images from a single patient with NTM-PD resulting in near-total lung destruction requiring a pneumonectomy.

resection, the same incision is often used and rib removal, commonly the fifth or sixth rib, can be helpful to optimize exposure and identify the extrapleural plane in the setting of an extrapleural pneumonectomy. Care should be taken upon entry to preserve muscle, typically an intercostal or latissimus dorsi muscle, for coverage of the bronchial stump and to allow for muscle transposition to manage residual space.[21]

Use of minimally invasive surgery, whether it be using a video-assisted thoracoscopic surgery (VATS) or robotic-assisted approach, is becoming more commonplace for patients with NTM-PD. Favorable results with minimally invasive techniques have been published previously[22] and at experienced centers like ours, comprise the majority of resections for NTM-PD. Standard incisions as one would use for an anatomic cancer resection are typically well-suited for these cases without the need for rib spreading in the majority of patients. For VATS cases, our standard set up includes two 10 mm ports as well as a 3 cm utility incision with a wound protector at the utility incision where the specimen is removed. It is important to note that in the setting of *Mycobacterium abscessus*, wound protectors are recommended to minimize the risk of wound infection at all port sites. For robotic cases, we use two to three 8 mm ports and one to two 12 mm ports depending on the planned anatomic resection for a total of 4 ports. The ports are placed in approximately the eighth intercostal space, but special attention is paid to choosing the widest interspaces as these are most favorable for port placement and are least likely to cause postoperative neuropathic pain. Determining adequate port placement may be a particular challenge in NTM-PD patients, as the most common phenotype is a petite female with narrow intercostal spaces. We use a 12 mm assistant port placed just medial and inferior to the camera port. At the conclusion of the case, the specimen is placed in a bag and removed through this incision.

Regardless of the approach, there are important differences between surgery for NTM-PD and pulmonary resection for other pathologies. Before an incision is made, intraoperative bronchoscopy may be useful to clear the airways and define segmental anatomy. Once the chest is entered, the first noticeable difference the surgeon encounters is adhesions, which are typically greatest in density surrounding the area of diseased parenchyma but may encompass the entire hemithorax (**Fig. 4**). Lysing the adhesions should proceed carefully as to avoid injury to critical structures and perseverance is often rewarded. Adhesions may be divided using a variety of techniques,

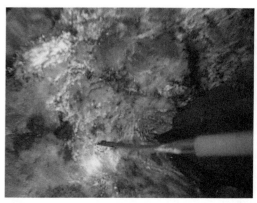

Fig. 4. Adhesions are common in patients with NTM-PD and chronic inflammation may lead to obliteration of tissue planes necessitating careful dissection. In this image, the diseased lung is freed from the overlying parietal pleura.

including blunt dissection or with the use of available energy devices. Interestingly, a minimally invasive video-based approach often facilitates adhesion management in patients with focal bronchiectasis or cavitary lesions. However, for cases in which the surgeon is dubious as to the success of a minimally invasive resection, exploratory thoracoscopy may be advantageous before committing to either technique.

The same care should be taken during hilar dissection. In contrast to cancer cases, patients with NTM-PD often have hypertrophy of the bronchial circulation, calcified nodes, and significant inflammation within the hilum of the lung. This may add a particular challenge to the hilar dissection due to increased bleeding and loss of clear tissue planes. In contrast to oncologic resections in which thorough nodal dissection is paramount to accurate staging, in NTM cases it is often safer to leave lymph nodes in situ. Furthermore, chronic inflammation may result in fusion of the fissures making fissural dissection potentially treacherous for the low-volume NTM surgeon. Once structures are identified, vascular and bronchial division is performed using standard stapling devices. We do not routinely buttress the bronchial stump in minimally invasive cases. These important differences, while manageable by an experienced surgeon, may be hazardous for surgeons not accustomed to this pathology. Careful dissection is essential and referral to a high-volume center is strongly encouraged.

Once the specimen has been removed, cultures of the affected areas should be immediately obtained on a back table within the operating room. We routinely send cultures to 2 different laboratories to optimize culture findings and minimize sampling error. The remainder of the case proceeds as would any lung resection with placement of chest drains and closure of incisions in the standard fashion.

Patients with NTM-PD are predisposed to issues with residual space after resection due to underlying poor lung compliance that prevents the remaining lung from adequately expanding to fill the hemithorax. Surgical options to minimize ipsilateral intrathoracic space include use of autologous tissue and a limited thoracoplasty. Autologous tissue, typically transposed latissimus dorsi or pectoralis major muscle, may be harvested at the time of initial incision in either minimally invasive or open cases. These transposed muscles (based on the appropriate neurovascular pedicle) may be used to fill intrathoracic space and promote healing of raw lung surfaces. Buttressing of the bronchial closure, important in cases of pneumonectomy or poorly controlled infection, is achieved with an intercostal muscle flap. While the serratus anterior muscle is an option in other patient populations, it is not commonly used in NTM patients who are typically very thin and prone to a "winged scapula" that results from harvest of this muscle, leading to wound issues. Use of an omental flap may be advantageous in patients requiring a pneumonectomy or in the setting of poorly controlled infection due to its excellent vascular supply and significant bulk and is typically reserved for the most severe cases. The omental flap is harvested by the thoracic surgeon via a mini laparotomy just prior to performing a thoracotomy and based on a vascular supply from the right gastroepiploic pedicle. The flap is transposed into the chest via a substernal tunnel into the mediastinal pleura or through an anterior diaphragmatic defect made near the costal attachments.[23] Thoracoplasty was originally developed in the management of tuberculosis in the late nineteenth century. The goal is to obliterate the pleural cavity with viable chest wall tissue and has been described as a total (11 ribs), partial (8–9 ribs), or tailored (fewer than 5 ribs) technique. Even in its most limited form, thoracoplasty is highly morbid and used in the setting of NTM-PD only in rare circumstances when severe space issues persist.

Open thoracostomy (Eloesser flap) is an important technique in the armamentarium of the NTM surgeon. This approach may be particularly useful in patients who have intraoperative spillage from thin-walled cavitary lesions or who already have involvement in the pleural space due to perforation. In these settings, our usual approach is to pack the chest daily at the bedside with dilute Dakin's (sodium hypochlorite)-soaked gauze and then perform a Clagett procedure (chest closure after filling the hemithorax with non-absorbable antimicrobial solution) in 6 to 12 weeks. If need for this approach is suspected, extensive preoperative counseling with the patient and family is imperative.

Postoperative Considerations

For most patients who undergo a segmentectomy or lobectomy for focal disease, the immediate postoperative care is very similar to that of a patient undergoing the same procedure for a non-infectious indication. Chest tubes are removed following resolution of air leaks and patients are maintained on standard deep vein thrombosis and atrial fibrillation prophylaxis. Good pulmonary hygiene is critical. The distinguishing feature of immediate postoperative management of NTM patients is that we typically continue their multidrug antibiotic regimen throughout the perioperative period. Intraoperative culture data are used to tailor antimicrobial therapy under the guidance of an infectious disease/pulmonary medicine specialist and many patients are able to stop parenteral (but not all) therapy within 1 to 2 months of surgery.

Postoperative Outcomes and Review of Recent Literature

Available data suggest that anatomic pulmonary resection for NTMPD may be performed safely with a high success rate of "culture conversion" postoperatively. At our institution, we have published results of minimally invasive resections for patients with NTM-PD with no mortality and minimal morbidity. Patients not only had similar rates of complications but comparable length of stay compared to those who underwent anatomic resection for lung cancer.[22] However, it is important to note that these outcomes are achieved in carefully selected patients in the setting of multidisciplinary care at a high-volume institution.

While these findings are certainly encouraging, surgery for NTM-PD is not without complications. Bronchopleural fistula (BPF), particularly after a right-sided pneumonectomy, is a dreaded but unfortunately not uncommon complication in this patient population. Rates of postpneumonectomy BPF have been reported in the literature ranging from 25% to 60%[23–25] Interestingly, development of BPF appears to be more common following pneumonectomy for NTM-PD as compared to multidrug-resistant tuberculosis.[26] Possible explanations for this discrepancy include presence of large cavitary lesions, poorly controlled infection, and a predilection for right-sided disease in the setting of NTM-PD.

Outcomes data dating back to the 1980s for patients undergoing surgery for NTM-PD have historically been limited to small, single-center studies contributing to discrepancies in the literature regarding postoperative results. However, recent studies provide data to support pushing the boundaries of surgical resection and offer updated statistics on postoperative outcomes. We will review several of the most recent additions to the literature.

In 2021, Yamada and colleagues[27] published a retrospective study in the Annals of Thoracic Surgery examining the safety and feasibility of surgery for patients with NTM-PD requiring extensive lung resection (ELR). In this report, the authors examined outcomes for 146 patients who underwent adjuvant resection between 2008 and 2019 at 2 major hospitals in Japan. Outcomes were compared between those undergoing simple anatomic lung resection (SALR) defined as resection isolated to a single lobe, as opposed to ELR in which the disease extended to multiple lobes. All patients received both preoperative and postoperative antimicrobial therapy and were selected for adjuvant surgery based on the decision of a multidisciplinary committee. Seventy three percent of the study population was female and the mean age was 56 years. There were no significant differences in age, gender, body mass index (BMI), time from initial treatment to surgery, or antimicrobial therapy between groups. Cases were completed using a minimally invasive approach in over 90% of patients, and interestingly rates of conversion to open did not differ based on extent of the disease. In the SALR group, most common operations included lobectomy (71%) and segmentectomy (29%). In the ELR group, 26% of the patients underwent lobectomy and wedge resection, 22% received a bilobectomy, and the 19% underwent lobectomy in addition to segmentectomy. Not surprisingly, operative times were significantly longer in the ELR group. In addition, ELR was associated with significantly higher complication rate (24 vs 7.6%), days requiring an indwelling chest tube (4.6 vs 3.0 days), and longer length of stay (8.8 vs 7.3 days). However, there was no significant difference in 30- and 90-day mortality, rates of culture conversion, microbiological recurrence, or rates of BFP between groups. The authors conclude that the safety of ELR is similar to that of SALR and is feasible to perform in a minimally invasive fashion. While ELR is associated with longer operative times and increased incidence of prolonged air leak, this may be a viable alternative to pneumonectomy for patients with multilobar disease.

In 2020, Yotsumoto and colleagues[28] reported outcomes of 100 patients with NTM-PD and examined postoperative outcomes and risks of disease recurrence. This Japanese retrospective analysis reported no postoperative deaths and found prolonged air leak to be the most common complication. Only 1 patient required a conversion to an open procedure; this was due to a pulmonary artery injury. The authors report a recurrence rate of 9%. A positive preoperative sputum culture and positive preoperative sputum stain ($\geq 2 +$) were significant risk factors for disease recurrence in the univariate analysis (sputum culture, $P = .038$; sputum stain, $P = .011$). Sputum stain ($\geq 2 +$) remained significant in the multivariate analysis. However, age, causative organism, CT findings, and extent of resection were not found to impact recurrence rates in this study. These findings build upon prior work by Asakura and colleagues[29] who followed 125 patients for a median of 7.1 years. These authors report an overall postoperative complication rate of 22%, no operative mortality, and 91% of patients achieved sputum conversion. In contrast to the cohort described by Yotsumoto and colleagues,[28] in this study the majority of resections were performed by thoracotomy and 25% of the patients received a pneumonectomy. Survival was 94% at 1 year and declined to 76% by 10 years. Receipt of pneumonectomy, presence of residual cavitary lesions, older age, and low BMI were found to be associated with poor prognosis while pneumonectomy and residual cavitary lesions were also associated with microbiological disease recurrence. Finally, Kim and colleagues[30] recently performed a similar analysis of 67 patients who underwent surgery between 2006 and 2020 at a university hospital in South Korea to examine factors associated with disease recurrence and poor postoperative outcomes. These authors found a lower rate of culture conversion, 71.7%, and 17% of the patients suffered disease recurrence. Postoperative complications occurred in 13.4% of the patients in this cohort. Similar to prior reports, the authors determined the presence of preoperative positive cultures as well as residual pulmonary disease after surgery to be associated with both recurrence and failure to achieve culture conversion.

While the bulk of recent data on surgical resection for NTM-PD remains the product of small single-institution investigation, we are fortunate to benefit from the publication of a systematic review and meta-analysis, which was released in Chest in 2022.[17] This analysis included 15 studies published prior to 2022 for a pooled total of 1071 patients. Of these patients, 93% achieved postoperative sputum culture negative conversion. The patients were followed for a median length of 34 months and during this time 9% (95% CI 6%–14%) experienced disease recurrence. Postoperative complications occurred in 17% of patients, and of those with complications 8.2% developed a BPF. In subgroup analyses, complication rates were similar between studies that included greater than 30% of patients undergoing ELR (16%) compared to studies in which ELR was performed in less than 30% of the cohort. Furthermore, complication rates in studies performed at Asian institutions (17%) were comparable to those performed in North America (20%). Across studies, the in-hospital mortality was 0% (95% CI 0%–2%). These findings support adjunctive surgery as an effective treatment modality for patients with NTM-PD with an acceptable morbidity and mortality profile. While this study provides the best available safety and efficacy data, important questions remain regarding the optimal timing of surgical resection. While there is agreement that it is optimal to delay surgery until after smear conversion, the specific duration one should wait before operating remains elusive. In fact, the duration of preoperative antibiotics ranged widely across studies from 2 to 24.5 months. In addition, there is a paucity of data regarding quality of life measures after pulmonary resection in this patient population.

SUMMARY

As rates of NTM-PD continue to rise across the globe, it is likely that surgery will play a significant role in the multimodal management of these patients. In selected patients, pulmonary resection has been shown to be both effective and safe in this patient population but is imperative that patients undergo a rigorous review by a multidisciplinary committee and are referred to a surgeon experienced in the management of this disease. While key intraoperative differences characterize surgery for NTM-PD, resection may be successfully and safely performed using minimally invasive techniques. Ongoing research is needed to clarify the optimal timing of surgery and postoperative quality of life measures.

CLINICS CARE POINTS

- In selected patients, the use of surgical resection may provide an important adjunct in the treatment of patients with pulmonary NTM infection.

DISCLOSURE

Dr J.D. Mitchell: Consultant, Intuitive Surgical, Inc Dr L.J. Taylor does not have any commercial or financial conflicts of interest.

REFERENCES

1. Griffith DE, Aksamit T, Brown-Elliott BA, et al. An official ATS/IDSA statement: diagnosis, treatment, and prevention of nontuberculous mycobacterial diseases. Am J Respir Crit Care Med 2007;175(4):367–745. https://doi.org/10.1164/rccm.200604-571ST [published correction appears in Am J Respir Crit Care Med. 2007 Apr 1;175(7):744-745. Dosage error in article text].

2. Diel R, Jacob J, Lampenius N, et al. Burden of nontuberculous mycobacterial pulmonary disease in Germany. Eur Respir J 2017;49(4):1602109. https://doi.org/10.1183/13993003.02109-2016.

3. Lee H, Myung W, Lee EM, et al. Mortality and prognostic factors of nontuberculous mycobacterial infection in Korea: a population-based comparative study. Clin Infect Dis 2021;72(10):e610–9. https://doi.org/10.1093/cid/ciaa1381.

4. Ballarino GJ, Olivier KN, Claypool RJ, et al. Pulmonary nontuberculous mycobacterial infections: antibiotic treatment and associated costs. Respir Med 2009;103(10):1448–55. https://doi.org/10.1016/j.rmed.2009.04.026.

5. Shah NM, Davidson JA, Anderson LF, et al. Pulmonary Mycobacterium avium-intracellulare is the main driver of the rise in non-tuberculous mycobacteria incidence in England, Wales and Northern Ireland, 2007-2012. BMC Infect Dis 2016;16:195. https://doi.org/10.1186/s12879-016-1521-3.

6. Learn About NTM Lung Disease. https://www.lung.org/lung-health-diseases/lung-disease-lookup/nontuberculous-mycobacteria/learn-about-nontuberculosis-mycobacteria. Published 2022. Accessed February 17, 2023.

7. Namkoong H, Kurashima A, Morimoto K, et al. Epidemiology of pulmonary nontuberculous mycobacterial disease. Japan. Emerg Infect Dis 2016;22(6):1116–7. https://doi.org/10.3201/eid2206.151086.

8. Daley CL, Iaccarino JM, Lange C, et al. Treatment of nontuberculous mycobacterial pulmonary disease: an official ATS/ERS/ESCMID/IDSA clinical practice guideline. Clin Infect Dis 2020;71(4):905–13. https://doi.org/10.1093/cid/ciaa1125.

9. Diel R, Nienhaus A, Ringshausen FC, et al. Microbiologic outcome of interventions against Mycobacterium avium complex pulmonary disease: a systematic review. Chest 2018;153(4):888–921. https://doi.org/10.1016/j.chest.2018.01.024.

10. Diel R, Ringshausen F, Richter E, et al. Microbiological and clinical outcomes of treating non-

Mycobacterium avium complex nontuberculous mycobacterial pulmonary disease: a systematic review and meta-analysis. Chest 2017;152(1):120–42. https://doi.org/10.1016/j.chest.2017.04.166.

11. Kwak N, Dalcolmo MP, Daley CL, et al. *Mycobacterium abscessus* pulmonary disease: individual patient data meta-analysis. Eur Respir J 2019;54(1): 1801991. https://doi.org/10.1183/13993003.01991-2018.

12. Kwak N, Park J, Kim E, et al. Treatment outcomes of Mycobacterium avium complex lung disease: a systematic review and meta-analysis. Clin Infect Dis 2017;65(7):1077–84. https://doi.org/10.1093/cid/cix517.

13. Moon SM, Jhun BW, Baek SY, et al. Long-term natural history of non-cavitary nodular bronchiectatic nontuberculous mycobacterial pulmonary disease. Respir Med 2019;151:1–7. https://doi.org/10.1016/j.rmed.2019.03.014.

14. Shin SH, Jhun BW, Kim SY, et al. Nontuberculous mycobacterial lung diseases caused by mixed infection with Mycobacterium avium complex and Mycobacterium abscessus complex. Antimicrob Agents Chemother 2018;62(10):e01105–18. https://doi.org/10.1128/AAC.01105-18.

15. Haworth CS, Banks J, Capstick T, et al. British Thoracic Society guidelines for the management of non-tuberculous mycobacterial pulmonary disease (NTM-PD). Thorax 2017;72(Suppl 2):ii1–64.

16. Mitchell JD. Surgical approach to pulmonary nontuberculous mycobacterial infections. Clin Chest Med 2015;36(1):117–22. https://doi.org/10.1016/j.ccm.2014.11.004.

17. Kim JY, Lee HW, Yim JJ, et al. Outcomes of adjunctive surgery in patients with nontuberculous mycobacterial pulmonary disease: a systematic review and meta-analysis (published online ahead of print, 2022 Oct 5). Chest. 2022;S0012-3692(22)03907-1. doi:10.1016/j.chest.2022.09.037

18. Yu JA, Pomerantz M, Bishop A, et al. Lady Windermere revisited: treatment with thoracoscopic lobectomy/segmentectomy for right middle lobe and lingular bronchiectasis associated with nontuberculous mycobacterial disease. Eur J Cardio Thorac Surg 2011;40(3):671–5. https://doi.org/10.1016/j.ejcts.2010.12.028.

19. Yen YT, Wu MH, Cheng L, et al. Image characteristics as predictors for thoracoscopic anatomic lung resection in patients with pulmonary tuberculosis. Ann Thorac Surg 2011;92(1):290–5. https://doi.org/10.1016/j.athoracsur.2011.02.039.

20. Mitchell JD. Surgical treatment of pulmonary nontuberculous mycobacterial infections. Thorac Surg Clin 2019;29(1):77–83. https://doi.org/10.1016/j.thorsurg.2018.09.011.

21. Sherwood JT, Mitchell JD, Pomerantz M. Completion pneumonectomy for chronic mycobacterial disease. J Thorac Cardiovasc Surg 2005;129(6):1258–65. https://doi.org/10.1016/j.jtcvs.2004.12.053.

22. Mitchell JD, Yu JA, Bishop A, et al. Thoracoscopic lobectomy and segmentectomy for infectious lung disease. Ann Thorac Surg 2012;93(4):1033–40. https://doi.org/10.1016/j.athoracsur.2012.01.012.

23. Mitchell JD, Bishop A, Cafaro A, et al. Anatomic lung resection for nontuberculous mycobacterial disease. Ann Thorac Surg 2008;85(6):1887–93. https://doi.org/10.1016/j.athoracsur.2008.02.041.

24. Koh WJ, Kim YH, Kwon OJ, et al. Surgical treatment of pulmonary diseases due to nontuberculous mycobacteria. J Kor Med Sci 2008;23(3):397–401. https://doi.org/10.3346/jkms.2008.23.3.397.

25. Shiraishi Y, Nakajima Y, Katsuragi N, et al. Pneumonectomy for nontuberculous mycobacterial infections. Ann Thorac Surg 2004;78(2):399–403. https://doi.org/10.1016/j.athoracsur.2004.02.103.

26. Shiraishi Y, Katsuragi N, Kita H, et al. Different morbidity after pneumonectomy: multidrug-resistant tuberculosis versus non-tuberculous mycobacterial infection. Interact Cardiovasc Thorac Surg 2010;11(4):429–32. https://doi.org/10.1510/icvts.2010.236372.

27. Yamada K, Seki Y, Nakagawa T, et al. Extensive lung resection for nontuberculous mycobacterial lung disease with multilobar lesions. Ann Thorac Surg 2021;111(1):253–60. https://doi.org/10.1016/j.athoracsur.2020.05.067.

28. Yotsumoto T, Inoue Y, Fukami T, et al. Pulmonary resection for nontuberculous mycobacterial pulmonary disease: outcomes and risk factors for recurrence. Gen Thorac Cardiovasc Surg 2020;68(9):993–1002. https://doi.org/10.1007/s11748-020-01326-1.

29. Asakura T, Hayakawa N, Hasegawa N, et al. Long-term outcome of pulmonary resection for nontuberculous mycobacterial pulmonary disease. Clin Infect Dis 2017;65(2):244–51. https://doi.org/10.1093/cid/cix274.

30. Kim JY, Park S, Park IK, et al. Outcomes of adjunctive surgery for nontuberculous mycobacterial pulmonary disease. BMC Pulm Med 2021;21(1):312. https://doi.org/10.1186/s12890-021-01679-0.

UNITED STATES POSTAL SERVICE® Statement of Ownership, Management, and Circulation
(All Periodicals Publications Except Requester Publications)

1. Publication Title	2. Publication Number	3. Filing Date
CLINICS IN CHEST MEDICINE	000 – 706	9/18/2023

4. Issue Frequency	5. Number of Issues Published Annually	6. Annual Subscription Price
MAR, JUN, SEP, DEC	4	$420.00

7. Complete Mailing Address of Known Office of Publication (Not printer) (Street, city, county, state, and ZIP+4®)

ELSEVIER INC.
230 Park Avenue, Suite 800
New York, NY 10169

Contact Person
Malathi Samayan
Telephone (Include area code)
91-44-4299-4507

8. Complete Mailing Address of Headquarters or General Business Office of Publisher (Not printer)

ELSEVIER INC.
230 Park Avenue, Suite 800
New York, NY 10169

9. Full Names and Complete Mailing Addresses of Publisher, Editor, and Managing Editor (Do not leave blank)

Publisher (Name and complete mailing address)

DOLORES MELONI ELSEVIER INC.
1600 JOHN F KENNEDY BLVD. SUITE 1600
PHILADELPHIA, PA 19103-2899

Editor (Name and complete mailing address)

JOANNA COLLETT, ELSEVIER INC.
1600 JOHN F KENNEDY BLVD. SUITE 1600
PHILADELPHIA, PA 19103-2899

Managing Editor (Name and complete mailing address)

PATRICK MANLEY, ELSEVIER INC.
1600 JOHN F KENNEDY BLVD. SUITE 1600
PHILADELPHIA, PA 19103-2899

10. Owner (Do not leave blank. If the publication is owned by a corporation, give the name and address of the corporation immediately followed by the names and addresses of all stockholders owning or holding 1 percent or more of the total amount of stock. If not owned by a corporation, give the names and addresses of the individual owners. If owned by a partnership or other unincorporated firm, give its name and address as well as those of each individual owner. If the publication is published by a nonprofit organization, give its name and address.)

Full Name	Complete Mailing Address
WHOLLY OWNED SUBSIDIARY OF REED/ELSEVIER, US HOLDINGS	1600 JOHN F KENNEDY BLVD. SUITE 1600 PHILADELPHIA, PA 19103-2899

11. Known Bondholders, Mortgagees, and Other Security Holders Owning or Holding 1 Percent or More of Total Amount of Bonds, Mortgages, or Other Securities. If none, check box → ☐ None

Full Name	Complete Mailing Address
N/A	

12. Tax Status (For completion by nonprofit organizations authorized to mail at nonprofit rates) (Check one)
The purpose, function, and nonprofit status of this organization and the exempt status for federal income tax purposes:
☒ Has Not Changed During Preceding 12 Months
☐ Has Changed During Preceding 12 Months (Publisher must submit explanation of change with this statement)

PS Form 3526, July 2014 [Page 1 of 4 (see instructions page 4)]   PSN: 7530-01-000-9931   PRIVACY NOTICE: See our privacy policy on www.usps.com.

---

13. Publication Title	14. Issue Date for Circulation Data Below
CLINICS IN CHEST MEDICINE	JUNE 2023

15. Extent and Nature of Circulation		Average No. Copies Each Issue During Preceding 12 Months	No. Copies of Single Issue Published Nearest to Filing Date
a. Total Number of Copies (Net press run)		294	271
b. Paid Circulation (By Mail and Outside the Mail)	(1) Mailed Outside-County Paid Subscriptions Stated on PS Form 3541 (Include paid distribution above nominal rate, advertiser's proof copies, and exchange copies)	192	178
	(2) Mailed In-County Paid Subscriptions Stated on PS Form 3541 (Include paid distribution above nominal rate, advertiser's proof copies, and exchange copies)	0	0
	(3) Paid Distribution Outside the Mails Including Sales Through Dealers and Carriers, Street Vendors, Counter Sales, and Other Paid Distribution Outside USPS®	84	76
	(4) Paid Distribution by Other Classes of Mail Through the USPS (e.g. First-Class Mail®)	15	16
c. Total Paid Distribution (Sum of 15b (1), (2), (3), and (4))	▶	291	270
d. Free or Nominal Rate Distribution (By Mail and Outside the Mail)	(1) Free or Nominal Rate Outside-County Copies included on PS Form 3541	2	0
	(2) Free or Nominal Rate In-County Copies Included on PS Form 3541	0	0
	(3) Free or Nominal Rate Copies Mailed at Other Classes Through the USPS (e.g. First-Class Mail)	0	0
	(4) Free or Nominal Rate Distribution Outside the Mail (Carriers or other means)	1	1
e. Total Free or Nominal Rate Distribution (Sum of 15d (1), (2), (3) and (4))	▶	3	1
f. Total Distribution (Sum of 15c and 15e)	▶	294	271
g. Copies not Distributed (See instructions to Publishers #4 (page #3))	▶	0	0
h. Total (Sum of 15f and g)	▶	294	271
i. Percent Paid (15c divided by 15f times 100)		98.98%	99.63%

* If you are claiming electronic copies, go to line 16 on page 3. If you are not claiming electronic copies, skip to line 17 on page 3.

PS Form 3526, July 2014 (Page 2 of 4)

16. Electronic Copy Circulation		Average No. Copies Each Issue During Preceding 12 Months	No. Copies of Single Issue Published Nearest to Filing Date
a. Paid Electronic Copies	▶		
b. Total Paid Print Copies (Line 15c) + Paid Electronic Copies (Line 16a)	▶		
c. Total Print Distribution (Line 15f) + Paid Electronic Copies (Line 16a)	▶		
d. Percent Paid (Both Print & Electronic Copies) (16b divided by 16c × 100)	▶		

☒ I certify that 50% of all my distributed copies (electronic and print) are paid above a nominal price.

17. Publication of Statement of Ownership

☒ If the publication is a general publication, publication of this statement is required. Will be printed   ☐ Publication not required.
in the ___DECEMBER 2023___ issue of this publication.

18. Signature and Title of Editor, Publisher, Business Manager, or Owner

Malathi Samayan

Malathi Samayan - Distribution Controller

Date
9/18/2023

I certify that all information furnished on this form is true and complete. I understand that anyone who furnishes false or misleading information on this form or who omits material or information requested on the form may be subject to criminal sanctions (including fines and imprisonment) and/or civil sanctions (including civil penalties).

PS Form 3526, July 2014 (Page 3 of 4)   PRIVACY NOTICE: See our privacy policy on www.usps.com.

Printed and bound by CPI Group (UK) Ltd, Croydon, CR0 4YY

08/05/2025

01864715-0007